Practical Approaches to Controversies in Obstetric Care

Guest Editors

SEAN C. BLACKWELL, MD
GEORGE R. SAADE, MD

OBSTETRICS AND GYNECOLOGY CLINICS OF NORTH AMERICA

www.obgyn.theclinics.com

Consulting Editor
WILLIAM F. RAYBURN, MD, MBA

June 2011 • Volume 38 • Number 2

SAUNDERS an imprint of ELSEVIER, Inc.

W.B. SAUNDERS COMPANY

A Division of Elsevier Inc.

Elsevier, Inc. ● 1600 John F. Kennedy Blvd. ● Suite 1800 ● Philadelphia, PA 19103-2899

http://www.theclinics.com

OBSTETRICS AND GYNECOLOGY CLINICS OF NORTH AMERICA Volume 38, Number 2
June 2011 ISSN 0889-8545, ISBN-13: 978-1-4557-0474-3

Editor: Stephanie Donley

Obstetrics and Gynecology Clinics (ISSN 0889-8545) is published quarterly by Elsevier Inc., 360 Park Avenue South, New York, NY 10010-1710. Months of issue are March, June, September, and December. Periodicals postage paid at New York, NY, and additional mailing offices. Subscription price per year is $275.00 (US individuals), $474.00 (US institutions), $137.00 (US students), $331.00 (Canadian individuals), $598.00 (Canadian institutions), $201.00 (Canadian students), $402.00 (foreign individuals), $598.00 (foreign institutions), and $201.00 (foreign students). To receive student/resident rate, orders must be accompanied by name of affiliated institution, date of term, and the signature of program/residency coordinator on institution letterhead. Orders will be billed at individual rate until proof of status is received. Foreign air speed delivery is included in all *Clinics* subscription prices. All prices are subject to change without notice. POSTMASTER: Send address changes to *Obstetrics and Gynecology Clinics*, Elsevier Health Sciences Division, Subscription Customer Service, 3251 Riverport Lane, Maryland Heights, MO 63043. **Customer Service: Telephone: 1-800-654-2452 (U.S. and Canada); 314-447-8871 (outside U.S. and Canada). Fax: 314-447-8029. E-mail: journals customerservice-usa@elsevier.com (for print support); journalsonlinesupport-usa@elsevier.com (for online support).**

Reprints. For copies of 100 or more of articles in this publication, please contact the Commercial Reprints Department, Elsevier Inc., 360 Park Avenue South, New York, New York 10010-1710. Tel.: 212-633-3818; Fax: 212-462-1935; E-mail: reprints@elsevier.com.

Obstetrics and Gynecology Clinics of North America is also published in Spanish by McGraw-Hill Interamericana Editores S.A., P.O. Box 5-237, 06500, Mexico; in Portuguese by Reichmann and Affonso Editores, Rio de Janeiro, Brazil; and in Greek by Paschalidis Medical Publications, Athens, Greece.

Obstetrics and Gynecology Clinics of North America is covered in MEDLINE/PubMed (Index Medicus), Excerpta Medica, Current Concepts/Clinical Medicine, Science Citation Index, BIOSIS, CINAHL, and ISI/BIOMED.

Printed and bound by CPI Group (UK) Ltd, Croydon, CR0 4YY

Transferred to Digital Print 2011

GOAL STATEMENT
The goal of *Obstetrics and Gynecology Clinics of North America* is to keep practicing physicians up to date with current clinical practice in OB/GYN by providing timely articles reviewing the state of the art in patient care.

ACCREDITATION
The *Obstetrics and Gynecology Clinics of North America* is planned and implemented in accordance with the Essential Areas and Policies of the Accreditation Council for Continuing Medical Education (ACCME) through the joint sponsorship of the University of Virginia School of Medicine and Elsevier. The University of Virginia School of Medicine is accredited by the ACCME to provide continuing medical education for physicians.

The University of Virginia School of Medicine designates this educational activity for a maximum of 15 *AMA PRA Category 1 Credits*™ for each issue, 60 credits per year. Physicians should only claim credit commensurate with the extent of their participation in the activity.

The American Medical Association has determined that physicians not licensed in the US who participate in this CME activity are eligible for a maximum of 15 *AMA PRA Category 1 Credits*™ for each issue, 60 credits per year.

Category 1 credit can be earned by reading the text material, taking the CME examination online at http://www.theclinics.com/home/cme, and completing the evaluation. After taking the test, you will be required to review any and all incorrect answers. Following completion of the test and evaluation, your credit will be awarded and you may print your certificate.

FACULTY DISCLOSURE/CONFLICT OF INTEREST
The University of Virginia School of Medicine, as an ACCME accredited provider, endorses and strives to comply with the Accreditation Council for Continuing Medical Education (ACCME) Standards of Commercial Support, Commonwealth of Virginia statutes, University of Virginia policies and procedures, and associated federal and private regulations and guidelines on the need for disclosure and monitoring of proprietary and financial interests that may affect the scientific integrity and balance of content delivered in continuing medical education activities under our auspices.

The University of Virginia School of Medicine requires that all CME activities accredited through this institution be developed independently and be scientifically rigorous, balanced and objective in the presentation/discussion of its content, theories and practices.

All authors/editors participating in an accredited CME activity are expected to disclose to the readers relevant financial relationships with commercial entities occurring within the past 12 months (such as grants or research support, employee, consultant, stock holder, member of speakers bureau, etc.). The University of Virginia School of Medicine will employ appropriate mechanisms to resolve potential conflicts of interest to maintain the standards of fair and balanced education to the reader. Questions about specific strategies can be directed to the Office of Continuing Medical Education, University of Virginia School of Medicine, Charlottesville, Virginia.

The faculty and staff of the University of Virginia Office of Continuing Medical Education have no financial affiliations to disclose.

The authors/editors listed below have identified no professional or financial affiliations for themselves or their spouse/partner:
Giuseppe Barilaro, MD; Sean C. Blackwell, MD (Guest Editor); D. Ware Branch, MD; Shannon M. Clark, MD; Maged M. Costantine, MD; Nathan Drever, MD; Alfredo F. Gei, MD; Nicole Ruddock Hall, MD; Carla Holloway (Acquisitions Editor); William Irvin, MD (Test Author); Julio Mateus, MD; Mary B. Munn, MD; Ramsey Nakad, MD; Gayle Olson, MD; Luis D. Pacheco, MD; William F. Rayburn, MD, MBA (Consulting Editor); Jerrie S. Refuerzo, MD; George R. Saade, MD (Guest Editor); Alex C. Vidaeff, MD, MPH; and Rohan Willis, MD.

The authors/editors listed below identified the following professional or financial affiliations for themselves or their spouse/partner:
Robert H. Allen, PhD is a stock and patent holder with Birth Injury Prevention, LLC.
Edith D. Gurewitsch, MD is a stock and patent holder with Birth Injury Prevention, LLC.
Benjamin Leader, MD, PhD is employed and owns stock with ReproSource, Inc.
Silvia S. Pierangeli, PhD is the owner and technical director of Louisville APL Diagnostics, Inc.
Mildred M. Ramirez, MD is an industry funded research/investigator for Cytokine Pharmaceutical.

Disclosure of Discussion of non-FDA approved uses for pharmaceutical products and/or medical devices:
The University of Virginia School of Medicine, as an ACCME provider, requires that all faculty presenters identify and disclose any off-label uses for pharmaceutical and medical device products. The University of Virginia School of Medicine recommends that each physician fully review all the available data on new products or procedures prior to clinical use.

TO ENROLL
To enroll in the Obstetrics and Gynecology Clinics of North America Continuing Medical Education program, call customer service at 1-800-654-2452 or visit us online at www.theclinics.com/home/cme. The CME program is available to subscribers for an additional fee of $180.00.

Contributors

CONSULTING EDITOR

WILLIAM F. RAYBURN, MD, MBA
Randolph Seligman Professor and Chair, Department of Obstetrics and Gynecology;
Chief of Staff, University Hospital, University of New Mexico Health Science Center,
Albuquerque, New Mexico

GUEST EDITORS

SEAN C. BLACKWELL, MD
Associate Professor, Director, Larry C. Gilstrap M.D. Center for Perinatal and Women's
Health Research; Assistant Dean for Quality in Perinatal and Women's Health, Department
of Obstetrics, Gynecology and Reproductive Sciences, University of Texas Health
Science Center at Houston, Houston, Texas

GEORGE R. SAADE, MD
Chief, Division of Maternal Fetal Medicine; Professor, Department of Obstetrics and
Gynecology, University of Texas Medical Branch, Galveston, Texas

AUTHORS

ROBERT H. ALLEN, PhD
Associate Research Professor, Departments of Gynecology and Obstetrics and
Biomedical Engineering, Johns Hopkins University School of Medicine, Baltimore,
Maryland

GIUSEPPE BARILARO, MD
Antiphospholipid Standardization Laboratory, Division of Rheumatology, Department
of Internal Medicine, University of Texas Medical Branch, Galveston, Texas

SEAN C. BLACKWELL, MD
Associate Professor, Director, Larry C. Gilstrap M.D. Center for Perinatal and Women's
Health Research; Assistant Dean for Quality in Perinatal and Women's Health, Department
of Obstetrics, Gynecology and Reproductive Sciences, University of Texas Health
Science Center at Houston, Houston, Texas

D. WARE BRANCH, MD
Department of Obstetrics and Gynecology, University of Utah Health Sciences Center and
Intermountain Healthcare, Salt Lake City, Utah

SHANNON M. CLARK, MD
Assistant Professor, Division of Maternal-Fetal Medicine, Department of Obstetrics and
Gynecology, University of Texas Medical Branch, Galveston, Texas

MAGED M. COSTANTINE, MD
Assistant Professor, Division Maternal-Fetal Medicine, Department of Obstetrics and Gynecology, The University of Texas Medical Branch, Galveston, Texas

NATHAN DREVER, MD
Fellow, Division Maternal Fetal-Medicine, Department of Obstetrics and Gynecology, The University of Texas Medical Branch, Galveston, Texas

ALFREDO F. GEI, MD
Associate Professor, Clinical Obstetrics and Gynecology, Weil-Cornell Medical College; Director, Division of Maternal-Fetal Medicine, Department of Obstetrics and Gynecology, The Methodist Hospital of Houston, Houston, Texas

EDITH D. GUREWITSCH, MD
Associate Professor, Departments of Gynecology and Obstetrics and Biomedical Engineering, Johns Hopkins University School of Medicine, Baltimore, Maryland

NICOLE RUDDOCK HALL, MD
Associate Professor, Division of Maternal-Fetal Medicine, Department of Obstetrics, Gynecology, and Reproductive Sciences, University of Texas Health Science Center at Houston, Houston, Texas

BENJAMIN LEADER, MD, PhD
Clinical Research Division, Reprosource, Inc, Woburn, Massachusetts

JULIO MATEUS, MD
Assistant Professor, Division of Maternal Fetal Medicine, Department of Obstetrics and Gynecology, The University of Texas Medical Branch at Galveston, Galveston, Texas

MARY B. MUNN, MD
Assistant Professor, Director of Ultrasound and Prenatal Diagnosis, Division of Maternal-Fetal Medicine, University of Texas Medical Branch, Galveston, Texas

RAMZY NAKAD, MD
Fellow, Division of Maternal-Fetal Medicine, Department of Obstetrics and Gynecology, University of Texas Medical Branch, Galveston, Texas

GAYLE OLSON, MD
Director, Maternal Fetal Medicine Fellowship Program, Division of Maternal Fetal Medicine, Department of Obstetrics and Gynecology, The University of Texas Medical Branch, Galveston, Texas

LUIS D. PACHECO, MD
Assistant Professor, Division of Maternal Fetal Medicine, Department of Obstetrics and Gynecology; Division of Surgical Critical Care, Department of Anesthesiology, The University of Texas Medical Branch at Galveston, Galveston, Texas

SILVIA S. PIERANGELI, PhD
Antiphospholipid Standardization Laboratory, Division of Rheumatology, Department of Internal Medicine, University of Texas Medical Branch, Galveston, Texas

MILDRED M. RAMIREZ, MD
Professor, Maternal-Fetal Medicine Division, Department of Obstetrics, Gynecology and Reproductive Sciences, University of Texas Medical School at Houston

JERRIE S. REFUERZO, MD
Associate Professor, Division of Maternal Fetal Medicine, Department of Obstetrics, Gynecology and Reproductive Sciences, University of Texas Health Science Center at Houston, Houston, Texas

ALEX C. VIDAEFF, MD, MPH
Professor of Obstetrics and Gynecology, Division of Maternal-Fetal Medicine, Department of Obstetrics, Gynecology and Reproductive Sciences, University of Texas Medical School at Houston, Houston, Texas

ROHAN WILLIS, MD
Antiphospholipid Standardization Laboratory, Division of Rheumatology, Department of Internal Medicine, University of Texas Medical Branch, Galveston, Texas

Contents

The antepartum administration of fluorinated corticosteroids for fetal maturation represents the most important clinical contribution in the battle against prematurity. This treatment reduces the risk of neonatal death and handicap. It is also known that on corticosteroid exposure, fetuses are subjected to transiently increased physiologic and metabolic demands. Healthy fetuses are able to cope, although emerging evidence suggests this may not be the case with severely growth-restricted fetuses. This review presents evidence of efficacy and safety pertaining to corticosteroid administration in fetal growth restriction–affected pregnancies, offers guidance to clinicians, and points out questions that still need answers.

This article reviews the essential criteria for inductions of labor, weighing both the advantages and disadvantages of labor induction, and the various mechanical and pharmacologic agents available for cervical ripening. At the end of this article, one should be able to counsel women about the potential risks and benefit of labor induction and understand the neonatal consequences of elective induction of labor before 39 weeks of gestation. This article also discusses the different mechanical and pharmacologic agents available for cervical ripening.

Multiple studies have been published illustrating the use of oral hypoglycemic agents in pregnancy. Glyburide and metformin have been shown to be as effective as insulin for the treatment of gestational diabetes. Both are safe with breastfeeding. Although both glyburide and metformin appear safe for the treatment of type 2 diabetes mellitus, more studies are needed to support this practice.

Preterm birth has increased over the last decade. In 2006, 12.5% of all births in the United States occurred at fewer than 37 weeks gestation.

This is associated with significant health care costs as well as related neo-natal morbidity and mortality. In 2003, costs related to care for infants with preterm-birth or low-birth weight exceeded 11 billion dollars. This article reviews the literature on 17 alpha-hydroxyprogesterone caproate (17-P) and natural progesterone and concludes that 17-P is indicated for prevention of preterm birth in women with a documented history of a preterm birth before 37 weeks.

Obstetric hemorrhage is one of the most common causes of maternal morbidity and mortality worldwide, and abnormal placentation, including placenta accreta, is currently the most common indication for peripartum hysterectomy. Prenatal identification of these cases and early referral to centers with the capability to manage them will likely result in improved outcomes. Interventions that may limit transfusion requirements include normovolemic hemodilution, selective embolization of pelvic vessels by interventional radiology, conservative management of accretism in a few selected cases, and the use of the cell saver intraoperatively. Current understanding of the mechanisms of acute coagulopathy has questioned the current transfusion guidelines, leading to a tendency to apply massive transfusion protocols based on hemostatic resuscitation. Prospective trials are required to validate the efficacy of this approach. Obstetricians should be familiar with current transfusion protocols, as the incidence of placental accretism is expected to increase in the future.

Forceps, vacuum, and cesarean sections are relatively recent additions to the obstetrician's armamentarium. The art of modern obstetrics is one that mandates from obstetricians the attentive vigilance of the development of natural processes and an active intervention when such processes fall outside normally accepted standards. What constitutes the "normal process" and the "accepted standard" is subject to discussion, and international variations in obstetric practice are in part the reflection of such controversies. This article presents a practical approach to the contemporary issue of instrumental deliveries, outlining supporting evidence (when available) and the most current position of professional colleges in obstetrics and gynecology.

Cerebral palsy is a leading cause of childhood neuromotor disability and is strongly associated with preterm delivery. Basic science research and some observational studies have suggested a neuroprotective benefit from antenatal exposure to magnesium sulfate. Recent randomized controlled studies and meta-analyses suggest that antenatal exposure to magnesium sulfate before anticipated preterm birth is associated with reduction in the risk of developing cerebral palsy or its associated neurologic disabilities in surviving infants. More importantly. this benefit has been achieved without increasing the risk of perinatal mortality.

Cervical cerclage is associated with prolongation of gestation in singleton pregnancies with prior spontaneous preterm delivery and a short cervix on vaginal ultrasonography in the mid-trimester. Ultrasound screening of cervical length is not indicated in low-risk singleton pregnancies and in women with multiple gestations. 17α-Hydroxyprogesterone does not prevent preterm delivery in twin gestations with a short cervix. Cervical cerclage may cause detrimental effects in twin gestations. Vaginal pessary for the prevention of preterm birth in women with a short cervix is currently under active investigation.

FORTHCOMING ISSUES

September 2011
Perimenopause
Nanette Santoro, MD, *Guest Editor*

December 2011
Advances in Laparoscopy and Minimally
Invasive Surgery
Michael Traynor, MD, MPH, *Guest Editor*

March 2012
Management of Preterm Birth
Alice Goepfert, MD, *Guest Editor*

RECENT ISSUES

March 2011
Diagnostic Imaging in Women's Health
Douglas W. Laube, MD, MEd,
Guest Editor

December 2010
Cosmetic Procedures in Gynecology
Douglas W. Laube, MD, MEd,
Guest Editor

September 2010
Prevention and Management of
Complications from Gynecologic Surgery
Howard T. Sharp, MD, *Guest Editor*

RELATED INTEREST

Clinics in Perinatology March 2011 (Vol. 38, Issue 1)
Fetal Assessment
Anthony O. Odibo, MD and George A. Macones, MD, *Guest Editors*
www.derm.theclinics.com

THE CLINICS ARE NOW AVAILABLE ONLINE!

Access your subscription at:
www.theclinics.com

Foreword

This issue of the *Clinics*, with Dr Sean Blackwell and Dr George Saade as Guest Editors, provides a timely update on topics of active interest in obstetrics. Highlighted are chapters which deal with labor and delivery, management of select medical preterm disorders, and conditions that affect fetal growth and placental integrity. This issue highlights those areas where problems can occur, their warning signs, and ways to prevent or reduce additional risks.

The demand for evidence-based medicine and documentation of clinical outcomes are major driving forces in clinical obstetrics. Although there is no doubt that obstetrics remains an art, it is also a science, and many of the changes described in this issue were long overdue. The authors' mandate was to chronicle scientific and medical advances, along with applying their clinical insights for improved care of mother and fetus.

Although definitive management recommendations are often not possible, the reader can still become familiar with the state of the current literature. To elucidate important problems that plague the mother and fetus, the authors drew heavily from reported experiences of multi-center collaboratives and national organizations to provide "the best available evidence." Clinical management schemata in each chapter are not the only acceptable ones but may be employed to hopefully obtain excellent clinical outcomes.

Information in this issue represents the opinions of several qualified experts in obstetrics. Each endeavored to provide to the practitioner of obstetrics clinical data that underlie recommendations for clinical practice. While not being absolute, views expressed here should be considered as flexible guidelines based on rational medical advice and on available local resources.

William F. Rayburn, MD, MBA
Department of Obstetrics and Gynecology
University of New Mexico School of Medicine
MSC10 5580, 1 University of New Mexico
Albuquerque, NM 87131-0001

E-mail address:
wrayburn@salud.unm.edu

doi:10.1016/j.ogc.2011.04.002
0889-8545/11/$ – see front matter
obgyn.theclinics.com

Preface

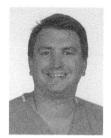 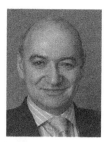

Sean C. Blackwell, MD   George R. Saade, MD
Guest Editors

A large proportion of clinical decision-making related to the care and treatment of pregnant women is not based on level I evidence (eg, RCTs). Although progress is being made by increasing the involvement and access of RCTs to pregnant women, it is likely that this disparity will continue for quite some time. In the meantime, what should clinicians do when there are limited data or significant controversy for a specific condition or treatment? What should guide their practice?

This volume of *Obstetrics and Gynecology Clinics* is meant to address this specific dilemma. Thirteen controversial but clinically relevant topics have been chosen for review by experts in order to summarize the best available information and provide some guidance in the absence of high-quality data. In each article, although definitive management recommendations are rarely able to be provided, readers will become familiar with the state of the current literature and the "best available evidence." Remarkably, the majority of the topics reviewed involve scenarios commonly confronted by clinicians such as preterm birth prevention, labor induction, gestational weight gain targets, fetal growth restriction, decreased amniotic fluid volume, and smoking cessation. As guest editors of this volume of the *Clinics*, we are quite proud of the contributions of these authors as they educate us regarding the controversial aspects of each subject and, even in the absence of intellectual consensus, offer some assistance regarding rational clinical practice.

Sean C. Blackwell, MD
Department of Obstetrics, Gynecology and Reproductive Sciences
University of Texas Health Science Center at Houston
6431 Fannin Street, Suite 3.283
Houston, TX 77030, USA

George R. Saade, MD
Department of Obstetrics and Gynecology
University of Texas Medical Branch
Galveston, TX, USA

E-mail addresses:
sean.blackwell@uth.tmc.edu (S.C. Blackwell)
gsaade@UTMB.edu (G.R. Saade)

Obstet Gynecol Clin N Am 38 (2011) xvii
doi:10.1016/j.ogc.2011.04.001
0889-8545/11/$ – see front matter © 2011 Elsevier Inc. All rights reserved.

Potential Risks and Benefits of Antenatal Corticosteroid Therapy Prior to Preterm Birth in Pregnancies Complicated by Severe Fetal Growth Restriction

Alex C. Vidaeff, MD, MPH[a],*, Sean C. Blackwell, MD[b]

KEYWORDS

- Antenatal corticosteroids • Fetal growth restriction
- Preterm birth

The antepartum administration of fluorinated corticosteroids (betamethasone [BTM] and dexamethasone [DXM]) for fetal maturation represents the most important clinical contribution so far in the battle against prematurity. This treatment reduces the risk of neonatal death and handicap. It is also known that on corticosteroid exposure, fetuses are subjected to transiently increased physiologic and metabolic demands. Healthy fetuses are able to cope, although emerging evidence suggests that this may not be the case with severely growth-restricted fetuses. Severe preterm fetal growth restriction (FGR) is frequently associated with chronic hypoxia and acidosis. Concerns have been raised that corticosteroid administration when preterm delivery is anticipated could be harmful in this setting.[1] This review presents evidence of

---

[a] Division of Maternal-Fetal Medicine, Department of Obstetrics, Gynecology and Reproductive Sciences, University of Texas Medical School at Houston, 6431 Fannin Street, Suite 3.283, Houston, TX 77030, USA
[b] Department of Obstetrics, Gynecology and Reproductive Sciences, University of Texas Health Science Center at Houston, 6431 Fannin Street, Suite 3.283, Houston, TX 77030, USA
* Corresponding author.
E-mail address: alex.c.vidaeff@uth.tmc.edu

Obstet Gynecol Clin N Am 38 (2011) 205–214
doi:10.1016/j.ogc.2011.02.011
0889-8545/11/$ – see front matter © 2011 Elsevier Inc. All rights reserved.

efficacy and safety pertaining to corticosteroid administration in FGR-affected pregnancies, offers guidance to clinicians, and points out questions that still need answers.

Data originating from the pioneering study on antenatal corticosteroids conducted by Liggins and Howie[2] suggested an excess of fetal death in cases of pregnancy-related hypertension and FGR treated with corticosteroids. Consequently, many of the subsequent clinical trials on the effect of antenatal corticosteroids excluded pregnancies with such complications. More recently, however, the indication for antenatal corticosteroids has been expanded to almost all pregnancies at risk for delivery before 32 to 34 weeks' gestation. The cumulative evidence so far has served to alleviate the concerns specifically related to pregnancy-related hypertension,[3] but the potential adverse effects of corticosteroid administration in growth-restricted fetuses continue to be debated. Severely growth-restricted fetuses in particular may have a poor response to the immediate physiologic demands imposed by corticosteroids.[4] A hypoxic growth-restricted fetus with diminished reserves may be barely coping when unchallenged, but exposure to corticosteroids may tip the balance.

BENEFITS OF ANTENATAL CORTICOSTEROIDS IN FGR

In the absence of randomized studies specifically designed to assess the effects of antenatal corticosteroids in preterm growth-restricted fetuses, the efficacy considerations are based on observational and retrospective data. Further complicating the interpretation are the frequently inconsistent results published in the literature. For instance, a large study in preterm infants born between 25 and 30 weeks' gestation seemed to document benefit with antenatal corticosteroids, even in growth-restricted cases, at a level comparable to that observed in appropriately grown infants.[5] Another study of growth-restricted babies born between 26 and 32 weeks' gestation suggested increased intact survival at 2-year follow-up in those babies who had received BTM compared with untreated controls.[6] Torrence and colleagues, in a systematic review of all available reports (as of 2007) on antenatal corticosteroid treatment in small-for-gestational-age fetuses or growth-restricted preterm fetuses, concluded, however, that the corticosteroids had no effect on neonatal morbidity or mortality.[7] The same lack of short-term neonatal benefit was noted in a retrospective cohort of severely growth-restricted fetuses with abnormal Doppler ultrasound evaluation analyzed by a nested case-control approach contrasting 54 corticosteroid-treated babies with 34 untreated babies.[8] Only cases of reduced diastolic velocities in the umbilical arteries were included in this study for a more accurate ascertainment of FGR and distinction from constitutionally small-for-gestational-age fetuses. The focus on hemodynamic changes as inclusion criterion, however, resulted in a study population with birthweight above the 10th percentile for gestational age in 34% of cases, deviating from the classical definition of FGR. As another limitation, no power calculation was provided to exclude the consequence of a too-small sample size. These limitations notwithstanding, the investigators suggested that in the absence of demonstrable benefit and given the potential for long-term adverse effects, corticosteroids should not be administered routinely in growth-restricted fetuses. They also called for a randomized controlled trial.

For a long time it has been speculated that the already elevated endogenous corticosteroid levels in growth-restricted fetuses would interfere and dampen any demonstrable beneficial effect of the additional exogenous corticosteroids.[9] Although such an opinion may be supported by the observation that increased endogenous corticosteroids lead to accelerated lung maturation in experimental animals, in human growth-restricted fetuses, elevated endogenous corticosteroid levels may not necessarily translate into accelerated pulmonary maturation.[10]

RISKS OF ANTENATAL CORTICOSTEROIDS IN FGR

Corticosteroids are key regulators of maturation and growth of fetal organ systems throughout pregnancy. They act in different ways, exercising both genomic and non-genomic effects. The genomic effects are dependent on the nuclear steroid receptors, whereas the nongenomic mechanisms are mediated by membrane steroid receptors or direct physicochemical interactions with the cellular membranes. Corticosteroids stimulate tissular maturation and differentiation essentially through genomic effects but may depress tissular growth in different organs via dose-dependent nongenomic effects. An example of corticosteroid nongenomic effect is the modification of bioenergetics of cellular metabolism; corticosteroids have been shown to inhibit the concanavalin A–stimulated cellular respiration and the ATP-consuming processes.[11] Besides the interference with cellular metabolism, the negative corticosteroid nongenomic effects on growth include increased apoptosis and inhibition of mitosis. According to Buttgereit and colleagues,[12] low doses of corticosteroids produce exclusively genomic effects, whereas with increasing doses, the additional nongenomic effects become evident.

In the clinical context of antenatal corticosteroid administration, with brief exposures to either DXM or BTM, the fetal maturational effects are most likely genomic in nature. With increased doses or a more prolonged exposure, the relative contribution of the nongenomic effects increases, enhancing the risk for iatrogenic harm. Although DXM and BTM are similar in pharmacologic activity, they are not identical, due to differences in spatial configuration and affinity for the steroid receptors. It seems that DXM is more potent than BTM in eliciting nongenomic effects.[11,12] Ozdemir and colleagues[13] have demonstrated a greater reduction in lung and liver weight in mice with repetitive doses of DXM rather than BTM.

As discussed previously, FGR may be associated with elevated endogenous corticosteroid levels. In addition, growth-restricted fetuses frequently become exposed to exogenous corticosteroids when preterm delivery is anticipated, the practice of administering corticosteroids that exaggerates the magnitude of exposure. FGR and exogenous corticosteroids individually and in combination have profound effects on fetal hemodynamics and neurologic development (discuss later).

Antenatal Corticosteroids and the Placental Barrier Function

The experimental model of single umbilical artery ligation induces extensive placental infarction and insufficiency, reducing oxygen and substrate transfer and subsequently resulting in asymmetric FGR, without effect on brain weight.[14] The experimental models of corticosteroid-induced FGR, however, suggest a different pathogenic mechanism. The uteroplacental perfusion is increased by the administration of corticosteroids and growth restriction cannot, therefore, be attributed to a reduction in placental perfusion. Furthermore, the pattern of growth restriction is symmetric, not sparing the head. It has been speculated that FGR is a consequence of intrauterine corticosteroids excess, which in turn is the result of reduced expression and function of 11β-hydroxysteroid dehydrogenase type 2 (11β-HSD 2) in the placenta.[15] Preeclampsia and severe FGR are conditions associated with reduced 11β-HSD 2 activity and mRNA expression, consequently with less cortisol to cortisone conversion, favoring excessive fetal transplacental exposure to maternal endogenous corticosteroids.[15–17] The addition of pharmacologic doses of fluorinated corticosteroids increases the degree of exposure and may also have a further impact on the activity of 11β-HSD 2. Although the evidence for that impact is still limited, Benediktsson and colleagues[18] have reported that exogenous corticosteroid administration decreases the activity of placental 11β-HSD 2 and Vackova and colleagues,[19] in a rat model, have demonstrated a considerably impaired placental barrier function mediated by 11β-HSD 2 after the antenatal administration of both DXM and BTM.

An observation has been made with direct weight-adjusted fetal administration of corticosteroids to the ovine fetus. In spite of the higher plasma corticosteroid levels obtained in fetuses with direct fetal administration, a separation was noted between the enhanced fetal lung maturational effects and the depression of tissular growth. After direct fetal administration, even repetitive, there was no FGR, in contrast to the decrement in growth noted with an equivalent maternal (transplacental) administration.[20] It seems that the fetal somatic growth depressor effect observed with maternal administration is mediated through the co-intervention of a placental factor or event, possibly the down-regulation of 11β-HSD 2.

In rodents, impaired placental 11β-HSD 2 function has been linked to reduced birthweight and long-term unfavorable programming, leading to hypertension and altered behavior.[21] The sustained action of 11β-HSD 2 late in pregnancy is important to maintain fetal cortisol concentrations several times lower than the maternal ones.[22] The hypocortisolic fetal milieu is presumed to be crucial for the development of the fetal hypothalamic-pituitary-adrenal (HPA) axis and may also be neuroprotective.[23] The HPA axis functional balance can be affected by corticosteroid exposure in a dose-dependent and time-dependent manner[24] and the concern is that severe FGR fetuses exposed to larger doses of corticosteroids may have greater potential for adverse effects of early HPA axis programming.

Antenatal Corticosteroids and Fetoplacental Hemodynamics

Corticosteroids are powerful regulators of vascular function. They increase the sympathetic tone in part via increased catecholamine levels and increased sensitivity to catecholamines after enhancing the intracellular secondary messenger systems via adenylate cyclase.[25] In addition, antenatal administration of corticosteroids has been shown to up-regulate placental expression and secretion of corticotropin-releasing hormone (CRH),[26] although it suppresses CRH secretion from the hypothalamus. Placental secretion of CRH increases within 3 hours of corticosteroid administration.[27] The up-regulation of placental CRH may be involved in the local regulation of placental blood flow, most likely as a vasodilator.[28] Corticosteroids have a vasodilatory effect on the human umbilical artery in vitro,[29] and the same effect is supposed to occur in vivo, presumably decreasing fetal vascular resistance. Hemodynamic studies focused on uteroplacental circulation or umbilical artery that are reflective of downstream vascular resistance in the placental bed may not be sensitive at all to upstream determinants, frequently missing the actual changes in fetal circulation.[30] Conclusions or observations based on umbilical artery Doppler indices are limited with regard to fetal circulation.

Initial invasive monitoring of healthy term sheep fetuses, preterm baboons, and growth-restricted sheep fetuses demonstrated that for 12 hours after direct fetal BTM infusion at doses equivalent to those used in clinical practice there is generalized vasoconstriction with increased fetal vascular resistance and systemic hypertension,[1,31,32] increased cerebral vascular resistance with 50% reduction in cerebral blood flow,[33] hypoxemia, and increased fetal lactate levels.[34] The hypertensive reaction is not demonstrable in the cerebral circulation, presumably because of autoregulatory mechanisms.

Pregnant sheep, the species in which corticosteroids' ability to accelerate fetal lung maturation was first shown, is a useful model to study the effects of corticosteroids on the fetus, with reasonable applicability to the human fetus.[35] More recent sheep experiments have indicated that maternally administered corticosteroids have distinctly different effects on cardiovascular function in normally grown and growth-restricted fetuses, most likely reflecting a fundamental difference in the regulation of vascular tone even in cases of only mild fetal hypoxia.[36] Where vasoconstriction with decreased total cardiac output was seen in healthy controls, vasodilatation with reduced cardiac after load and higher cardiac output was noted in growth-restricted fetuses. The blood flow increased to all major organs, particularly to the heart (4-fold increase). The increased cardiac output, especially if sustained, may actually overload the fetal heart, which works close to the upper limit of the ventricular function curve and has only limited functional reserve available to increase stroke volume via the Frank-Starling mechanism.

In healthy fetuses and in growth-restricted human fetuses, provided that diastolic flow in umbilical artery is present, corticosteroids are considered to have no major effect on Doppler blood flow in the umbilical and fetal vessels and do not induce fetal hypoxemia or acidemia.[37–39] In severely growth-restricted fetuses with Doppler evaluation indicative of absent end-diastolic flow in the umbilical artery, however, the Doppler flow changes may be similar to those observed in the sheep FGR experiments.[36] Reduced diastolic velocities in the umbilical arteries are suggestive of increased impedance in the fetoplacental circulation, causing reduced placental oxygen transfer, chronic fetal hypoxia, possibly lactic acidosis, and impaired myocardial function. These growth-restricted fetuses with abnormal Doppler flow patterns and altered responses to corticosteroids may be a group of significant concern. Unfortunately, the group is nonhomogeneous and a precise identification of growth-restricted fetuses with increased risk of adverse neonatal outcomes after maternal corticosteroid administration is not achievable at the current level of knowledge.

Researchers from Australia first reported, in 1999, in a small retrospective human study, that in a majority of FGR cases of increased placental vascular resistance, as evidenced by absent end-diastolic flow in the umbilical artery, the flow throughout diastole is temporarily regained after corticosteroid administration.[40] They confirmed the finding in a subsequent prospective cohort study,[41] and other investigators have independently verified the same phenomenon in Canada,[4] Germany,[42] and Brazil.[43] The cumulative evidence so far, from 161 cases, indicates that the return of end-diastolic flow may be expected to occur within 24 hours after corticosteroid injection in approximately 62% of cases, lasting for a median of 3 days (range up to 10 days). Even in multiple pregnancies discordant for absent end-diastolic flow, the administration of BTM was associated with return of umbilical artery end-diastolic flow in 50% of cases for a median of 5 days.[44] The mechanisms underlying these changes and their impact—beneficial versus deleterious—are still unknown. As early as 1999, Adamson and Kingdom[45] warned that the return of end-diastolic flow does not necessarily equate with improved gas exchange. Several researchers,[42,46] although not all,[43] have found that the return of end-diastolic flow in the umbilical artery is accompanied by a decrease in the middle cerebral artery velocity, change that is consistent with blood redistribution to the brain as part of the fetal response to a more advanced stage of hypoxia.

In a prospective study, Simchen and colleagues[4] confirmed the changes in umbilical artery Doppler waveforms in a majority of cases of FGR after corticosteroid administration. The investigators observed a better perinatal outcome in fetuses showing return of end-diastolic flow after corticosteroids compared with those with persistent absent or reverse end-diastolic flow, a subgroup that may include sicker fetuses with more extensive placental damage. In the latter subgroup, 4 of 9 fetuses had reverse end-diastolic flow, 2 of 9 had umbilical vein pulsations, and, ultimately, 2 died, and 2 were severely acidotic at birth. No such outcomes (death or severe acidosis) occurred in the subgroup with transient return of end-diastolic flow, in spite of the fact that the numbers of reverse flow waveforms (3 of 10) and umbilical vein pulsations (2 of 10) were almost equivalent. More recently, Robertson and colleagues[47] confirmed, in a larger study group (92 cases), the higher risk of neonatal morbidity associated with lack of return of end-diastolic flow after corticosteroid administration in growth-restricted fetuses. Clinicians should be particularly wary of growth-restricted fetuses that fail to show the transient return of diastolic flow in response to corticosteroids.[47] The rate of acute deterioration noted by Simchen and colleagues[4] in this subgroup may be as high as 89%, although even in the subgroup with end-diastolic flow return, there is still a 40% acute deterioration rate, suggesting an overall poor tolerance to corticosteroids.

The efforts to identify prognostic categories based on different fetal Doppler responses after corticosteroid administration are hampered by the observational nature of the reported studies and lack of a comparison group unexposed to cortico-steroids. Based on available data, it is challenging to differentiate over time the presumed corticosteroid-attributable effects from gradual deterioration of fetal condi-tion in a severely an affected fetus unrelated to corticosteroids. In Simchen and colleagues'[4] report, even cases of reverse end-diastolic flow in the umbilical artery continued to be managed expectantly, and delivery was not effected unless florid umbilical vein pulsations were noted. This would not necessarily be the approach in most clinical settings.

Antenatal Corticosteroids and the Brain of Growth-Restricted Fetuses

There is both experimental and clinical evidence that the brain of growth-restricted fetuses is particularly at risk of damage. Healthy fetuses are estimated to acquire an average of 173 million cells per day in the cerebral cortex in the second half of preg-nancy. Growth-restricted fetuses acquire only half of that cell estimate in the same period.[48] The subsequent smaller cortical volume may explain the decreased academic and professional abilities in adulthood of former FGR infants. An intriguing question that warrants further investigation is whether antenatal corticosteroids contribute to neuronal injury in growth-restricted fetuses affected by hypoxia. It has been suggested that corticosteroids may affect the ability of the brain to withstand hypoxia-ischemia,[49] and experiments conducted in fetal rat hippocampal cultures have demonstrated that exposure to corticosteroids may enhance both hypoxic and hypoglycemic neuronal and astroglial injury.[50]

Miller and colleagues,[1] in a sheep experimental model of FGR, showed that admin-istration of BTM was associated with disturbed neuronal integrity and enhanced cell death in the brain due to increased cerebral oxidative stress. This study used twin pregnancies to provide internal age-matched controls and provided the first in vivo experimental evidence that maternally administered corticosteroids may have detri-mental effects on the brain of growth-restricted fetuses. Three hours after BTM admin-istration, a decline in brain perfusion in both control and growth-restricted fetuses was first noted lasting for 3 hours. After that, a significant rebound reperfusion, persisting for 4 hours, was noted only in growth-restricted fetuses. It has been hypothesized that this exaggerated reperfusion would lead to overproduction of reactive oxygen species in mitochondria, causing lipid peroxidation. In metabolically compromised cells, such as those of the hypoxic growth-restricted fetal brain, lipid peroxidation results in generation of excess free radicals, with possible brain injury.[51] The brain is particularly vulnerable to oxidative damage due to its high lipid composition and relatively low content of antioxidant enzymes. The increased oxidative stress also increases apoptosis in the fetal brain.

Similar brain hyperperfusion and oxidative stress may be present after antenatal corticosteroid administration in the severely growth-restricted human fetus,[36] placing the developing brain at risk for profound neurologic deficits. Unfortunately, the effects of antenatal corticosteroids on the brain of human growth-restricted fetuses remain largely understudied.

SUMMARY

The effects of corticosteroids on growth-restricted fetuses are necessary future research directions not only from the perspective of efficacy but also, most importantly, from that of safety. Until more relevant information becomes available to guide the clinical use of antenatal corticosteroids in pregnancies complicated by FGR, based on available evidence, the authors suggest the following precautions be observed:

- In preterm pregnancies complicated by severe FGR, if corticosteroids are administered, fetal hemodynamic evaluation with Doppler ultrasound should be performed prior to or shortly thereafter receiving corticosteroids to evaluate for the presence of abnormal umbilical artery patterns.
- Due to the known effects of corticosteroids on umbilical and placental blood flow in severely growth-restricted fetuses, close fetal surveillance (eg, continuous electronic monitoring) may be considered for up to 48 to 72 hours after treatment depending on fetal heart rate and biophysical parameters.
- Because DXM is more potent than BTM in eliciting potentially unfavorable non-genomic effects, when available, BTM should be preferred to DXM.
- Because pregnancies complicated by FGR were not included in the original randomized controlled trials of antenatal corticosteroids and there is ample evidence from basic science and observational studies for potential fetal harms, placebo-controlled RCTs of antenatal corticosteroids in severely growth-restricted fetuses are both scientifically justified and ethical.

REFERENCES

1. Miller SL, Chai M, Loose J, et al. The effects of maternal betamethasone administration on the intrauterine growth restricted fetus. Endocrinology 2007;148: 1288–95.
2. Liggins GC, Howie RN. A controlled trial of antepartum glucocorticoid treatment for prevention of the respiratory distress syndrome in premature infants. Pediatrics 1972;50:515–25.
3. Jobe AH. Indications for and questions about antenatal steroids. Adv Pediatr 2002;49:227–43.
4. Simchen MJ, Alkazaleh F, Adamson SL, et al. The fetal cardiovascular response to antenatal steroids in severe early-onset intrauterine growth restriction. Am J Obstet Gynecol 2004;190:296–304.
5. Bernstein IM, Horbar JD, Badger GJ, et al. Morbidity and mortality among very-low-birth-weight neonates with intrauterine growth restriction: the Vermont Oxford Network. Am J Obstet Gynecol 2000;182:198–206.

6. Schaap AH, Wolf H, Bruinse HW, et al. Effects of antenatal corticosteroid administration on mortality and long-term morbidity in early preterm, growth-restricted infants. Obstet Gynecol 2001;97:954–60.

7. Torrance HL, Derks JB, Scherjon SA, et al. Is antenatal steroid treatment effective in preterm IUGR fetuses? Acta Obstet Gynecol Scand 2009;88:1068–73.

8. van Stralen G, van der Bos J, Lopriore E, et al. No short-term benefit of antenatal corticosteroid treatment in severely preterm growth restricted fetuses: a case-control study. Early Hum Dev 2009;85:253–7.

9. Schaap AH, Wolf H, Bruinse HW, et al. Fetal distress due to placental insufficiency at 26 through 31 weeks: a comparison between an active and a more conservative management. Eur J Obstet Gynecol Reprod Biol 1996;70:61–8.

10. Tyson JE, Kennedy K, Broyles S, et al. The small for gestational age infant: accelerated or delayed pulmonary maturation? increased or decreased survival? Pediatrics 1995;95:534–8.

11. Schmid D, Burmester GR, Tripmacher R, et al. Bioenergetics of human peripheral blood mononuclear cell metabolism in quiescent, activated, and glucocorticoid-treated states. Biosci Rep 2000;20:289–302.

12. Buttgereit F, Brand MD, Burmester GR. Equivalent doses and relative drug potencies for non-genomic glucocorticoid effects: a novel glucocorticoid hierarchy. Biochem Pharmacol 1999;58:363–8.

13. Ozdemir H, Guvenal T, Cetin M, et al. A placebo-controlled comparison of effects of repetitive doses of betamethasone and dexamethasone on lung maturation and lung, liver, and body weights of mouse pups. Pediatr Res 2003;53:98–103.

14. Supramaniam VG, Jenkin G, Loose J, et al. Chronic fetal hypoxia increases activin A concentrations in the late-pregnant sheep. BJOG 2006;113:102–9.

15. Kajantie E, Dunkel L, Turpeinen U, et al. Placental 11 beta-hydroxysteroid dehydrogenase-2 and fetal cortisol/cortisone shuttle in small preterm infants. J Clin Endocrinol Metab 2003;88:493–500.

16. Schoof W, Girstl M, Frobenius W, et al. Decreased gene expression of 11β-hydroxysteroid dehydrogenase type 2 and 15-hydroxyprostaglandin dehydrogenase in human placenta of patients with preeclampsia. J Clin Endocrinol Metab 2001;86:1313–7.

17. McTernan Cl, Draper N, Nicholson H, et al. Reduced placental 11beta-hydroxysteroid dehydrogenase type 2 mRNA levels in human pregnancies complicated by intrauterine growth restriction: an analysis of possible mechanisms. J Clin Endocrinol Metab 2001;86:4979–83.

18. Benediktsson R, Lindsay RM, Noble J, et al. Glucocorticoid exposure in utero: a new model for adult hypertension. Lancet 1993;341:339–41.

19. Vackova Z, Vagnerova K, Libra A, et al. Dexamethasone and betamethasone administration during pregnancy affects expression and function of 11β-hydroxysteroid dehydrogenase type 2 in the rat placenta. Reprod Toxicol 2009;28:46–51.

20. Jobe AH, Newnham J, Willet K, et al. Fetal versus maternal and gestational age effects of repetitive antenatal glucocorticoids. Pediatrics 1998;102:1116–25.

21. Bertram C, Trowern AR, Copin N, et al. The maternal diet during pregnancy programs altered expression of the glucocorticoid receptor and type 2 11β-hydroxysteroid dehydrogenase: potential molecular mechanisms underlying the programming of hypertension in utero. Endocrinology 2001;142:2841–53.

22. Lockwood CJ, Radunovic N, Nastic D, et al. Corticotropin-releasing hormone and related pituitary-adrenal axis hormones in fetal and maternal blood during the second half of pregnancy. J Perinat Med 1996;24:243–51.

23. Stewart PM, Rogerson FM, Mason JI. Type 2 11β-hydroxysteroid dehydrogenase messenger ribonucleic acid and activity in human placenta and fetal membranes: its relationship to birth weight and putative role in fetal adrenal steroidogenesis. J Clin Endocrinol Metab 1995;80:885–90.

24. Wellberg LA, Seckl JR. Prenatal stress, glucocorticoids and the programming of the brain. J Neuroendocrinol 2001;13:113–28.

25. Slotkin TA, Lau C, McCook EC, et al. Glucocorticoids enhance intracellular signaling via adenylate cyclase at three distant loci in the fetus: a mechanism for heterologous teratogenic sensitization? Toxicol Appl Pharmacol 1994;127:64–75.

26. Robinson BG, Emanuel RL, Frim DM, et al. Glucocorticoids stimulate expression of corticotropin-releasing hormone gene in human placenta. Proc Natl Acad Sci U S A 1988;85:5244–8.

27. Challis JRG. Effect of betamethasone in vivo on placental corticotropin-releasing hormone in human pregnancy. Am J Obstet Gynecol 1998;178:770–8.

28. Challis JRG, Matthews SG, Van Meir C, et al. The placental corticotropin-releasing hormone-adrenocorticotrophin axis. Placenta 1995;16:481–502.

29. Potter SM, Dennedy MC, Morrison JJ. Corticosteroids and fetal vasculature: effects of hydrocortisone, dexamethasone and betamethasone on human umbilical artery. BJOG 2002;109:1126–31.

30. Adamson SL. Arterial pressure, vascular input impedance, and resistance as determinants of pulsatile blood flow in the umbilical artery. Eur J Obstet Gynecol Reprod Biol 1999;84:119–25.

31. Derks JB, Giussani DA, Jenkins SL, et al. A comparative study of cardiovascular, endocrine and behavioural effects of betamethasone and dexamethasone administration to fetal sheep. J Physiol 1997;499:217–26.

32. Koenen SU, Mecenas CA, Smith GS, et al. Effects of maternal betamethasone administration on fetal and maternal blood pressure and heart rate in the baboon at 0.7 of gestation. Am J Obstet Gynecol 2002;186:812–7.

33. Schwab M, Roedel M, Anwar MA, et al. Effects of betamethasone administration to the fetal sheep in late gestation on fetal cerebral blood flow. J Physiol 2000; 528:619–32.

34. Bennet L, Kozuma S, McGarrigle HHG, et al. Temporal changes in fetal cardiovascular, behavioural, metabolic and endocrine response to maternally administered dexamethasone in the late gestation fetal sheep. BJOG 1999; 106:331–9.

35. Sloboda DM, Challis JR, Moss TJ, et al. Synthetic glucocorticoids: antenatal administration and long-term implications. Curr Pharm Des 2005;11:1459–72.

36. Miller SL, Supramaniam VG, Jenkin G, et al. Cardiovascular responses to maternal betamethasone administration in the intrauterine growth-restricted ovine fetus. Am J Obstet Gynecol 2009;201:613.e1–8.

37. Cohlen BJ, Stigter RH, Derks JB, et al. Absence of significant haemodynamic changes in the fetus following betamethasone administration. Ultrasound Obstet Gynecol 1996;8:252–5.

38. Senat MV, Ville Y. Effect of steroids on arterial Doppler in intrauterine growth retardation fetuses. Fetal Diagn Ther 2000;15:36–40.

39. Mulder EJ, de Heus R, Visser GH. Antenatal corticosteroid therapy: short-term effects on fetal bahaviour and haemodynamics. Semin Fetal Neonatal Med 2009;14:151–6.

40. Wallace EM, Baker LS. Effect of antenatal betamethasone administration on placental vascular resistance. Lancet 1999;353:1404–7.

41. Edwards A, Baker LS, Wallace EM. Changes in umbilical artery flow velocity waveforms following maternal administration of betamethasone. Placenta 2003; 24:12–6.
42. Muller T, Nanan R, Dietl J. Effect of antenatal corticosteroid administration on Doppler flow velocity parameters in pregnancies with absent or reverse end-diastolic flow in the umbilical artery. Acta Obstet Gynecol Scand 2003;82:794–6.
43. Nozaki AM, Francisco RP, Fonseca ES, et al. Fetal hemodynamic changes following maternal betamethasone administration in pregnancies with fetal growth restriction and absent end-diastolic flow in the umbilical artery. Acta Obstet Gynecol Scand 2009;88:350–4.
44. Barkehall-Thomas A, Thompson M, Baker LS, et al. Betamethasone associated changes in umbilical artery flow velocity waveforms in multiple pregnancies with umbilical artery absent end diastolic flow. Aust N Z J Obstet Gynaecol 2003;43:360–3.
45. Adamson SL, Kingdom J. Antenatal betamethasone and fetoplacental blood flow [letter]. Lancet 1999;354:255–6.
46. Edwards A, Baker LS, Wallace EM. Changes in fetoplacental vessel flow velocity waveforms following maternal administration of betamethasone. Ultrasound Obstet Gynecol 2002;20:240–4.
47. Robertson MC, Murila F, Tong S, et al. Predicting perinatal outcome through changes in umbilical artery Doppler studies after antenatal corticosteroids in the growth-restricted fetus. Obstet Gynecol 2009;113:636–40.
48. Samuelsen GB, Pakkenberg B, Bogdanovic N, et al. Severe cell reduction in the future brain cortex in human growth-restricted fetuses and infants. Am J Obstet Gynecol 2007;197:56.e1–7.
49. Whitelaw A, Thoresen M. Antenatal steroids and the developing brain. Arch Dis Child Fetal Neonatal Ed 2000;83:F154–7.
50. Tombaugh GC, Yang SH, Swanson RA, et al. Glucocorticoids exacerbate hypoxic and hypoglycaemic hippocampal injury in vitro. J Neurochem 1992;59:137–46.
51. Nita DA, Nita V, Spulber S, et al. Oxidative damage following cerebral ischemia depends on reperfusion—a biochemical study in rat. J Cell Mol Med 2001;5: 163–70.

Labor Induction: A Review of Current Methods

Mildred M. Ramirez, MD

KEYWORDS

• Induction of labor • Neonatal • Oxytocin • Prostaglandin

For centuries, physicians have been intrigued by the process of parturition. Through the ages, concerns for maternal well-being and timing of the birth have generated multiple approaches to initiate labor. Some of the methods or approaches are still used in current practices. Other methods such as vaginal or uterine douches, stimulant injections thrown into the rectum, and the use of secale cornutum (ergot alkaloid) have been abandoned because of their "ineffectiveness or poisonous effects on the infant."[1]

In the United States, there is an alarming increase in the rate of induction of labor in this era. From 1990 to 2006, the rate of induction of labor has doubled.[2] In 2006, more than 22% of gravid women underwent induction of labor. More disturbing is that the rate of elective induction of labor seems to be increasing at a more rapid rate than that of the overall induction of labor.[3] The reasons for this increase are both complex and multifactorial. The most commonly cited reasons are timing of birth by either the patient or the physician. How much of this increase is because of pressures from demanding patients or recommendations by their physician is disputable. An additional factor is the prevailing relaxed attitude toward elective inductions. The availability of cervical ripening agents and the perceived ease of induction is another contributing component. How much the presumed medical liability and financial gain of the provider contribute to this increase is debatable.

Without robust evidence that induction of labor causes harm to the pregnant woman or neonate and without a clear understanding of the effects of induction of labor on maternal and neonatal outcomes, we are left unarmed to reduce this increasing trend in labor inductions. On the other hand, if induction of labor reduces complications and costs, elective induction of labor would be a reasonable clinical practice.

This article reviews the essential criteria for inductions of labor, weighing both the advantages and disadvantages of labor induction, and the various mechanical and pharmacologic agents available for cervical ripening. At the end of this article, one should be able to counsel women about the potential risks and benefit of labor

Department of Obstetrics, Gynecology and Reproductive Sciences, University of Texas Health Science Center at Houston, 6410 Fannin Street, Suite 210, Houston, TX 77030, USA
E-mail address: mildred.m.ramirez@uth.tmc.edu

Obstet Gynecol Clin N Am 38 (2011) 215–225
doi:10.1016/j.ogc.2011.02.012
0889-8545/11/$ – see front matter © 2011 Published by Elsevier Inc.

obgyn.theclinics.com

induction and understand the neonatal consequences of elective induction of labor before 39 weeks of gestation. This article also discusses the different mechanical and pharmacologic agents available for cervical ripening.

The indications for induction of labor are not absolute. Medical induction of labor includes conditions that may increase maternal or fetal/neonatal morbidity and mortality, if undelivered. Induction of labor is defined as elective when a medical indication cannot be identified. What is medically indicated is sometimes debatable between experts. When reviewing the literature, it is important to determine the source document. The indications for delivery can vary depending on whether information is extracted from birth certificates, electronic records, or prenatal records. For example, Donovan and colleagues[4] found that the rate of late preterm induction was overestimated by 11-fold if birth certificates were used. The condition of the cervix is an important predictor of labor outcome. Cervical remodeling is critical in the process of parturition. This remodeling may include movement of an inflammatory infiltrate into the cervix; release of metalloproteases that break down collagen, changing the structure of the cervix; alterations in the level of glycosaminoglycans; and increased production of cytokines.[5] A variety of techniques have been developed to quantify cervical ripening. One of the more commonly used methods to evaluate cervical ripening is the Bishop score. The scoring system includes evaluation of the cervical dilation, effacement, consistency, position, and fetal station. A numerical value from 0 to 3 is assigned to each parameter.[6] Twelve observational studies measuring the Bishop score as a predictor of cesarean delivery in women undergoing induction of labor reported an inverse relationship between cesarean delivery rate and Bishop score, the lower the Bishop score the higher the cesarean delivery rate. In women undergoing elective induction of labor, there is moderate evidence that a low Bishop score (ie, unfavorable cervix) is a predictor of cesarean delivery.[7] Most studies define an unfavorable cervix as a Bishop score of 6 or less.[8] Cervical dilation is also inversely associated with cesarean delivery. In nulliparous women, a closed cervix is associated with a 50% cesarean delivery rate, whereas a 4-cm cervical dilation has a less than 10% risk of cesarean delivery. The same relationship is also reported in multiparous women but with a smaller magnitude of effect.

When counseling women regarding elective induction of labor, possible maternal, fetal, and neonatal risks and benefits should be included. However, most of the observational studies that evaluate these risks compare induction of labor to spontaneous labor and therefore are flawed by design.[7] When elective induction is considered, the alternative option is expectant management or to continue pregnancy until spontaneous labor occurs, and induction is again considered at a later gestational age.

The most concerning risk of induction of labor in nulliparous women is the doubling of risk of cesarean delivery reported in most retrospective and observational studies that compared induction of labor with spontaneous labor. When compared with expectant management, in a systematic review of the literature, Caughey and colleagues[7] reported that the risk of cesarean delivery is decreased in women at 41 weeks of gestation. There were 9 randomized controlled trials (RCTs) included in this analysis but only 3 trials that included women whose gestation period was less than 41 weeks, therefore, there was limited information to draw recommendations for women at this gestational age.

A retrospective study of 115,528 singleton deliveries after 34 weeks' gestation from 2002 through 2008 using electronic medical records at 10 institutions across the United States analyzed deliveries by the labor onset type (spontaneous, elective induction, indicated induction, or unlabored cesarean). The cesarean delivery rate was the lowest in spontaneous labor at each gestational age except at 39 weeks' gestation, at which elective induction was lower (5.9% vs 6.9%). Overall, the cesarean delivery rate was 8% for spontaneous and elective induction. In contrast, indicated induction of labor had a 24% cesarean delivery rate.[9] It is important to stress that this study represents current clinical practices; however, no randomizations were performed. Further, patient characteristics that caused physicians to offer elective inductions were not described. However, it is encouraging that the cesarean delivery rate did not seem to be increased compared with that of spontaneous labor. The absence of an increased cesarean delivery rate in women whose labor was induced is also supported by other studies. In a retrospective design, Caughey and colleagues[10] compared induction of labor to expectant management after 38 weeks of gestation. The cesarean delivery rate was not increased in the induction group (11.9% compared with 13.3%). The study did include all women induced for medical indications.[10] Osmundson and colleagues[11] compared elective induction of labor with expectant management of labor in nulliparous women with a favorable cervix. In this retrospective study, they compared women with known cervical status and a modified Bishop score of at least 5. The primary outcome was cesarean delivery rate. The study was powered to detect a 10% increase in cesarean delivery rate from 20% to 30%. The cesarean delivery rate was 20.1% in the expectantly managed group compared with 20.8% in the electively induced group ($P = .84$).

In addition to the potential increase in cesarean delivery, other maternal morbidities may include the rate of operative vaginal delivery, intra-amniotic infection, blood loss, and hysterectomy. There is limited information on the rate of operative vaginal delivery in women undergoing elective induction of labor. Both RCTs[6] and observational studies did not find a statistical difference in the rate of operative vaginal delivery, including vacuum or forceps delivery.[7] There was insufficient evidence to conclude the effect on women whose gestation period was less than 41 weeks.[7] More recent retrospective studies are consistent with previous reports that failed to demonstrate an increased risk of operative vaginal delivery in women who underwent induction of labor.[12]

In terms of maternal infection, the few reports that provided information of the maternal risks of infection did not uncover an increased risk of chorioamnionitis or endometritis. In a large retrospective cohort study, the rate of chorioamnionitis was statistically higher in spontaneous and indicated inductions when compared with elective inductions at 38 to 39 weeks.[9] In addition, indicated inductions, but not elective inductions, were associated with an increased risk for endometritis.[9] Therefore it seems that elective induction is not associated with an increased risk of maternal infection.

There are no large RCTs published that evaluate the risk of elective induction of labor and maternal blood loss (postpartum hemorrhage and blood transfusions). One trial reported (N = 440) no association between maternal transfusion and elective induction of labor (0.75%) and expectant management (1.7%).[13]

Al-Zirqi and colleagues[13] reported on the incidence of severe postpartum hemorrhage defined as estimated blood loss greater than 1500 mL in 24 hours or need for transfusion as reported in Norway's Medical Birth Registry that included more than 300,000 deliveries and contained detailed information on the delivery and postpartum period. Induction of labor carried a significantly higher risk of severe postpartum hemorrhage (odds ratio [OR], 1.71; 95% confidence interval [CI], 1.56–1.88), compared with spontaneous labor. Emergency cesarean after induction of labor had the highest risk of severe postpartum hemorrhage (OR, 6.57; 95% CI, 4.25–10.00). The investigators concluded that induction of labor should be practiced with caution because of the increased risk of postpartum hemorrhage.

More concerning is the recent report of increased risk of maternal hysterectomy associated with elective induction of labor.[9] The large sample size allowed for estimation of rare outcomes. The risk of hysterectomy was 3.21 adjusted odds ratio (95% CI, 1.08–9.54) when compared with spontaneous labor. Even though the rate of hysterectomy is low, only 24 reported in the cohort; the consequences are irrevocable. Other outcomes not frequently reported are serious perineal lacerations, risk of injury to internal organs, or wound complications after elective induction of labor.

The literature regarding women's perception and satisfaction of induction of labor is sparse. In a questionnaire-based study, compared with women who had spontaneous labor, women undergoing induction of labor were less satisfied about the induction process. In addition, 35% were not satisfied with the information received before induction. The duration of induction, route of agent administration, number of pelvic examinations, and complications associated with the induction were a few of their concerns.[14]

In terms of neonatal outcomes, it seems that meconium-stained amniotic fluid is observed more frequently in nulliparous women undergoing expectant management of labor than elective induction. Analysis of 6 combined RCTs revealed an odds ratio of 2.04 (95% CI, 1.34–3.09; $P = .001$). In contrast, the risk of meconium aspiration syndrome was not observed more frequently in the expectant management group. Analysis of 5 RCTs reported an odds ratio of 1.39 (95% CI, 0.71–2.72; $P = .34$). There was no statistical significance in the 5-minute Apgar score less than 7 between expectant management and elective induction of labor in the 4 RCTs that reported this outcome (OR, 1.18; 95% CI, 0.67–2.06). Admission to neonatal intensive care unit was reported in 3 RCTs, with no difference in the odds ratio between the expectant and induction group. Other neonatal outcomes including need for resuscitation, transient tachypnea, sepsis, jaundice, and hypoglycemia were reported in fewer studies.[7] Without large RCTs evaluating neonatal morbidity, the large multicenter cohort of the Consortium of Safe labor confirmed in other smaller studies that some neonatal outcomes improve until 39 weeks, regardless of the labor onset type.[9]

Regarding resources used, Caughey and colleagues[7] reported on an exploratory model-based analyses that suggests that elective induction of labor at 41 weeks was not only cost-effective but also improved maternal and fetal outcomes. Because of less evidence available, elective induction of labor before 41 weeks' gestation (39–40 weeks), in theory, may improve outcomes and could reach thresholds for cost-effectiveness, but at present, it is only hypothesis generating. Most of these studies support the American College of Obstetricians and Gynecologists guidelines of discouraging elective induction of labor before 39 weeks. Furthermore, the author supports Dr Rayburn's statement that "Until prospective clinical trials can better validate reasons for the liberal use of labor induction, it would seem prudent to maintain a cautious approach, especially among nulliparous women."[15] In particular, elective induction of labor in nulliparous women with a low Bishop score or a closed cervix should be prevented.

Several centers have reported on their outcomes after guidelines were developed to reduce elective inductions before 39 weeks. Fisch and colleagues[16] reported during a 3-year period a 30% reduction in elective inductions at their institution, which translated to a 60% reduction in cesarean delivery in nulliparous women. Oshiro reported that 6 years after initiation of their program to reduce late preterm birth the incidence of elective induction before 39 weeks continues to be less than 3%. This reduction was associated with a reduction in length of stay in labor and delivery.[17]

MECHANICAL AGENTS FOR INDUCTION OF LABOR

When induction of labor is indicated and the status of the cervix is unfavorable, several methods may be used to ripen the cervix.

Mechanical methods include hygroscopic dilators, osmotic dilators, the Foley catheter, and extra-amniotic saline infusion (EASI). Various studies have shown mechanical methods to be safe and efficacious. When compared with induction of labor with oxytocin alone, mechanical methods except EASI have been associated with a reduction in cesarean delivery rate.[18]

In the last 2 decades, there has been a reduction in the use of hygroscopic and osmotic dilators for the induction of labor in favor of other mechanical and pharmacologic agents. The increased risk of maternal and fetal infections with hygroscopic and osmotic dilators when compared with that associated with the use of other pharmacologic agents[19,20] and the ease of pharmacologic administration may be reasons for the decline. Placement of dilators also requires additional training and may be associated with rupture of membranes, vaginal bleeding, and patient discomfort or pain.

The use of the Foley catheter during induction of labor was first described in 1967 by Embrey and Mollison.[21] Use of a 26F catheter with a 50 mL insufflation was originally reported. Since then, 14F to 26F Foley catheters with inflation volumes of 30 to 80 mL, the Atad ripener device, and the EASI with infusion rates of 30 to 40 mL/h have been shown to be safe and efficacious. Potential advantages of the Foley catheter when compared with prostaglandins include lower cost, stability at room temperature, reduced risk of uterine tachysystole with or without fetal heart rate (FHR) changes, and appropriateness in an outpatient setting.[22] It seems that higher insufflation volumes (80 mL) may be more efficacious than lower volumes (30 mL).[23–25]

The Foley catheter has also been associated with a reduction in the duration of labor before oxytocin induction.[22] The concomitant use of oxytocin with the Foley catheter does not seem to shorten the duration of labor.[26]

When compared with misoprostol induction, Foley catheter trials produce inconsistent results because of the different regimens evaluated.[18,22]

A recent meta-analysis of 27 RCTs comparing Foley catheter balloon with locally applied prostaglandins concluded that the mode of delivery was not significantly different between these 2 methods of induction. Neither was there a difference in the proportion of women with unfavorable Bishop score, duration of induction, proportion of women who delivered before 12 or 24 hours, maternal fever, neonatal Apgar score of less than 5 at 7 minutes, or admission to neonatal intensive care unit. However, prostaglandins were associated with an increased risk of excessive uterine activity when compared with the Foley catheter.[27] The Foley catheter can be associated with risks of rupture of membranes, vaginal bleeding in women with a low-lying placenta, febrile morbidity, and displacement of the presenting part.[28,29]

When extra-amniotic saline is infused through the Foley catheter with concurrent oxytocin administration and is compared with the Foley catheter alone, contrasting results are observed. Karjane and colleagues reported a shorter duration of labor in women with Bishop score less than 5, 16.6 hours with EASI compared with 21.4 hours with the Foley catheter.[30] In contrast, studies by Guinn and colleagues[31] and Lin and colleagues[32] did not corroborate those findings. Neither study identified a difference in either duration of labor or cesarean delivery rate.

When EASI and concomitant oxytocin administration are compared with misoprostol, 50 µg every 4 hours with a maximum of 3 intravaginal doses, no difference in the duration of labor is noted between the groups. Of significance, there was a reported increase in the risk of uterine tachysystole.

As with other mechanical methods for cervical ripening, it is technically more difficult to introduce the Foley catheter through a nulliparous closed cervix. Other complications reported in approximately 8% of women from a large retrospective cohort who underwent cervical ripening with EASI that required removal of the Foley catheter included transient febrile reaction, nonreassuring FHR monitoring (2%), vaginal bleeding (1.8%), unbearable pain that required removal of the catheter (1.7%), and displacement from cephalic presentation to breech (1.3%). Displacement of the presenting part occurred only in women with unengaged fetal head.[33]

PHARMACOLOGIC AGENTS

Pharmacologic methods include prostaglandins, oxytocin, and the nitric oxide donor isosorbide mononitrate. Other methods include membrane stripping, amniotomy, castor oil, and unilateral breast stimulation.

There are 2 classes of prostaglandins available for cervical ripening and induction of labor. Prostaglandin E_2 (PGE_2) dinoprostone is available as a gel containing 0.5 mg dinoprostone and a vaginal insert that contains 10 mg of dinoprostone, which releases 0.3 mg/h. Both preparations are approved by the US Food and Drug Administration (FDA).

The synthetic analogue of prostaglandin E_1, misoprostol, has also been used for cervical ripening and induction of labor. Misoprostol can be administered via vaginal, oral, and sublingual route. It is available as unscored 100 and 200 μg tablets. In addition, a new misoprostol vaginal insert is being evaluated in the United States for FDA approval.

When intracervical or vaginal dinoprostone is compared with placebo, there is a significant difference in treatment success whether defined as improved Bishop score of 3 or more points, Bishop score of 6 or more points, or delivery during the first 12 hours of dosing. Time to onset of labor as well as median time to delivery was also shortened, 25.7 hours versus 34.5 hours in nulliparous women and 12.3 hours versus 24.6 hours in multiparous women.[34]

Hughes and colleagues[35] in a meta-analysis reported the outcomes of trials comparing the vaginal insert with other prostaglandin preparations. Seven studies compared the insert with the gel and 2 studies compared the insert with misoprostol. The primary outcomes that were analyzed included delivery within 24 hours, rate of uterine hypertonus with fetal heart changes, and cesarean delivery rate. There was no statistical difference in the primary outcome of delivery by 24 hours. The odds ratio was 0.80 with a 95% CI of 0.56 to 1.15. Similarly, there was no difference in the cesarean delivery rate, with an OR of 0.78 and a 95% CI of 0.56 to 1.08, or the reported rate of uterine hyperstimulation, with an OR of 1.19 and a 95% CI 0.56 of 2.54.

An updated meta-analysis reaffirms previous findings of no increase in cesarean delivery rate but concluded that PGE_2 is associated with increases in successful vaginal delivery rates by 24 hours and cervical favorability. In addition, although the vaginal insert seems superior to the vaginal gel in some outcomes measured, further studies are needed to determine the best vehicle for prostaglandin administration.[36] Factors that predict vaginal delivery in women undergoing induction of labor with PGE_2 preparations include multiparity (OR, 4.63; 95% CI, 3.39–6.32), Bishop score greater than 4 (OR, 2.15; 95% CI, 1.12–4.20), body mass index, defined as the weight in kilograms divided by the height in meters squared, less than 30 (OR, 1.69; 95% CI, 1.32–2.22), height of 5 ft5 in (OR, 1.47; 95% CI, 1.15–1.9), birthweight less than 4 kg (OR, 2.17; 95% CI, 1.51–3.13), maternal age less than 35 years (OR, 1.81; 95% CI, 1.15–2.86; $P = .01$) and Hispanic ethnicity (OR, 1.45; 95% CI, 1.02–2.05; $P = .036$).[37]

Despite the extensive clinical experience with the use of misoprostol as a cervical or induction agent, the drug is only approved for treatment of peptic ulcer by the FDA. In 2002, the FDA approved a new label on the use of misoprostol (Cytotec).

LABOR AND DELIVERY

Cytotec can induce or augment uterine contractions. Vaginal administration of Cytotec, outside of its approved indication, has been for cervical ripening, for the induction of labor, and for treatment of serious postpartum hemorrhage in the presence of uterine atony. A major adverse effect of the obstetric use of Cytotec is hyperstimulation of the uterus, which may progress to uterine tetany with marked impairment of uteroplacental blood flow, uterine rupture (requiring surgical repair, hysterectomy, and/or salpingo-oophorectomy), or amniotic fluid embolism. Pelvic pain, retained placenta, severe genital bleeding, shock, fetal bradycardia, and fetal and maternal death have been reported. There may be an increased risk of uterine tachysystole, uterine rupture, meconium passage, meconium staining of amniotic fluid, and cesarean delivery caused by uterine hyperstimulation with the use of higher doses of Cytotec, including the manufactured 100-μg tablet. The risk of uterine rupture increases with advancing gestational ages and with prior uterine surgery, including cesarean delivery. Grand multiparity also seems to be a risk factor for uterine rupture. The effect of Cytotec on the later growth, development, and functional maturation of the child when Cytotec is used for cervical ripening or induction of labor have not been established. Information on Cytotec's effect on the need for forceps delivery or other interventions is unknown."[38]

The labeling does not specify dose, dosing intervals, or safety or efficacy.

Misoprostol pharmacokinetics depends on the route of administration. The oral route has a faster increase, a higher peak, and a faster decline of plasma levels when compared with the vaginal route. The highest peak levels are observed when administered through the sublingual route.[39]

The ACOG practice bulletin recommends considering 25 μg as the initial dose for cervical ripening, repeated if needed not more than every 3- to 6-hour intervals.[8] Higher doses can be used and be appropriate in some clinical settings but are associated with an increased risk of complications. A systematic review of the use of misoprostol for labor induction concluded that misoprostol seemed to be safe and effective for induction of labor with unfavorable cervix. Misoprostol is associated with more vaginal deliveries within 24 hours when compared with either oxytocin or dinoprostone. The vaginal route seems more efficacious that the oral route and is associated with less use of epidural analgesia but at a disadvantage of an increased risk of abnormal FHR patterns and episodes of uterine tachysystole with associated FHR changes. The observed tachysystole does not seem to increase fetal adverse outcomes. The occurrence of these complications seems to be dose dependent.[40,41]

When higher doses of misoprostol are compared with lower doses, the former are not associated with a higher success of delivery by 24 hours but are associated with less oxytocin administration. Again, no differences are noted in the mode of delivery, meconium-stained fluid, or maternal side effects.

Because of the limited number of RCTs comparing the sublingual versus vaginal route of administration, the results of those trials do no show the sublingual route to be either superior or safer than the vaginal route at present. Hence, the use of sublingual misoprostol should be limited to clinical trials.

The use of misoprostol in women with prior cesarean delivery should be avoided because of the increased risk of uterine rupture.

OXYTOCIN

Since the discovery and use of the posterior pituitary extract in 1948, followed by its synthesis 5 years later, oxytocin is one of the most commonly used drugs in the United States.[8] More than 61 RCTs including 12,000 women have been reported evaluating the efficacy and safety of oxytocin for the induction of labor. When oxytocin is compared with placebo, it is superior to the placebo in the proportion of women delivering vaginally within 24 hours (53.8% vs 8.4%). Oxytocin administration is associated with an increased use of epidural analgesia. Two regimens of oxytocin administration are commonly practiced. The low-dose regimen includes a starting dose of 0.5 to 2 mU/min with an incremental increase of 1 to 2 mU/min every 15 to 40 minutes, and the high-dose regimen has a starting dose of 6 mU and an incremental increase of 3 to 6 mU/min every 15 to 40 minutes. What regimen of oxytocin is superior is debatable, with both regimens acceptable for the induction of labor.[8] Of the 6 RCTs comparing high with low dose, providers of only 1 study were blinded. The high-dose protocol was not only associated with significantly shorter labors but also associated a higher incidence of uterine hyperstimulation (61% vs 46%; P<.001) and need for oxytocin discontinuation.[42,43] In 1 trial, high-dose oxytocin resulted in a significantly higher cesarean delivery rate for fetal distress. The only double-blinded RCT, which included 816 women who received high-dose oxytocin (4.5 mU/min increased by 4.5 mU/min every 30 minutes), was associated with significant shortening of labor of 1.9 hours from oxytocin administration to complete cervical dilation (9.7 ± 0.3 hours vs 7.8 ± 0.2 hours, P<.001).[44] Whatever regimen is decided upon, each hospital should develop protocols for their administration. Oxytocin protocol checklists have been instituted in some settings in an effort to improve maternal safety. Results of this protocol checklist have reduced mean maximum oxytocin infusion rate and improved neonatal outcomes without increasing cesarean delivery rate.[44]

In 2007, a new notice for prescribing oxytocin was published by the FDA, which states that because available data are inadequate to evaluate the benefits-to-risks considerations, oxytocin (Pitocin) is not indicated for elective induction of labor (a women with no medical indication for induction of labor).[45]

NITRIC OXIDE DONORS

The use of vaginal nitric oxide donor isosorbide mononitrate for cervical ripening has been reported in a few publications.[46] Nitric oxide donors by increasing the expression of cyclooxygenase 2 in the cervix improve cervical distensibility without causing uterine contractions. Potential benefits include its potential use in the outpatient setting, low cost, and ease of administration. Side effects may include maternal hemodynamic changes associated with a vasodilator, including hypotension and tachycardia. Women reported headaches and palpitations as the most common side effects of intravaginal administration of isosorbide mononitrate, 40 mg.[47] A recent RCT comparing self-administered isosorbide mononitrate with placebo did not detect a difference in admission to delivery interval despite a clinical effect on cervical ripening.[48] Furthermore, the addition of misoprostol or dinoprostone to the isosorbide mononitrate does not reduce the time to vaginal delivery.[49,50] Therefore, at present, isosorbide mononitrate should not be use for cervical ripening except in clinical trials.

SUMMARY

This is an era of induction of labor. Data to support elective induction of labor before 39 weeks is lacking. Future research may shed light on the optimal timing for delivery that may result in a change of paradigm in the profession. Although multiple agents are available for induction of labor, no 1 agent is superior to the others. Mechanical methods, prostaglandins, and oxytocin are appropriate for labor induction. Clinical presentation, physician preference, and cost may be used in selecting the method of induction. In most agents, a trade-off from efficacy is safety. Cost, safety, and patient satisfaction should be included in future studies. Institutions should establish guideless to improve patient's safety during induction of labor.

REFERENCES

1. Radford Thomas observations on the caesarean section and on other obstetrics complications. Manchester: Bradley's Library Oxford; 1865.
2. Martin JA, Hamilton BE, Sutton PD, et al. Birth final data for 2006. Natl Vital Stat Rep 2009;57:1–102.
3. Zhang J, Yancey MK, Henderson CE. U.S. national trends in labor induction, 1989-1998. J Reprod Med 2002;47(2):120–4.
4. Donovan EF, Lannon C, Bailit J, et al, Ohio Perinatal Quality Collaborative Writing Committee. A statewide initiative to reduce inappropriate scheduled birth at 36 (0/7)-38 6/7 weeks' gestation. Am J Obstet Gynecol 2010;202(3):243.
5. Smith R. Parturition. N Engl J Med 2007;356:271–83.
6. Bishop EH. Pelvic scoring for elective inductions. Obstet Gynecol 1964;24:266–8.
7. Caughey AB, Sundaram V, Kaimai AJ, et al. Maternal and neonatal outcomes of elective induction of labor. Evidence report/technology assessment No. 176. AHRQ Publication No. 09-E005. Rockville (MD): Agency for Healthcare Research and Quality; 2009.
8. ACOG Committee on Practice Bulletins – Obstetrics. ACOG practice bulletin No. 107: induction of labor. Obstet Gynecol 2009;114(2 Pt 1):386–97.
9. Bailit JL, Gregory KD, Reddy UM, et al. Maternal and neonatal outcomes by labor onset type and gestational age. Am J Obstet Gynecol 2010;202:245.e1–245.e12.
10. Caughey AB, Nicholson JM, Cheng YW, et al. Induction of labor and cesarean delivery by gestational age. Am J Obstet Gynecol 2006;195:700–5.
11. Osmundson SS, Ou-Yang RJ, Grobman WA. Elective induction compared with expectant management in nulliparous women with a favorable cervix. Obstet Gynecol 2010;116(3):601–5.
12. Osmunson SS, Janakiraman V, Ecker J, et al. Comparing the second stage in induced and spontaneous labor. Obstet Gynecol 2010;116(3):606–11.
13. Al-Zirqi L, Vangen S, Forsen L, et al. Effects of onset of labor and mode of delivery on severe postpartum hemorrhage. Am J Obstet Gynecol 2009;201:273.e1–9.
14. Shetty A, Burt R, Templeton A. Women's perceptions, expectations and satisfaction with induced labor—a questionnaire-based study. Eur J Obstet Gynecol Reprod Biol 2005;123(1):56–61.
15. Rayburn WF. Minimizing the risks from elective induction of labor. J Reprod Med 2007;52(8):671–6.
16. Fisch JM, English D, Pedaline S, et al. Labor induction process improvement: a patient quality-of-care initiative. Obstet Gynecol 2009;113:797–803.
17. Oshiro BT, Henry E, Wilson J, et al. Decreasing elective deliveries before 39 weeks of gestation in an integrated health care system. Obstet Gynecol 2009; 113:804–11.
18. Boulvain M, Kelly A, Lohse C, et al. Mechanical methods for induction of labour. Cochrane Database Syst Rev 2001;4:CD001233.

19. Heinemann J, Gillen G, Sanchez-Ramos L, et al. Do mechanical methods of cervical ripening increase infectious morbidity? A systematic review. Am J Obstet Gynecol 2008;199:177–87.
20. Krammer J, Williams MC, Sawai SK, et al. Pre-induction cervical ripening: a randomized comparison of two methods. Obstet Gynecol 1995;85:614–8.
21. Embrey MP, Mollison BG. The unfavourable cervix and induction of labour using a cervical balloon. J Obstet Gynaecol Br Commonw 1967;74:44–8.
22. Gelber S, Sciscione A. Mechanical methods of cervical ripening and labor induction. Clin Obstet Gynecol 2006;49:642–57.
23. Levy R, Kanengiser B, Furman B, et al. A randomized trial comparing a 30-mL and an 80-mL Foley catheter balloon for preinduction cervical ripening. Am J Obstet Gynecol 2004;191:1632–6.
24. Kashanian M, Nazemi M, Malakzadegan A. Comparison of 30-mL and 80-mL Foley catheter balloons and oxytocin for preinduction cervical ripening. Int J Gynaecol Obstet 2009;105:174–5.
25. Delaney S, Shaffer BL, Cheng YW, et al. Labor induction with a Foley balloon inflated to 30 mL compared with 60 ml: a randomized controlled trial. Obstet Gynecol 2010;115(6):1239–45.
26. Pettker CM, Pocock SB, Smock DP, et al. Transcevical Foley catheter with and without oxytocin for cervical ripening: a randomized controlled trial. Obstet Gynecol 2008;111(6):1320–6.
27. Vaknin Z, Kurzweil Y, Sherman D. Foley catheter balloon vs locally applied prostaglandins for cervical ripening and labor induction: a systematic review and metaanalysis. Am J Obstet Gynecol 2010;203(5):418–29.
28. Chua S, Arulkumaran S, Vanaja K, et al. Preinduction cervical ripening: prostaglandin E2 gel vs hygroscopic mechanical dilator. J Obstet Gynaecol Res 1997;23:171–7.
29. Sherman DJ, Frenkel E, Tovbin J, et al. Ripening of the unfavorable cervix with extraamniotic catheter balloon: clinical experience and review. Obstet Gynecol Surv 1996;51:621–7.
30. Karjane NW, Brock EL, Walsh SW. Induction of labor using a Foley balloon, with and without extra-amniotic saline infusion. Obstet Gynecol 2006;107(2):234–9.
31. Guinn DA, Davies JK, Jones RO, et al. Labor induction in women with an unfavorable Bishop score: randomize controlled trial of intrauterine Foley catheter with concurrent oxytocin infusion versus Foley catheter with extra-amniotic saline infusion with concurrent oxytocin infusion. Am J Obstet Gynecol 2004;191:225–9.
32. Lin MG, Reid KJ, Treaster MR, et al. Transcervical Foley catheter with and without extra amniotic saline infusion for labor induction: a randomized controlled trial. Obstet Gynecol 2007;110(3):558–65.
33. Maslovitz S, Lessing JB, Many A. Complications of trans-cervical Foley catheter for labor induction among 1,083 women. Arch Gynecol Obstet 2010;281(3):473–7.
34. Witter FR, Rocco LE, Johnson TR. A randomized trial of prostaglandin E2 in a controlled-release vaginal pessary for cervical ripening at term. Am J Obstet Gynecol 1992;166:830–4.
35. Hughes EG, Kelly AJ, Kavanagh J. Dinoprostone vaginal insert for cervical ripening and labor induction: a meta-analysis. Obstet Gynecol 2001;97:847–55.
36. Kelly AJ, Malik S, Smith L, et al. Vaginal prostaglandin (PGE2 and PGF2a) for induction of labour at term. Cochrane Database Syst Rev 2003;(4):CD003101.
37. Pevzner L, Rayburn WF, Rumney P, et al. Factors predicting successful labor induction with dinoprostone and misoprostol vaginal inserts. Obstet Gynecol 2009;114(2 Pt 1):261–7.

38. FDA. Available at: http://www.fda.gov/Drugs/DrugSafety/PostmarketDrugSafety InformationforPatientsandProviders/ucm111315.htm. Accessed February 28, 2011.
39. Tang OS, Schweer H, Seyberth HW, et al. Pharmacokinetics of different routes of administration of misoprostol. Hum Reprod 2002;17(2):332–6.
40. Hofmeyr GJ, Gülmezoglu GJ. Vaginal misoprostol for cervical ripening and induction of labour. Cochrane Database Syst Rev 2003;1:CD000941.
41. Toppozada MK, Anwar MY, Hassan HA, et al. Oral or vaginal misoprostol for induction of labor. Int J Gynaecol Obstet 1997;56:135–9.
42. Satin AJ. High- versus low-dose oxytocin for labor stimulation. Obstet Gynecol 1992;80:111–6.
43. Merrill DC, Zlatnik FJ. Randomized, double-masked comparison of oxytocin dosage in induction and augmentation of labor. Obstet Gynecol 1999;94:455–63.
44. Clark S. Implementation of a conservative checklist-based protocol for oxytocin administration: maternal and newborn outcomes. AJOG 2007;197(5):480.e1–5.
45. FDA oxytocin labelling. Available at: http://www.jhppharma.com/products/pitocin. html. Accessed February 28, 2011.
46. Chanrachakul B, Herabutya Y, Punyavachira P. Potential efficacy of nitric oxide for cervical ripening in pregnancy at term. Int J Gynaecol Obstet 2000;71:217–9.
47. Ekerhovd E, Bullarbo M, Andersch B, et al. Vaginal administration of the nitric oxide donor isosorbide mononitrate for cervical ripening at term: a randomized controlled study. Am J Obstet Gynecol 2003;189(6):1692–7.
48. Bollapragada SS, MacKenzie F, Norrie JD, et al. Randomised placebo-controlled trial of outpatient (at home) cervical ripening with isosorbide mononitrate (IMN) prior to induction of labour–clinical trial with analyses of efficacy and acceptability. The IMOP study. BJOG 2009;116(9):1185–95.
49. Collingham JP, Fuh KC, Caughey AB, et al. Oral misoprostol and vaginal isosorbide mononitrate for labor induction: a randomized controlled trial. Obstet Gynecol 2010;116(1):121–6.
50. Wölfler MM, Facchinetti F, Venturini P, et al. Induction of labor at term using isosorbide mononitrate simultaneously with dinoprostone compared to dinoprostone treatment alone: a randomized, controlled trial. Am J Obstet Gynecol 2006; 195(6):1617–22.

Oral Hypoglycemic Agents in Pregnancy

Jerrie S. Refuerzo, MD

KEYWORDS

• Pregnancy • Diabetes mellitus • Hypoglycemic agents

Diabetes mellitus (DM) affects approximately 3% to 5% of pregnancies.[1] Diabetes that begins before the onset of pregnancy is divided into type 1 DM and type 2 DM. Approximately 10% of pregestational diabetics have type 1 DM and require exogenous insulin to avoid ketoacidosis. The onset of disease usually occurs during childhood, and these women are of normal weight. In contrast, 90% of pregestational diabetics have type 2 DM. These women may require insulin, but can often be controlled with oral hypoglycemic agents. The onset of their DM is usually in adulthood, and most of these women are obese. Gestational DM (GDM) is carbohydrate intolerance first recognized in pregnancy. The prevalence of GDM in the United States is between 1% and 14%.[2] Most women with GDM are obese and have excessive gestational weight gain. After delivery, carbohydrate intolerance is expected to resolve gradually.

Adverse pregnancy outcomes in diabetic pregnancies are related to fetal hyperinsulinemia, which arises as a response to increased levels of maternal glucose crossing the placenta.[3] Fetal hyperinsulinemia is associated with increased fetal growth, fat deposition, and demand for oxygen. Women with DM are at significantly increased risk of spontaneous abortions, congenital birth defects, preeclampsia, and intrauterine fetal death.[1,2] Poor pregnancy outcomes are also due to macrosomia, increasing the rate of shoulder dystocia, leading to neonatal birth injury and potential need for cesarean section. Moreover, most of these women are obese. Obesity itself independently increases the rate of cesarean section.[4,5] Offspring born to women with type 2 DM have a higher rate of developing obesity and insulin resistance later in life.[6–8] These pregnancy complications and the process of fetal programming in utero are directly related to the level of glycemic control during pregnancy. Pregnancy management aims to reduce pregnancy complications by returning maternal glucose levels to normal.[1,3,9]

The HAPO study (Hyperglycemia and Adverse Pregnancy Outcome), published in 2008, demonstrated an association between maternal glucose levels and pregnancy outcomes.[10] This study included 25,505 pregnant women in 15 different centers

Division of Maternal Fetal Medicine, Department of Obstetrics, Gynecology, and Reproductive Sciences, University of Texas Health Science Center at Houston, 6431 Fannin Street, Room 3.270A, Houston, TX 77030, USA
E-mail address: jerrie.s.refuerzo@uth.tmc.edu

Obstet Gynecol Clin N Am 38 (2011) 227–234
doi:10.1016/j.ogc.2011.02.013
0889-8545/11/$ – see front matter © 2011 Elsevier Inc. All rights reserved.

who underwent a 75 g glucola screen between 24 and 32 weeks of pregnancy. Data was blinded to allow clinicians to management free of bias. Women with higher fasting, 1-hour and 2-hour postprandial glucose levels had higher odds ratios for a neonatal birth weight greater than the 90th percentile. In addition, there were similar increased odds ratios for cord blood serum C-peptide levels, a marker for fetal/neonatal hyperinsulinemia. These findings suggest benefit in achieving optimal glycemic control during pregnancy.

Optimal glycemic control can be achieved with medications. Over the last decade, several studies have offered oral hypoglycemic agents as options for medical therapy for the treatment of diabetes during pregnancy. For the purposes of this article, the focus will concentrate on glyburide and metformin, since these 2 oral hypoglycemic agents are the most commonly used during pregnancy.

GOALS FOR MEDICAL THERAPY

The decision to administer medication during pregnancy must take into consideration the benefits and risks to both the pregnant woman and her fetus. The primary risks of medications are affected by the transplacental passage of medications, association with fetal anomalies, potential for maternal adverse effects, and after delivery of the newborn, the safety of the medications during breastfeeding.

INSULIN

Historically, insulin has been the therapeutic agent of choice for controlling hyperglycemia in pregnant women. However, difficulty in medication administration with multiple daily injections, potential for hypoglycemia, and increase in appetite and weight make this therapeutic option cumbersome for the pregnant patient.[3] Moreover, hypoglycemia occurs in approximately 71% of women who take insulin during some time during their pregnancy.

GLYBURIDE
Glyburide as an Oral Hypoglycemic Agent

Glyburide is a second-generation oral sulfonylurea hypoglycemic agent. Its chemical name is 1-[p-[2-(5-chloro-o-anisamido) ethyl] phenyl] sulfonyl]-3-cy-clohexylurea. Sulfonylureas are effective only in patients who have retained some degree of pancreatic insulin-releasing function (type 2 DM). Glyburide acts by enhancing the release of insulin from the pancreatic beta cells in normal and type 2 DM patients in response to stimulation by insulin. Extrapancreatic effects include improvement in glucose use and reversal of early diabetic microangiopathy.[11] Pharmacologically, glyburide is well absorbed following oral administration and independent of food intake. The time to peak concentration ranges from 2 to 3 hours; the volume of distribution is 9 to 40 L, and the half-life is 7 to 10 hours. Glyburide is metabolized by the liver. The initial dose of glyburide is 2.5 to 5.0 mg once or twice a day with a maximum dose of 20 mg/day.[11,12]

The use of oral sulfonylureas is attractive in pregnancy. The ease and relatively infrequent administration of glyburide make this medication much more favorable to patients than insulin. Also, the potential adverse effects of glyburide are minimal compared with insulin. The overall incidence of hypoglycemia from glyburide is 1% to 5%. Thus, prescribing glyburide rather than insulin during pregnancy may increase patient compliance, satisfaction, and overall maternal and neonatal outcome.

Unlike other sulfonylureas, there is substantial evidence demonstrating the lack of transplacental passage of glyburide to the fetus. Although studies have detected glyburide concentrations in the fetuses of pregnant rats comparable to maternal concentrations, this is not true in people.[13] Using a single-cotyledon placental model, Elliott demonstrated 0.47% to 1.1% transport of glyburide from mother to fetus.[14] He later compared the transport of glyburide with glipizide, chlorpropamide and tolbutamide. In contrast to the other oral hypoglycemic medications, the maternal-to-fetal transport of second-generation sulfonylureas is significantly lower than the first-generation drugs, suggesting that greatly reduced or insignificant fetal exposure may occur with these newer agents, particularly glyburide.[15] Possible explanations for such lack of placental transport of glyburide include the extensive plasma protein binding and short elimination half-life.[16,17] From a clinical perspective, in the randomized study of glyburide versus insulin in gestational diabetes conducted by Langer, glyburide was not detected in the cord blood of any infant.[18] Thus, the lack of transplacental transport of glyburide suggests that this newer sulfonylurea is safe in pregnancy.

Studies of Glyburide in Pregnancy

There have been a few studies involving the use of glyburide in pregnancy. The outcomes of pregnant women on glyburide for gestational diabetes was first reported in 1997 by Lim.[19] There was no difference in pregnancy outcomes between women who received glyburide (33 patients) versus those on insulin (21 patients). Of the 33 patients, 21.2% (n = 7) of women failed glyburide treatment and were eventually switched to insulin therapy. The birth weights were higher in the glyburide patients, and there were 2 neonatal mortalities. One neonatal death was associated with severe cardiac anomalies and the other due to intraventricular hemorrhage and neonatal sepsis, both of which were not attributed to the glyburide. Overall, they claimed that most women with gestational diabetes can be managed effectively and safely with glyburide.

In a landmark randomized trial by Langer, glyburide was compared with insulin in the treatment of gestational diabetes.[18] The daily blood glucose concentrations and glycosylated hemoglobin values were similar between patients on glyburide (n = 201) compared with insulin (n = 203). The failure rate was 4% (n = 8) in the glyburide patients, thus requiring the need to switch to insulin. There were no differences in the infants with large for gestational age, macrosomia, lung complications, hypoglycemia, admission to the neonatal intensive care unit (NICU), or fetal anomalies. Also, the cord insulin concentrations were similar between groups. In contrast, glyburide was not detected in the cord serum of infants of the glyburide group. Langer concluded that glyburide was a clinically effective alternative to insulin therapy in women with gestational diabetes.

A cost analysis was then performed by Goetzl to compare the costs associated with glyburide versus insulin for the treatment of gestational diabetes.[20] They found that glyburide was significantly less costly than insulin. The average cost savings per patient based on wholesale drug costs and hospital costs was $165.84. Thus, it appears that glyburide is more cost-effective than insulin in the treatment of gestational diabetes.

To assess the comparative effectiveness of glyburide versus insulin, a meta-analysis has been performed of randomized controlled trials of glyburide versus insulin in the treatment of gestational diabetes.[21] There have been 3 randomized controlled trials with a total of 478 participants conducted in the United States, India, Brazil, New Zealand and Australia. There were no differences in glycemic control including fasting blood glucose or 2-hour postprandial. There were similar rates of cesarean delivery, with a range between 23% and 52%. Some investigators reported a higher rate of maternal hypoglycemia in the women who received insulin (20%) compared with glyburide (4%),[18] although other investigators reported similar hypoglycemia rates.[22,23] In contrast, neonatal hyperglycemia was reported to be higher among those women who received glyburide (33%) compared with insulin (4%),[23] whereas others did not find such differences.[18] Newborn birth weights were similar between groups, (weighted mean difference −93 g, 95% confidence interval −191 to 5 g). Overall, maternal and neonatal outcomes appear to be similar in women treated with glyburide compared with insulin in these studies.

Risks of Glyburide in Pregnancy

Glyburide is a category C medication in pregnancy. Hypoglycemia may occur with all sulfonylureas. The incidence of hypoglycemia with glyburide ranges from 1% to 5%. The overall incidence of adverse effects ranges from 3.2 to 4.1%. The most common adverse effects are (GI) (nausea, vomiting, dyspepsia) and dermatologic (pruritus, urticaria, erythema, and morbilliform or maculopapular eruptions). Elevations of liver function tests have been reported, but jaundice is rare.[11]

Identifying those women who fail glyburide therapy in pregnancy is important when deciding medical therapy for the treatment of gestational diabetes. An observational trial was conducted by Conway examining factors that predict failure of glyburide treatment in gestational diabetes.[24] Of the 75 patients, there was a 16% failure rate. Patients who failed glyburide therapy were compared with those treated successfully with glyburide. Conway found that among women with high fasting plasma glucose levels greater than or equal to 110 mg/dL, 24% failed to respond to glyburide compared with 12% who did respond to glyburide. Overall, glyburide was successful in achieving good glycemic control in women with gestational diabetes.[24]

Glyburide and Breastfeeding

Studies focusing on the transfer of glyburide into the milk of lactating mothers have been performed.[25,26] In 8 women who received a single dose of glyburide, the mean maximum theoretical infant dose as a percent of the weight-adjusted maternal dose was less than 1.5% and less than 0.7% for the 5 mg dose and 10 mg dose, respectively.[25] In 5 women receiving daily doses, glyburide levels could not be detected in the breast milk. In addition, there were no neonatal cases of hypoglycemia. Thus, it appears that breastfeeding is safe in women receiving glyburide.

METFORMIN
Metformin as an Oral Hypoglycemic Agent

Metformin is a biguanide that improves insulin sensitivity by reducing fasting plasma glucose and insulin concentrations. It functions by decreasing hepatic glucose output by inhibition of gluconeogenesis and enhanced peripheral glucose uptake.[3] It also decreases intestinal glucose absorption and increases insulin sensitivity. It is metabolized by the CYP450 pathway, is excreted in the urine, and has a half-life of 6.2 hours. Metformin is available in 500 mg, 850 mg, and 1000 mg tablets in both regular-release and extended-release forms. The usual starting dose is usually 500 to 850 mg/d, which can be increased gradually to a maximum dose of 2500 mg/day.

Studies of Metformin During Pregnancy

Metformin has been used by women throughout pregnancy. The first studies were performed by Coetzee and colleagues[27] during the 1970s. Women with insulin-independent diabetes were prospectively followed throughout gestation; 22 women received metformin compared with 42 women who received insulin. The perinatal mortality rate was 50 deaths per 1000 population for those on metformin versus 51 deaths per 1000 population on insulin. Neonatal birth weight greater than 4000 g occurred in only 10% of women on metformin. There were no cases of maternal hypoglycemia or lactic acidosis. In addition, metformin use in the first trimester was not associated with congenital anomalies.[28] In a follow-up study, Coetzee was able to achieve glycemic control in women on metformin within 24 hours compared with 2 to 3 weeks for insulin.[29]

In 2000, Hellmuth and colleagues[30] performed a cohort study of type 2 DM pregnant women on metformin (n = 50) versus glyburide (n = 68) versus insulin (n = 42). His findings suggest concern for the use of metformin due to the increased rate of preeclampsia, (32% metformin vs 7% glyburide vs 10% insulin) and intrauterine fetal death (8% vs 0% vs 2.3%). Critics of his study claim that women in the study were not well matched. Those women who received the metformin were morbidly obese and started the medication later in the pregnancy. Thus, the women were inherently at risk for adverse pregnancy outcomes unrelated to metformin.[3,31] In contrast, in a series of 90 women with polycystic ovarian syndrome (PCOS) who conceived on 1.5 to 2.55 g/d of metformin, treatment with metformin was not associated with preeclampsia in pregnancy (5.2% metformin vs 3.6% no metformin).[32]

Others studies have been conducted primarily in women with PCOS treated for infertility. In an observation trial of 72 women who conceived on 2.55 g/d of metformin, there was a higher live birth rate in those who received metformin compared with those without metformin, 75% versus 34%. The spontaneous abortion rate was lower with metformin, (17% vs 62%). Again, there were no cases of lactic acidosis, fetal anomalies, or maternal or neonatal hypoglycemia.[33] The neonates whose mothers received metformin were also followed prospectively and displayed normal weight and social and motor skills at 6 months. At 18 months, there were no differences in height, weight, motor, or social skills between neonatal groups.[34]

A randomized, double-blinded controlled pilot study was performed on 18 PCOS women who conceived on metformin compared with 22 women who received a placebo. Women who received the metformin had a lower rate of pregnancy complications (0% metformin vs 32% placebo) including preterm birth, sepsis, deep venous thrombosis, or adult respiratory distress syndrome. There were no differences in neonatal outcomes such as birth weight.[35] Another study involving PCOS women who conceived on metformin showed a lower rate of developing gestational diabetes later in pregnancy (3% metformin vs 31% no metformin).[36]

A meta-analysis revealed 1 randomized controlled trial of metformin compared with insulin for the treatment of gestational diabetes.[21] This Australian study conducted by Rowan and colleagues[37] and included 751 women (371 received metformin, and 378 received insulin) who were randomized between 20 and 33 weeks of pregnancy. The metformin failure rate was 7.4%, in which a second diabetic agent was needed to maintain controlled glucose levels. Although there was no difference in mean fasting blood glucose levels between groups, those on metformin had lower 2-hour postprandial glucose levels. There was no difference in the rate of preeclampsia. Infants of women randomized to metformin experienced a lower rate of hypoglycemia compared with insulin, (insulin 8.1% vs metformin 3.3%, $P = .008$). There was no difference in infant birth weight, the proportion of infants with birth trauma, shoulder dystocia, 5-minute Apgar score less than 7, or admission to a NICU between groups.

Risks of Metformin During Pregnancy

Metformin is a category B medication in pregnancy. The risks from metformin in pregnancy include the potential for neonatal hypoglycemia. In ex vivo placental perfusion model studies, metformin had a maternal-to-fetal transfer rate of 10% to 16%.[38,39] Neonatal hypoglycemia is always a concern postnatally. In several reports on the infants in the immediate neonatal period, there was not an increase in the rate of neonatal hypoglycemia after delivery compared with women who received insulin. In those who did develop neonatal hypoglycemia, it was determined that this outcome was related to maternal hyperglycemia at the time of delivery.[27–29,33,36,40] There were no cases of neonatal lactic acidosis.

Regarding teratogenicity, metformin has been used in primarily 2 groups of women during pregnancy: (1) pregnant women with polycystic ovary syndrome during organogenesis in the first trimester and (2) pregnant women with diabetes, both pregestational and gestational diabetes.[27–29,33,36,40] In these reports, there was not an increased risk of congenital anomalies compared with those who received insulin or compared with the general population. The development of congenital anomalies that did occur in these studies was attributed to the presence of hyperglycemia during organogenesis and not to metformin itself. Therefore, metformin is not considered teratogenic.

From a maternal perspective, hypoglycemia related to metformin occurs in 0% to 21% of patients.[41] There are some adverse effects including GI upset, including diarrhea, flatulence, nausea, and vomiting. The rate of these symptoms can occur with a rate of 2% to 63%, with many reporting approximately a 5% to 15% rate.[41,42] These adverse effects can be minimized by gradually increasing metformin over several days. In a systematic review, there was little or no elevated risk of lactic acidosis in diabetics who received metformin compared with those on other oral anti-hyperglycemic agents.[41]

Breastfeeding and Metformin

Multiple studies have demonstrated that breastfeeding is safe for the infant in women who breastfeed. The mean infant exposure to drug ranged from 0.11% to 0.65% of the weight-normalized maternal dose.[43–45] This is below the 10% level of concern for breastfeeding.[43] In addition, the blood glucose concentrations in infants 4 hours after a feeding were within the normal limit, ranging from 47 to 77 mg/dL serum. Based on these findings metformin use by breastfeeding mothers is safe.

SUMMARY

In summary, multiple studies have been published illustrating the use of oral hypoglycemic agents in pregnancy. Glyburide and metformin have been shown to be as effective as insulin for the treatment of gestational diabetes. Both are safe with breastfeeding. Although both glyburide and metformin appear safe for the treatment of type 2 DM, more studies are needed to identify risks and benefits of oral hypoglycemic for the treatment of pregestational diabetes.

REFERENCES

1. Gabbe S, Graves CR. Management of diabetes mellitus complicating pregnancy. Obstet Gynecol 2003;102(4):857–68.
2. American College of Obstetricians and Gynecologists. ACOG practice bulletin 30. Washington, DC: ACOG; 2001.
3. Norman RJ, Wang JX, Hague W. Should we continue or stop insulin-sensitizing drugs during pregnancy? Curr Opin Obstet Gynecol 2004;16(3):245–50.

4. Ehrenberg HM, Durnwald CP, Catalano P, et al. The influence of obesity and diabetes on the risk of cesarean delivery. Am J Obstet Gynecol 2004;191(3):969–74.
5. Ehrenberg HM, Mercer BM, Catalano PM. The influence of obesity and diabetes on the prevalence of macrosomia. Am J Obstet Gynecol 2004;191(3):964–8.
6. Martorell S, Schroeder DG. Early nutrition and later adiposity. J Nutr 2001;131: 874S–80S.
7. Strauss R. Effects of intrauterine environment on childhood growth. Br Med Bull 1997;53(1):85–95.
8. Whitaker R, Dietz WH. Role of the prenatal environment in the development of obesity. J Pediatr 1998;135(5):768–76.
9. Jovanovic R, Jovanovic L. Obstetric management when normaolgycemia is maintained in diabetic pregnant women with vascular compromise. Am J Obstet Gynecol 1984;149(6):617–23.
10. Metzger BE, Lowe LP, Dyer AR, et al. Hyperglycemia and adverse pregnancy outcomes. N Engl J Med 2008;358(19):1991–2002.
11. Prendergast BD. Glyburide and glipizide, second-generation oral sulfonylurea hypoglycemic agents. Clin Pharm 1984;3(5):473–85.
12. Merlob P, Levitt O, Stahl B. Oral antihyperglycemic agents during pregnancy and lactation: a review. Paediatr Drugs 2002;4(11):755–60.
13. Sivan E, Feldman B, Dolitzki M, et al. Glyburide crosses the placenta in vivo in pregnant rats. Diabetologia 1995;38(7):753–6.
14. Elliott BD, Langer O, Schenker S, et al. Insignificant transfer of glyburide occurs across the human placenta. Am J Obstet Gynecol 1991;165:807–12.
15. Elliott BD, Schenker S, Langer O, et al. Comparative placental transport of oral hypoglycemic agents in humans: a model of human placental drug transfer. Am J Obstet Gynecol 1994;171(3):653–60.
16. Koren G. Glyburide and fetal safety; transplacental pharmacokinetic considerations. Reprod Toxicol 2001;15(3):227–9.
17. Garcia-Bournissen F, Feig DS, Koren G. Maternal-fetal transport of hypoglycaemic drugs. Clin Pharmacokinet 2003;42(4):303–13.
18. Langer O, Conway DL, Berkus MD, et al. A comparison of glyburide and insulin in women with gestational diabetes mellitus. N Engl J Med 2000;343(16):1134–8.
19. Lim JM, Tayob Y, O'Brien PM, et al. A comparison between the pregnancy outcome of women with gestation diabetes treated with glibenclamide and those treated with insulin. Med J Malaysia 1997;52(4):377–81.
20. Goetzl L, Wilkins I. Glyburide compared to insulin for the treatment of gestational diabetes mellitus: a cost analysis. J Perinatol 2002;22(5):403–6.
21. Nicholson W, Bolen S, Witkop CT, et al. Benefits and risks of oral diabetes agents compared with insulin in women with gestational diabetes: a systematic review. Obstet Gynecol 2009;113(1):193–205.
22. Anjalakshi C, Balaji V, Balaji MS, et al. A prospective study comparing insulin and glibenclamide in gestational diabetes mellitus in Asian Indian women. Diabetes Res Clin Pract 2007;76(3):474–5.
23. Bertini AM, Silva JC, Taborda W, et al. Perinatal outcomes and the use of oral hypoglycemic agents. J Perinat Med 2005;33(6):519–23.
24. Conway D, Gonzales O, Skiver D. Use of glyburide for the treatment of gestational diabetes: the san antonio experience. Obstet Gynecol Surv 2004;59(7):491–3.
25. Feig DS, Briggs GG, Kraemer JM, et al. Transfer of glyburide and glipizide into breast milk. Diabetes Care 2005;28(8):1851–5.
26. Glatstein MM, Djokanovic N, Garcia-Bournissen F, et al. Use of hypoglycemic drugs during lactation. Can Fam Physician 2009;55(4):371–3.

27. Coetzee EJ, Jackson WP. Pregnancy in established non-insulin-dependent diabetics. A five-and-a-half year study at Groote Schuur Hospital. S Afr Med J
1980;58(20):795–802.

28. Coetzee EJ, Jackson WP. Oral hypoglycaemics in the first trimester and fetal
outcome. S Afr Med J 1984;65(16):635–7.

29. Coetzee EJ, Jackson WP. The management of non-insulin-dependent diabetes
during pregnancy. Diabetes Res Clin Pract 1986;1:281–7.

30. Hellmuth E, Damm P, Molsted-Pedersen L. Oral hypoglycaemic agents in 118
diabetic pregnancies. Diabet Med 2000;17(7):507–11.

31. Checa MA, Requena A, Salvador C, et al. Insulin-sensitizing agents: use in pregnancy and as therapy in polycystic ovary syndrome. Hum Reprod Update 2005;
11(4):375–90.

32. Glueck CJ, Bornovali S, Pranikoff J, et al. Metformin, preeclampsia, and pregnancy outcomes in women with polycystic ovary syndrome. Diabet Med 2004;
21(8):829–36.

33. Glueck CJ, Wang P, Goldenberg N, et al. Pregnancy outcomes among women
with polycystic ovary syndrome treated with metformin. Hum Reprod 2002;
17(11):2858–64.

34. Glueck CJ, Goldenberg N, Pranikoff J, et al. Height, weight, and motor–social
development during the first 18 months of life in 126 infants born to 109 mothers
with polycystic ovary syndrome who conceived on and continued metformin
through pregnancy. Hum Reprod 2004;19(6):1323–30.

35. Vanky E, Salvesen KA, Heimstad R, et al. Metformin reduces pregnancy
complications without affecting androgen levels in pregnant polycystic ovary
syndrome women: results of a randomized study. Hum Reprod 2004;19(8):
1734–40.

36. Glueck CJ, Wang P, Kobayashi S, et al. Metformin therapy throughout pregnancy
reduces the development of gestational diabetes in women with polycystic ovary
syndrome. Fertil Steril 2002;77(3):520–5.

37. Rowan JA, Hague WM, Gao W, et al. Metformin versus insulin for the treatment of
gestational diabetes. N Engl J Med 2008;358(19):2003–15.

38. Kovo M, Haroutiunian S, Feldman N, et al. Determination of metformin transfer
across the human placenta using a dually perfused ex vivo placental cotyledon
model. Eur J Obstet Gynecol Reprod Biol 2008;136(1):29–33.

39. Nanovskaya TN, Nekhayeva IA, Patrikeeva SL, et al. Transfer of metformin across
the dually perfused human placental lobule. Am J Obstet Gynecol 2006;195(4):
1081–5.

40. Glueck CJ, Goldenberg N, Streicher P, et al. Metformin and gestational diabetes.
Curr Diab Rep 2003;3(4):303–12.

41. Bolen S, Feldman L, Vassy J, et al. Systematic review: comparative effectiveness
and safety of oral medications for type 2 diabetes mellitus. Ann Intern Med 2007;
147(6):386–99.

42. Asche CV, McAdam-Marx C, Shane-McWhorter L, et al. Association between oral
antidiabetic use, adverse events, and outcomes in patients with type 2 diabetes.
Diabetes Obes Metab 2008;10(8):638–45.

43. Briggs GG, Ambrose PJ, Nageotte MP, et al. Excretion of metformin into breast
milk and the effect on nursing infants. Obstet Gynecol 2005;105(6):1437–41.

44. Gardiner SJ, Kirkpatrick CM, Begg EJ, et al. Transfer of metformin into human
milk. Clin Pharmacol Ther 2003;73(1):71–7.

45. Hale TW, Kristensen JH, Hackett LP, et al. Transfer of metformin into human milk.
Diabetologia 2002;45(11):1509–14.

What Agent Should be Used to Prevent Recurrent Preterm Birth: 17-P or Natural Progesterone?

Nicole Ruddock Hall, MD

KEYWORDS

- Preterm birth • 17 alpha-hydroxyprogesterone caproate
- Natural progesterone • Prevention

Preterm birth is an important public health issue with an increasing incidence over the last decade. According to the March of Dimes, there has been a 20% increase in the preterm birth rate between 1990 and 2006. In 2006, 12.5% of all births in the United States occurred at fewer than 37 weeks gestation. The majority of this increase has occurred in births between 32 to 36 weeks gestation (March of Dimes, 2006). This has been associated with significant health care costs as well as related neonatal morbidity and mortality.[1] It is the leading cause of neonatal mortality in neonates without anomalies and is responsible for approximately 50% of cerebral palsy, 33% of visual impairment, 20% of mental retardation and an increased risk of long-term cardiovascular morbidity.[2] In 2003, costs related to care for infants with preterm-birth or low-birth weight exceeded 11 billion dollars.[3]

RISK FACTORS

Low socioeconomic status, infection or inflammation, multiple gestation, short cervix, African American race, and genetic factors have all been associated with a higher risk of spontaneous preterm birth.[4–6] There are significant racial, ethnic, and socio-economic disparities in the rates of preterm birth. The highest rates of preterm birth are among African American and Hispanic women, with lower rates in Asian and Caucasian women.[7] However, the risk of preterm birth is highest in women with a prior preterm birth, especially if it occurred in the penultimate pregnancy.[8]

Division of Maternal Fetal Medicine, Department of Obstetrics/Gynecology, University of Texas Health Science Center, 5656 Kelley Street, Houston, TX 77026, USA
E-mail address: nicole.r.hall@uth.tmc.edu

Obstet Gynecol Clin N Am 38 (2011) 235–246
doi:10.1016/j.ogc.2011.02.014
0889-8545/11/$ – see front matter © 2011 Elsevier Inc. All rights reserved.

TREATMENT
Tocolysis

Although there has been some improvement in the approach to treatment of preterm neonates with the use of antenatal corticosteroids, surfactant, and improved neonatal care, fewer advances have been made in primary prevention of preterm birth and effective tocolysis. Numerous studies have focused on the prevention of preterm birth and its effect on reducing neonatal morbidity and mortality. Recent clinical trials using 17 alpha-hydroxyprogesterone caproate (17-P) and natural progesterone have shown benefit in prevention of recurrent preterm birth in patients with a history of a preterm delivery before 37 weeks gestation.[9,10] In clinical studies, progestational agents are most beneficial for patients with either an early preterm birth or a short cervix.

PROPOSED MECHANISMS OF PROGESTERONE ACTION

Progesterone has been shown to support gestation and inhibit uterine activity. In human parturition, the corpus luteum produces progesterone in early pregnancy; its production is mainly by the placenta in the remaining two thirds of pregnancy. Its mode of action includes relaxation of uterine smooth muscle, immunosuppression against the activation of T lymphocytes, inhibition of oxytocin effects on the myometrium, and the formation of gap junctions between myometrial cells.[11,12] Progesterone has also been shown to regulate uterine contractility[13] and promote cervical ripening,[14] which culminates in the onset and progression of labor.

PROGESTERONE WITHDRAWAL

Csapo[13] proposed that labor is initiated by progesterone withdrawal, that is, a physiologically regulated decrease in progesterone levels. This has been validated in animal models but has not been confirmed in human pregnancy. In the sheep model of parturition, the onset of labor is triggered by activation of the fetal pituitary-adrenal axis and increased secretion of fetal cortisol, which initiates an enzyme cascade resulting in a decrease in progesterone levels and an increase in estrogen levels at the onset of labor.[15] Although findings of lower serum progesterone levels have not been reproduced in human studies, the current hypothesis proposes a "functional" withdrawal of progesterone that initiates labor.[16] A study examined the changes in nuclear progesterone receptors PR-A and PR-B with advancing gestation to determine how changes in the PR-A to PR-B ratio affects myometrial responsiveness to progesterone. PR-B is thought to promote uterine quiescence, whereas PR-A, which is upregulated with the onset of labor, is thought to promote myometrial contractility. The PR-A to PR-B protein ratio is increased in myometrial tissues from term versus preterm deliveries, and is further increased in tissue from term-laboring patients. This suggests that functional progesterone withdrawal is mediated by the change in PR-A to PR-B ratio. Expression of PR-A decreases the PR-B-mediated progesterone responsiveness.[17]

EFFECTS ON MYOMETRIUM

Because the human placenta produces large quantities of progesterone, it seems unlikely that exogenous progesterone compounds given in pregnancy would have any effect on plasma concentrations or on any actions of progesterone upon the myometrium or other tissues. However, modest changes of progesterone to estrogen ratio at the tissue level may have significant effects. Progesterone is postulated to affect gap junction formation in human myometrium. Gap junctions are specialized regulated channels that propagate action potentials and facilitate exchange between cells. Its expression in human myometrium is inhibited by progesterone and upregulated by estrogen.[18] The regulation of the gap junction gene in human gestation is characterized by a steady increase in gene message in late pregnancy. Relatively minor changes in the progesterone-to-estrogen ratio in decidua or fetal membranes could have large effects on gap junction formation in the myometrium. Progesterone serves to inhibit gap junction formation and, thus, labor.

EFFECTS ON CERVICAL RIPENING

Inhibition of premature cervical ripening, either primarily or as an adjunct to inhibition of myometrial contractility, has not been adequately investigated. Antiprogestins have long been known to induce cervical ripening.[19] Studies have shown that progesterone inhibits, whereas antiprogestin promotes, cervical ripening through an effect on a number of enzymes (eg, inducible nitric oxide synthase, cyclooxygenase) involved in remodeling of cervical extracellular matrix.[20–22] Progesterone administration could exert an inhibitory effect on the biochemical changes that alter the extracellular matrix of the cervix, and lead to cervical shortening before the onset of premature labor. Shynlova and colleagues[22] found that fibronectin and laminar mRNA increased, but fibrillar collagen mRNA decreased, in pregnant rats as term labor approached. Treatment with a progesterone antagonist before term gestation accelerated these changes, leading to preterm labor. Conversely, administration of progesterone led to reductions in both fibronectin and laminar mRNA, the maintenance of collagen mRNA levels, and prolongation of pregnancy. Marx and colleagues[20] evaluated inducible nitric oxide synthase and cyclooxygenase-2 mRNA, two enzymes involved in cervical ripening, and found that progesterone antagonists increased expression of both enzymes' mRNA and caused preterm labor. Progesterone administration suppressed these enzymes' mRNA and led to pregnancy prolongation.

REGULATION OF THE IMMUNE RESPONSE

There have been several studies that have examined the role of progesterone in regulation of the immune response. Uterine levels of IL-1 α, a preterm-labor signaling protein, and Toll-like receptors, which are all associated with preterm delivery, are decreased by treatment with progesterone.[23–25] A short or dilated cervix has been associated with increased inflammation and, therefore, may be amenable to treatment with progesterone. A short or dilated cervix has been associated with an increased risk of intrauterine inflammation, as a shorter cervix is more likely to permit bacteria to ascend into the uterine cavity. Among pregnancies complicated by symptomatic preterm labor with intact membranes, cervicovaginal secretions had higher concentrations of IL-6 in women who delivered preterm compared with those who delivered at term.[26–28] IL-6 was elevated in 56.3% of preterm birth fewer than 37 weeks compared with 27.3% of term births.[26] The median value of IL-6 was significantly higher in pregnancies with preterm birth before 34 weeks or delivery within 7 days of preterm labor.[27] Those with elevated IL-6 had shorter latency to delivery (37.0 days vs 46.7 days).[26] There were also significantly higher cytokine levels in cervical secretion in the presence of intra-amniotic infection confirmed by amniocentesis among women with preterm labor and intact membrane.[28] Preterm delivery at the earliest gestational ages has also been associated with a greater prevalence of intrauterine inflammation.[29] Goldenberg and colleagues[30] demonstrated that even after inflammation occurs and the maternal-fetal interface has been disrupted, the risk for preterm delivery can be reduced if the extracellular matrix damage can be repaired.

HISTORY OF PROGESTERONE RESEARCH

Since the 1970s, studies have used varying doses and formulations of progesterone for different indications to demonstrate the effect on parturition. Several early studies suggested that progesterone, particularly 17-P, might be used to treat preterm labor. An analysis of all the early studies, conducted by Keirse.[31] supported the concept that 17-P treatment might be effective for preterm labor prevention. More recent studies by Meis and colleagues[9] and da Fonseca and colleagues[10] in 2003 have shown a reduction in preterm birth in patients with a prior history of preterm birth treated with 17-P and vaginal progesterone, respectively. 17-P has been proven effective for prevention of preterm delivery in five successful trials.[9,32–35] The optimal dose, formulation, and route of administration is still widely debated in the literature.

EARLY CLINICAL TRIALS OF 17-P

One of the first randomized trials of progestational agents for the prevention of preterm birth in women at increased risk was published in 1970 by Papiernik.[32] Ninety-nine women were randomized to 17-P or placebo in the third trimester. The incidence of preterm delivery was 4% in the 17-P treated group and 18% in the placebo group. This was followed by a study by Johnson and colleagues,[33] in 1975, using 17-P 250 mg weekly for women with recurrent spontaneous abortions and at least one preterm delivery. This was a prospective, randomized, double-blind, placebo-controlled study that enrolled 50 women with a history of two previous spontaneous abortions or preterm births before 36 weeks gestation. Study patients were treated with weekly intramuscular injections of 250 mg 17-P or placebo from enrollment until 24 weeks gestation. Patients with a history of cervical incompetence and multiple gestations were included. The objective of the study was to test the efficacy of a progestational agent in preventing the onset of preterm labor. The outcomes measured were delivery before 37 weeks gestation, birth weight less than 2500 g, and perinatal death. There was a 41% incidence of preterm delivery in the placebo group and none in the treatment group. These results were not statistically significant. The rate of preterm birth was 11% and 48% in the treatment and placebo groups, respectively, with an odds ratio of 0.14. The mean gestational age of delivery was 38.6 ($\pm$ 1.4) weeks in the treatment group and 35.3 ($\pm$ 6.2) weeks in the placebo group. In this trial, there was no uniform gestational age for starting therapy and the sample included patients with cerclage.

In 1985, Yemini and colleagues[35] randomized 79 women with history of two spontaneous abortions, two preterm deliveries, or one of each to 17-P 250 mg intramuscularly weekly versus placebo starting at 16 to 20 weeks gestation. The rate of preterm delivery was 16% in the 17-P treated group and 37.82% in the placebo group. Hauth and colleagues[29] used a relatively high dose of 1000 mg weekly in low-risk, active duty military recruits but no difference was noted in delivery outcome. In these early studies, there was no uniformity in the indication for treatment, gestational age at initiation, duration of treatment, or study outcomes.

RECENT CLINICAL TRIALS OF 17-P

The Meis and colleagues[9] trial was a prospective, double-blind, placebo-controlled trial including 463 women with a history of spontaneous preterm birth. Patients were treated with weekly intramuscular injections of 250 mg 17-P or placebo from 16 to 20 weeks of gestation until 36 weeks or birth. The primary outcome of the study was birth before 37 weeks gestation. Treatment with 17-P reduced the incidence of delivery before 37 weeks (36.3% in the 17-P group vs 54.9% in the placebo group). In addition, there was a reduction in delivery less than 35 weeks (20.6% in the 17-P group vs 30.7% in the control group) and at less than 32 weeks (11.4% in the 17-P group vs 19.6% in the control group). There was also a reduction in the rates of necrotizing enterocolitis, intraventricular hemorrhage, and need for supplemental oxygen in infants of women treated with 17-P. In the Meis and colleagues[9] trial, 250 mg of 17-P or inert oil (controls) were injected intramuscularly on a weekly basis in women with a history of preterm labor starting at 16 to 20 weeks of gestation. This landmark clinical trial showed that weekly injections of 17-P resulted in a substantial reduction in the rate of recurrent preterm delivery in women with a high risk of preterm delivery. A summary of clinical trials using 17-P is included in **Table 1**.

CURRENT RECOMMENDATIONS FOR USE

Current American College of Obstetricians and Gynecologists guidelines restrict progesterone use to women with a documented preterm delivery before 37 weeks.[36] There is no evidence to support the use of progestins in patients with multiple gestations,[37,38] but there may be some benefit for asymptomatic women with shortened cervical length less than 15 mm.[39] Tocolysis is useful for short-term prolongation

Table 1
Clinical trials involving 17-P to prevent preterm birth

Author (Year)	Intramuscular Dose (Frequency)	Indication	Gestational Age
Levine[34] 1964	500 mg q wk	≥ 3 SAB	<16–36 wk
Sherman[48] 1966	2000 mg q wk	≥ 2 SAB and low urine pregnanediol	Enrollment–24 wk
Papiernik[32] 1970	250 mg q 3 d	High preterm risk score	28–32 wk
Johnson et al,[33] 1975	250 mg q wk	≥ 2 SAB or preterm births	Enrollment–37 wk
Breart et al, 1979	2 doses 250 mg q wk	Risk of preterm labor	20–37 wk
Hartikainen-Sorri et al, 1980	250 mg q wk	Twin gestation	28–37 wk
Hauth et al,[29] 1983	1000 mg q wk	Active duty military women	16–36 wk
Yemini et al,[35] 1985	250 mg q wk	≥ 2 SAB or preterm birth	Enrollment–37 wk
Meis et al,[9] 2003	250 mg q wk	Preterm birth	16–36 wk
Rouse et al,[37] 2007	q wk	Twin gestation	16–36 wk
Facchinetti et al,[41] 2007	341 mg q 4 d	Acute preterm labor	25–36 wk
Caritis et al,[38] 2009	250 mg q wk	Triplet gestation	16–35 wk

Abbreviation: SAB, spontaneous abortions.

after the onset of labor, however, these treatments are associated with maternal side effects without the benefit of improved neonatal morbidity and mortality.[40]

LIMITATIONS OF USE
Threatened Preterm Labor

The use of progestins for patients who present with preterm labor has been studied, but there are currently no recommendations for its use in this group. Facchinetti and colleagues[41] evaluated the use of 17-P in patients admitted with an acute episode of preterm labor who were undelivered. They showed that cervical shortening is attenuated by treatment with 17-P in women admitted for threatened preterm labor. Undelivered patients were randomized to treatment with 17-P 341 mg intramuscularly twice weekly until 36 weeks versus placebo. The rationale for using a higher dose in this trial was the onset of preterm labor requiring tocolysis. In these patients, cervical ripening and the cascade of preterm labor was already initiated. Cervical shortening, as measured by ultrasound performed 7 and 21 days postrandomization, was significantly less in the 17-P–treated group as compared with placebo.

Almost 40% of patients who deliver preterm have had preterm labor during their pregnancy, therefore patients with threatened preterm labor have a higher risk of preterm delivery requiring more aggressive intervention.[42] Currently, there is insufficient evidence to advocate progestational agents as a tocolytic agent for women presenting with preterm labor.

MULTIPLE GESTATIONS

Rouse and colleagues[37] investigated the effects of 17-P in twin pregnancies. In these women, 250 mg of 17-P administered weekly from 20 to 34 weeks of gestation was ineffective as compared with placebo in reducing either the rate of delivery before 35 weeks or severe adverse fetal outcomes. On average, the women in the study delivered at 34.8 weeks, as compared with a national average of 35.2 weeks for women carrying twins. Similarly, Caritis and colleagues[38] demonstrated no reduction in preterm birth in women with triplet pregnancies treated with 17-P. Healthy women with triplets were randomly assigned to weekly intramuscular injections of either 250 mg of 17-P or placebo, starting at 16 to 20 weeks and ending at delivery or 35 weeks of gestation. The primary study outcome was delivery or fetal loss before 35 weeks. Eighty-three percent of women in the treatment group versus 84% in the placebo group delivered before 35 weeks. The study concluded that treatment with 17-P did not reduce the rate of preterm birth in women with triplet gestations.

VAGINAL PROGESTERONE

The use of naturally occurring progesterone has also been studied for preterm birth prevention. The use of vaginal versus intramuscular formulations for progesterone has been advocated because of the "uterine first-pass effect." The efficacy of progesterone is thought to be improved with an increase in the delivery to the endometrium with vaginal dosing. Studies of this formulation noted a 14-times greater increase in the ratio of endometrial-to-serum concentrations after vaginal dosing than after systemic, intramuscular administration.[43,44]

In 2003, da Fonseca and colleagues used 100 mg progesterone vaginal suppository daily versus placebo from 24 to 34 weeks in women with a prior spontaneous preterm birth. This was a prospective, randomized, double-blind, placebo-controlled study that included 142 high-risk pregnancies. The objective was to evaluate the effect of prophylactic vaginal progesterone on the incidence of preterm birth in a high-risk population. Study patients were given 100 mg progesterone vaginal suppositories or placebo from 24 to 28 weeks gestation, and underwent weekly home uterine monitoring. There was a statistically significant difference in uterine activity between the progesterone and placebo group (23.6% vs 54.3%, respectively). There was also a decreased incidence of preterm birth before 34 weeks in the treatment group versus placebo (2.7% vs 18.5%).

In 2007, Fonseca and colleagues[39] studied the effect of vaginal progesterone in asymptomatic women who were found to have a short cervix (15 mm or less) on routine transvaginal ultrasound at 20 to 25 weeks. In that study, daily vaginal administration of 200 mg of progesterone from 24 to 34 weeks of gestation reduced the rate of delivery before 34 weeks from 34% to 19%. There were no significant reductions in adverse fetal outcomes, but the trial was not powered to detect these. In a negative study by O'Brien and colleagues,[45] women with a prior history of preterm birth were treated with progesterone vaginal gel (90 mg) daily. Prophylactic treatment with vaginal progesterone did not reduce the frequency of recurrent preterm birth (≤32 weeks) in women with a history of spontaneous preterm birth. The administration of vaginal progesterone gel to women with a sonographic short cervix in the midtrimester is associated with a 45% reduction in the rate of preterm birth before 33 weeks of gestation, and improved neonatal outcomes.[46]

Borna and Sahabi[47] performed a randomized controlled trial to study whether supplementation of vaginal progesterone after an episode of threatened preterm labor resulted in an increased latency period and decreased recurrent episodes of preterm labor. The trial found a longer latency period preceding delivery but no significant reduction in recurrent preterm labor. A summary of clinical trials using progesterone is included in **Table 2**.

EFFICACY AND SAFETY OF PROGESTINS

17-P is a synthetic caproate ester of the progesterone metabolite. Several studies have evaluated the safety of 17-P in pregnancy.[9] The evidence for the safety of the use of 17-P hydroxyprogesterone in pregnancy is based on theoretical considerations, animal studies, and clinical studies. There has not been evidence of teratogenic effects, androgenic or glucocorticoid activity, or virilization of female fetuses. The safety of 17-P has been established in both animal and human studies. Higher doses, including 1000 mg weekly[29] and 2000 mg weekly,[48] have been used without adverse maternal or fetal side effects. The safety of progesterone supplementation is

Table 2
Clinical trials involving progesterone to prevent preterm birth

Author (Year)	Dose (Frequency)	Indication	Gestational Age
da Fonseca et al,[10] 2003	100 mg suppository q d	Prior preterm birth	24–34 wk
Fonseca et al,[39] 2007	200 mg suppository q d	Short cervix <15 mm	20–34 wk
O'Brien et al,[46] 2007	90 mg vaginal gel q d	Prior preterm birth	18–37 wk
Borna and Sahabi[47] 2008	400 mg suppository q d	Threatened preterm labor	24–34 wk

supported by a review of outcomes of pregnancies treated before 1990, by a review of animal studies, and, more recently, by a thorough neurodevelopmental evaluation of children at 4-years of age who were born to women treated in the National Institute of Child Health and Human Development trial.[48]

The effects of 17-P on pregnancy have been studied in rats, rabbits, mice, and monkeys.[49–53] Junkmann,[53] and Kessler and Borman,[49] studied 17-P in rabbits and rats and found that esterification amplified the progestational effects of hydroxyprogesterone but found no evidence of androgen or glucocorticoid activity. Johnstone and Franklin[50] studied virilizing effects of several steroid compounds in the fetal mouse model. Suchowsky and Junkmann[54] examined a number of progestogens for: (1) virilizing activity upon the female fetus in rats, (2) androgenic activity on the spayed rat seminal vesicle weight, and on the chick comb, and (3) progestational effect on the rabbit uterus. In both studies, 17-P demonstrated no virilizing effect and no androgenic properties, even at very high doses. Courtney and Valerio[51] examined effects of various compounds and found no effects of 17-P on the developing monkey fetus. Carbone and Brent[52] treated pregnant mice with doses of 17-P of up to 70 times the equivalent human dose and Seegmiller and colleagues[55] administered 17-P at 200 times the human dose. Neither study found any effects on embryonic or fetal development, cleft palate or endochondral ossification, or increase in congenital anomalies. Thus, animal studies of 17-P have found no evidence of any harmful or teratogenic effects on the fetus of a number of species, even when the drug was administered at very high doses.

A number of well-controlled clinical studies have reported on the safety of 17-P in human pregnancy. Varma and Morsman[56] compared 150 pregnancies with threatened abortion treated with hydroxyprogesterone to 150 patients with early-pregnancy bleeding who were not treated with the drug. They did not identify any evidence of adverse effect on the fetus or the outcome of the pregnancy. In a cohort study of 13,643 pregnancies with in utero exposure to 17-P, Michaelis and colleagues[57] found no increase in malformations in infants, compared with controls. A cohort of 24,000 pregnancies delivered in Olmstead County, Minnesota, had 649 offspring exposed to 17-P, and they did not show an increase in congenital anomalies or other ill effects compared with controls.[58] Kesler[59] performed a battery of psychological tests on a group of adolescent males who were exposed in utero to 17-P and on matched control subjects. They found no significant differences between the groups in psychological testing.

Several extensive reviews have established the safety of progestins in pregnancy. Schardein[60] found "no justification for undue concern over the induction of nongenital malformations through hormone use in pregnancy." They found that progesterone and 17-P have no such potential for masculinization of the female fetus. In a meta-analysis of 186 published articles, no association between first-trimester exposure to sex hormones and external genital malformations was identified.[61]

The safety of 17-P administration in pregnancy is well documented by animal and clinical studies. Despite absence of evidence for increased maternal or fetal risk from treatment with progestins, their safety remains a concern. The commercially available form of 17-P has been approved by the Food and Drug Administration as Makena. Its use is therefore limited because of lack of widespread availability.

PHARMACOKINETICS OR PHARMACODYNAMICS

The mechanism by which exogenous progestins decrease preterm birth is unclear because of limited pharmacokinetic studies of progestins. In 2008, Zhang and colleagues[62] developed a method to quantitate 17-P, 17α-hydroxyprogesterone, and progesterone in human plasma using high-performance liquid chromatography–mass spectrometry. Sharma and colleagues[63] evaluated the metabolism of 17-P in adult and fetal human hepatocytes and in expressed cytochrome P450 enzymes. The study demonstrated that the enzyme CYP3A is involved in the metabolism of 17-P by adult and fetal hepatocytes. There is no difference in the binding affinity of 17-P or progesterone for either progesterone or glucocorticoid receptors. Thus, there is presumably no difference in gene expression.[64]

COST

Treatment with 17-P or progesterone provides a significant reduction in the risk of recurrent preterm birth. In addition, there is a reduction in direct and indirect costs associated with preterm delivery.

For women with a prior preterm delivery treated with 17-P, the projected discounted lifetime medical costs of their offspring could be reduced by more than 2 billion dollars annually.[65] Odibo and colleagues[66] used a decision-analysis modeling to compare the cost-effectiveness of using 17-P in different high-risk groups. They found that use of 17-P for the prevention of preterm deliveries results in cost-savings in women with prior preterm deliveries less than 32 weeks and 32 to 37 weeks.

SUMMARY

Based on the studies presented, 17-P is indicated for prevention of preterm birth in women with a documented history of a preterm birth before 37 weeks. It has no proven benefit in twin and triplet pregnancies. Its use in patients with acute preterm labor has not been validated.

Vaginal progesterone has been used for preterm birth prevention in one successful randomized clinical trial and has been shown unsuccessful in another. It is recommended for use in asymptomatic women with a short cervix (<15 mm).

REFERENCES

1. Goldenberg RL, Culhane JF, Iams JD, et al. Epidemiology and causes of preterm birth. Lancet 2008;371:75–84.
2. Spong CY. Prediction and prevention of recurrent spontaneous preterm birth. Obstet Gynecol 2007;110(2 Pt 1):405–15.
3. 2000 Nationwide inpatient sample prepared by March of Dimes Perinatal Data Center. Agency for Healthcare Research and Quality; 2003.
4. Salafia CM, Vogel CA, Vintzileos AM, et al. Placental pathologic findings in preterm birth. Am J Obstet Gynecol 1991;165(4 Pt 1):934–8.
5. Bhattacharya S, Raja EA, Mirazo ER, et al. Inherited predisposition to spontaneous preterm delivery. Obstet Gynecol 2010;115(6):1125–33.
6. Kiely JL. What is the population-based risk of preterm birth among twins and other multiples? Clin Obstet Gynecol 1998;41(1):3–11.
7. Bryant AS, Worjoloh A, Caughey AB, et al. Racial/ethnic disparities in obstetric outcomes and care: prevalence and determinants. Am J Obstet Gynecol 2010; 202(4):335–43.
8. Bloom SL, Yost NP, McIntire DD, et al. Recurrence of preterm birth in singleton and twin pregnancies. Obstet Gynecol 2001;98(3):379–85.
9. Meis PJ, Klebanoff M, Thom E, et al. Prevention of recurrent preterm delivery by 17-alpha-hydroxyprogesterone caproate. N Engl J Med 2003;348:2379–85.

10. da Fonseca EB, Bittar RE, Carvalho MH, et al. Prophylactic administration of progesterone by vaginal suppository to reduce the incidence of spontaneous preterm birth in women at increased risk: a randomized placebo-controlled double blind study. Am J Obstet Gynecol 2003;188:419–24.

11. Siiteri PK, Seron-Ferre M. Some new thoughts on the feto-placental unit and parturition in primates. In: Novy JM, Reskko AJ, editors. Fetal endocrinology. New York: Academic Press; 1981.

12. Garfield RE, Dannan MS, Daniel EE. Gap junction formation in myometrium: control by estrogens, progesterone, and prostaglandins. Am J Physiol 1980;238:C81–9.

13. Csapo AI. Force of labor. New York: John Wiley and Sons; 1981. p. 761–99.

14. Chwalisz K, Hegele-Hartung C, Schulz R, et al. Progesterone control of cervical ripening. Perinatology Press; 1991. p. 119–31.

15. Bernal A. Overview. Preterm labour: mechanisms and management. BMC Pregnancy Childbirth 2007;7(Suppl 1):S2.

16. Zakar T, Hertelendy F. Progesterone withdrawal: key to parturition. Am J Obstet Gynecol 2007;196(4):289–96.

17. Merlino AA, Welsh TN, Tan H, et al. Nuclear progesterone receptors in the human pregnancy myometrium: evidence that parturition involves functional progesterone withdrawal mediated by increased expression of progesterone receptor-A. J Clin Endocrinol Metab 2007;92(5):1927–33.

18. Petrocelli T, Lye SJ. Regulation of transcripts encoding the myometrial gap junction protein, connexin-43, by estrogen and progesterone. Endocrinology 1993;133:284.

19. Clark K, Ji H, Feltovich H, et al. Mifepristone-induced cervical ripening: structural, biomechanical, and molecular events. Am J Obstet Gynecol 2006;194:1391–8.

20. Marx SG, Wentz MJ, Mackay LB, et al. Effects of progesterone on iNOS, COX-2, and collagen expression in the cervix. J Histochem Cytochem 2006;54:623–39.

21. Shi L, Shi SQ, Saade GR, et al. Studies of cervical ripening in pregnant rats: effects of various treatments. Mol Hum Reprod 2000;6:382–9.

22. Shynlova O, Mitchell JA, Tsampalieros A, et al. Progesterone and gravidity differentially regulate expression of extracellular matrix components in the pregnant rat myometrium. Biol Reprod 2004;70:986–92.

23. Melendez JA, Vinci JM, Jeffrey JJ, et al. Localization and regulation of IL-1alpha in rat myometrium during late pregnancy and the postpartum period. Am J Physiol Regul Integr Comp Physiol 2001;280(3):R879–88.

24. Suarez VR, Park ES, Hankins GD, et al. Expression of regulator of G protein signaling-2 in rat myometrium during pregnancy and parturition. Am J Obstet Gynecol 2003;188(4):973–7.

25. Elovitz MA, Mrinalini C. Can medroxyprogesterone acetate alter Toll-like receptor expression in a mouse model of intrauterine inflammation? Am J Obstet Gynecol 2005;193(3 Pt 2):1149–55.

26. Inglis SR, Jeremias J, Kuno K, et al. Detection of tumor necrosis factor-alpha, interleukin-6, and fetal fibronectin in the lower genital tract during pregnancy: relation to outcome. Am J Obstet Gynecol 1994;171:5–10.

27. Coleman MA, Keelen JA, McCowen LM. Predicting preterm delivery: comparison of cervicovaginal interleukins (IL)-1beta, IL-6 and IL-8 with fetal fibronectin and cervical dilation. Eur J Obstet Gynecol Reprod Biol 2001;95:154–8.

28. Rizzo G, Capponi A, Rinaldo D, et al. Interleukin-6 concentrations in cervical secretions identify microbial invasion of the amniotic fluid cavity in patients with preterm labor and intact membranes. Am J Obstet Gynecol 1996;175:812–7.

29. Hauth JC, Andrews WW, Goldenberg RL. Infection-related risk factors predictive of spontaneous preterm labor and birth. Prenat Neonatal Med 1983;88:233–8.

30. Goldenberg RL, Klebanoff M, Carey JC, et al. Vaginal fetal fibronectin measurements from 8 to 22 weeks' gestation and subsequent spontaneous preterm birth. Am J Obstet Gynecol 2000;183:469–75.

31. Keirse MJ. Progesterone administration in pregnancy may prevent preterm delivery. Br J Obstet Gynaecol 1990;97:149–54.

32. Papaiernik E. Double-blind study of an agent to prevent pre-term delivery among women at increased risk. In: Edition Schering, Serie IV, fiche 3; 1970. p. 65–68.

33. Johnson JW, Austin KL, Jones GS, et al. Efficacy of 17 alpha-hydroxyprogesterone caproate in the prevention of premature labor. N Engl J Med 1975;293:675–80.

34. Levine L. Habitual abortion: a controlled clinical study of progestational therapy. West J Surg Obstet Gynecol 1964;72:30–6.

35. Yemini M, Borenstein R, Dreazen E, et al. Prevention of premature labor by 17 alpha-hydroxyprogesterone caproate. Am J Obstet Gynecol 1985;151:574–7 p. 28–31.

36. American College of Obstetricians and Gynecologists. Use of progesterone to reduce preterm birth: ACOG committee opinion, no 291. Obstet Gynecol 2003; 102:1115–6.

37. Rouse DJ, Caritis SN, Peaceman AM, et al. A trial of 17 alpha-hydroxyprogesterone caproate to prevent prematurity in twins. N Engl J Med 2007;357:454–61.

38. Caritis SN, Rouse DJ, Peaceman AM, et al. Prevention of preterm birth in triplets using 17 alpha-hydroxyprogesterone caproate: a randomized controlled trial. Obstet Gynecol 2009;113(2 Pt 1):285–92.

39. Fonseca EB, Celik E, Parra M, et al. Progesterone and the risk of preterm birth among women with a short cervix. N Engl J Med 2007;357:462–9.

40. Gyetvai K, Hannah ME, Hodnett ED, et al. Tocolytics for preterm labor: a systematic review. Obstet Gynecol 1999;94:869–77.

41. Facchinetti F, Paganelli S, Comitini G, et al. Cervical length changes during preterm cervical ripening: effects of 17-alpha-hydroxyprogesterone caproate. Am J Obstet Gynecol 2007;196:453.e1–4.

42. McPheeters M, Miller W, Hartmann K, et al. The epidemiology of threatened preterm labor: a prospective cohort study. Am J Obstet Gynecol 2005;192: 1329–30.

43. De Ziegler D, Bulletti C, De Monstier B, et al. The first uterine pass effect. Ann N Y Acad Sci 1997;828:291–9.

44. Cicinelli E, De Ziegler D, Bulletti C, et al. Direct transport of progesterone from vagina to uterus. Obstet Gynecol 2000;95:403–6.

45. O'Brien JM, Defranco EA, Adair CD, et al; Progesterone Vaginal Gel Study Group. Effect of progesterone on cervical shortening in women at risk for preterm birth: secondary analysis from a multinational, randomized, double-blind, placebo-controlled trial. Ultrasound Obstet Gynecol 2007;34(6):653–9.

46. Hassan SS, Romero R, Vidyadhari D, et al. Vaginal progesterone reduces the rate of preterm birth in women with a sonographic short cervix: a multicenter, randomized, double-blind, placebo-controlled trial. Ultrasound in Obstetrics & Gynecology 2011, in press.

47. Borna S, Sahabi N. Progesterone for maintenance tocolytic therapy after threatened preterm labour: a randomised controlled trial. Aust N Z J Obstet Gynaecol 2008;48(1):58–63.

48. Sherman AI. Hormonal therapy for control of the incompetent os of pregnancy. Obstet Gynecol 1966;28:198–205.

49. Kessler W, Borman A. Some biological activities of certain progesterons. I. 17 alpha-hydroxyprogesterone 17-n-caproate. Ann N Y Acad Sci 1958;71:486–93.
50. Johnstone EE, Franklin RR. Assay of progestins for fetal virilizing properties using the mouse. Obstet Gynecol 1964;23:359–62.
51. Courtney KD, Valerio DA. Teratology in the Macaca mulatta. Teratology 1968;1: 163–72.
52. Carbone JP, Brent RL. Genital and nongenital teratogenesis of prenatal progesterone therapy: the effects of 17 alpha-hydroxyprogesterone caproate on embryonic and fetal development and endochondral ossification in the C57B1/6L mouse. Am J Obstet Gynecol 1993;169:1292–8.
53. Junkmann K. Estrogens with prolonged action. Naunyn Schmiedebergs Arch Exp Pathol Pharmakol 1953;220(5):358–64 [in Undetermined Language].
54. Suchowsky GK, Junkmann K. Research on the maintenance of pregnancy by 17 alpha-hydroxyprogesterone caproate in the castrated pregnant rabbit. Acta Endocrinol (Copenh) 1958;28(2):129–31 [in German].
55. Seegmiller RE, Nelson GW, Johnston CK. Evaluation of teratogenic potential of delalutin, (17 alpha-hydroxyprogesterone caproate) in mice. Teratology 1983; 28:201–8.
56. Varma T, Morsman J. Evaluation of the use of Proluton-Depot (hydroxyprogesterone hexanoate) in early pregnancy. Int J Gynaecol Obstet 1982;20:13–7.
57. Michaelis J, Michaelis H, Gluck E, et al. Prospective studies of suspected association between certain drugs administered in early pregnancy and congenital malformations. Teratology 1983;27:57–64.
58. Resseguie LJ, Hick JF, Bruen JA, et al. Congenital malformations among offspring exposed in utero to progestins. Olmstead County, Minnesota, 1936–1974. Fertil Steril 1985;43:514–9.
59. Kesler PA. Effects of prenatally administered 17 alpha-hydroxyprogesterone caproate in adolescent males. Arch Sex Behav 1984;13:441–55.
60. Schardein JL. Congenital abnormalities and hormones during pregnancy: a clinical review. Teratology 1980;22:251–70.
61. Raman-Wilms L, Tseng AL, Wighardt S, et al. Fetal genital effects of first-trimester sex hormone exposure: a meta-analysis. Obstet Gynecol 1995;85:141–9.
62. Zhang S, Mada SR, Sharma S, et al. Simultaneous quantitation of 17alpha-hydroxyprogesterone caproate, 17alpha-hydroxyprogesterone and progesterone in human plasma using high-performance liquid chromatography-mass spectrometry (HPLC-MS/MS). J Pharm Biomed Anal 2008;48(4):1174–80.
63. Sharma S, Ellis EC, Dorko K, et al. Metabolism of 17alpha-hydroxyprogesterone caproate, an agent for preventing preterm birth, by fetal hepatocytes. Drug Metab Dispos 2010;38(5):723–7.
64. Attardi Barbara J, Zeleznik Anthony, Simhan Hyagriv, et al. Comparison of progesterone and glucocorticoid receptor binding and stimulation of gene expression by progesterone, 17-alpha hydroxyprogesterone caproate (17-OHPC), and related progestins. Am J Obstet Gynecol 2007;197(6):599.e1–7.
65. Bailit JL, Votruba ME. Medical cost savings associated with 17 alpha-hydroxyprogesterone caproate. Am J Obstet Gynecol 2007;196(3):219.
66. Odibo AO, Stamilio DM, Macones GA, et al. 17alpha-hydroxyprogesterone caproate for the prevention of preterm delivery: a cost-effectiveness analysis. Obstet Gynecol 2006;108(3 Pt 1):492–9.

Reducing the Risk of Shoulder Dystocia and Associated Brachial Plexus Injury

Edith D. Gurewitsch, MD[a],*, Robert H. Allen, PhD[b]

KEYWORDS

• Shoulder dystocia • Brachial plexus • Injury • Delivery

The current American College of Obstetricians and Gynecologists (ACOG) and Royal College of Obstetricians and Gynecologists (RCOG) guidelines for shoulder dystocia, which were published in 2002 and 2005, respectively, offer useful guidelines for clinicians about shoulder dystocia incidence, risk factors, prevention, and management.[1,2] Considerable research on shoulder dystocia and its related injuries, some of it controversial, has been published on the topic since that time. In this review, the authors summarize some of the recent developments concerning incidence, risk factors, prevention, and management that may be useful to consider in future ACOG and RCOG guidelines.

Despite studies that suggest otherwise, considerable evidence can be found to recommend guidelines and interventions that would improve clinical practice and patient outcomes. The objective of this review is to offer health care providers information, practical direction, and advice on how to limit shoulder dystocia risk and, more importantly, to reduce anoxic and brachial plexus injury risk. The authors review such areas of controversy as prior shoulder dystocia and reducing recurrence, monitoring and counseling about maternal weight and weight gain during pregnancy to control macrosomia incidence, ultrasonographic assessment of fetal growth to detect asymmetric accelerated truncal growth and/or macrosomia, screening for glucose intolerance and maintenance of target glycemic control to reduce adverse pregnancy outcome (including shoulder dystocia), use of operative delivery in at-risk patients, a safe head-to-body interval, the etiology and natural

[a] Departments of Gynecology and Obstetrics and Biomedical Engineering, Johns Hopkins University School of Medicine, 600 North Wolfe Street, Phipps 217, Baltimore, MD 21287, USA
[b] Departments of Gynecology and Obstetrics and Biomedical Engineering, Johns Hopkins University School of Medicine, 3400 North Charles Street, Clark 118C, Baltimore, MD 21208, USA
* Corresponding author.
E-mail address: egurewi@jhmi.edu

Obstet Gynecol Clin N Am 38 (2011) 247–269
doi:10.1016/j.ogc.2011.02.015
0889-8545/11/$ – see front matter © 2011 Elsevier Inc. All rights reserved.

obgyn.theclinics.com

history of shoulder dystocia-associated neonatal brachial plexus injury, efficacy and safety of shoulder dystocia maneuvers, and provider training.

INCIDENCE

The ACOG bulletin reports a shoulder dystocia incidence range from 0.6% to 1.4% of deliveries.[2] The full range of reported shoulder dystocia incidence among vaginal deliveries is from 1 in 750 in a population-based study to 1 in 15 in studies totaling 61 vaginal deliveries.[3–5] Reasons for this wide variation in incidence include differences in study design, patient population, delivery volume, varying definitions, and, most importantly, the difficulty in diagnosis.[3,6,7]

Although few in number, prospective studies totaling about 2100 shoulder dystocia deliveries report higher incidence values, from 3.3% to 7% of term vaginal deliveries and are likely more accurate.[4,5,8–10] Irrespective of the true incidence range, the complication of shoulder dystocia is one that any obstetric provider is bound to encounter (likely more frequently than perceived) and must be adequately prepared to recognize and manage.

PREVENTION

The only alternative guaranteed to prevent shoulder dystocia in a specific patient is that of elective cesarean delivery without trial of labor. Yet, the potential for injury from shoulder dystocia, although undesirable and preferably avoided, does not justify the seemingly facile intervention of cesarean delivery for several reasons. Although considered an obstetric emergency, shoulder dystocia is usually managed properly and resolved uneventfully by a trained obstetric provider. Similarly, neonatal complications linked to shoulder dystocia (eg, neonatal depression, brachial plexus injury, and skeletal fractures) are infrequent and most often resolve in the neonatal period or soon thereafter. Cesarean delivery substitutes risks to the mother for risk to the neonate[11,12] at a ratio of more than 3500 cesarean deliveries performed to prevent 1 permanent brachial plexus injury and nearly $9 million in extra cost.[13] And, although far less likely, the abdominal route of delivery still poses a small (<4%) risk of brachial plexus injury, especially for macrosomic fetuses,[3,14–17] and thus is not guaranteed to prevent untoward fetal outcomes associated with shoulder dystocia. Furthermore, even if a policy of avoiding vaginal delivery in all at-risk patients were strictly enforced, shoulder dystocia cannot be averted entirely because it occurs, not infrequently, in women without risk factors and even in women with average and small-for-gestational-age (SGA) fetuses.[18,19]

Herein lies the quandary for any obstetric provider caring for patients at risk for shoulder dystocia: emphasizing fetal risk over maternal risk by favoring avoidance approaches (ie, scheduled elective cesarean delivery) is biased, costly, and ineffective.[20] Although lines for offering this intervention are drawn at specific estimated fetal weight (EFW) cutoffs (>5000 g in nondiabetic individuals or 4500 g for diabetic individuals),[2] more than 95% of women who are either at risk for or who actually experience shoulder dystocia never reach those cutoffs. How else can the remainder of women at risk for shoulder dystocia be best counseled and managed so as to reduce untoward outcome?

From a practical standpoint, there are 2 time frames afforded to the obstetric provider that can affect occurrence of shoulder dystocia and its associated complications: (1) before delivery occurs, when evidence-based preventive measures can be taken during the antenatal and intrapartum periods to reduce shoulder dystocia incidence, and (2) during shoulder dystocia, when evidence-based preventive measures can be taken to reduce risk of injury.

ANTENATAL RISK FACTORS FOR SHOULDER DYSTOCIA

The most consistent and highly significant antepartum risk factors for shoulder dystocia and its related neonatal complications are fetal macrosomia, maternal diabetes, and a history of shoulder dystocia in a prior pregnancy.[2,21–24] Within an index pregnancy for both multiparous and nulliparous women, classic antepartum risk factors for shoulder dystocia include baseline maternal obesity, excessive gestational weight gain, maternal diabetes, and postdatism.[2,25,26] Considered retrospectively, half the deliveries complicated by shoulder dystocia will have had one or several of these specific antecedents that could have been prospectively identified and managed prenatally. Considered prospectively, however, women with classic risk factors for shoulder dystocia are still more likely to deliver vaginally without encountering the complication. This conundrum tends to thwart the notion that shoulder dystocia is amenable to prospective preventive efforts. However, it is noteworthy that, although shoulder dystocia deliveries and associated neonatal brachial plexus injury involve "average-weight" infants as often as large-for-gestational-age (LGA) infants,[18] these infants tend to weigh more than 3000 g at birth and thus are in comparatively higher birth weight percentiles among appropriate-for-gestational-age (AGA) infants.[27] The incidence of shoulder dystocia increases steadily for each 500-g increment in birth weight, reaching a 10-fold increase, from an incidence of 2.3% in the median birth weight group (3500–3999 g) to 23.9% in the highest birth weight group ($\geq$4500 g); a marked jump in incidence of nearly 5-fold over the 3.5 to 3.9 kg birth weight group occurs beyond 4000 g.[26] Indeed, when birth weight is specifically controlled for, most other risk factors for shoulder dystocia, such as maternal weight, gestational weight gain, and increasing gestational age, drop out of logistic regression analyses.[28] Thus, unless women with classic risk factors for shoulder dystocia are actually carrying an LGA fetus, their deliveries are more likely to be uneventful. The onus for the provider is to screen, detect, and take measures to prevent accelerated fetal growth in all pregnant women, especially those with classic risk factors.

There are 2 major contributors to high shoulder dystocia incidence: increased birth weight and increased ponderal index; the former is mediated predominantly by gestational weight gain, the latter by varying degrees of relative maternal hyperglycemia (even below that of overt diabetes mellitus). Together, these comprise most shoulder dystocia events (**Fig. 1**). Evidence has been mounting that both these factors, gestational weight gain and maternal hyperglycemia, are amenable to screening and effective intervention. Thus, although shoulder dystocia itself may be neither predictable nor preventable in a specific patient, the phenomenon of accelerated fetal growth is potentially modifiable, which in turn decreases shoulder dystocia incidence and severity in a population.[29] Considered epidemiologically, high birth weight correlates with obesity in adulthood, as well as other determinants of cardiovascular disease and metabolic disease.[30,31] Thus, preventing macrosomia will not only reduce obstetric and neonatal complications but more importantly, it is likely to have significant impact on future pediatric and adult disease incidences.[30,31]

Maternal Weight and Gestational Weight Gain

Shoulder dystocia is at least twice as likely to occur among obese mothers compared with normal weight controls, yet most such women experience uncomplicated vaginal deliveries.[32–34] In the same manner that it generally impedes normal progress of labor

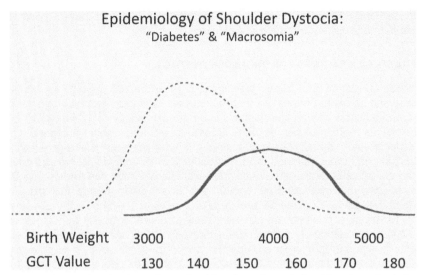

Fig. 1. Population distribution of nonshoulder dystocia and shoulder dystocia deliveries relative to birth weight and maternal glycemic concentration. In term cephalic vaginal deliveries, the distribution of both birth weight and maternal 50-g glucose challenge test (GCT) value among shoulder dystocia (*solid bell curve*) deliveries is shifted to the right relative to nonshoulder dystocia (*broken bell curve*) deliveries.

among obese women, excess soft tissue likely adds to the true bony obstruction that begets shoulder dystocia in any woman, thereby increasing the severity of shoulder dystocia if and when it occurs in an obese parturient. Indeed, among women who experience a shoulder dystocia, severity of shoulder dystocia and likelihood of neonatal injury are greater if the mother is obese.[35,36]

From the maternal perspective, preconceptional attainment of ideal body weight and within-target weight gain during pregnancy prevent not only fetal macrosomia and its attendant risks for obstetric complications and their potential injuries[37] but also other scourges of overnutrition for the mother herself.

Earlier fears of detrimental effects of caloric and nutrient restrictions on fetal growth, especially among obese gravidas, have recently been dispelled,[38] whereas excessive weight gain has been shown to increase the odds ratio (OR) for both primary cesarean delivery (OR, 1.17; confidence interval [CI], 1.01–1.35) and macrosomia, defined as 4 kg or more (OR, 1.23; CI, 1.04–1.45).[39] These results have led to modification of the Institute of Medicine's recommendations for gestational weight gain stratified by baseline weight category (**Table 1**). Among women with class II and III obesity (body mass index$\geq$35 cm/kg^2), gestational weight gain between -4.9 kg and $+4.9$ kg reduces the odds of fetal macrosomia, without increasing the odds of SGA birth weights.[40]

Maternal Hyperglycemia

Patients with a false-positive glucose screen (ie, elevated 1-hour glucose challenge test [GCT] followed by normal 3-hour glucose tolerance test [GTT]) have an OR for shoulder dystocia of 2.85 compared with normal (negative GCT) controls.[41,42] Such women with subclinical impaired glucose tolerance eventually deliver higher–birth-weight infants than women with overt gestational diabetes owing to comparatively

Table 1	
The Institute of Medicine recommendations for gestational weight gain	
Initial BMI	**Recommended Gain in Pounds (kg)**
<19.8 (low)	28–40 (12.5–18.0)
19.8–26.0 (normal)	25–35 (11.5–16.0)
26.1–29.0 (high, overweight)	15–25 (7.0–11.5)
>29 (obese)	11–20 (5–9)

Data from Institute of Medicine. Weight gain in pregnancy: reexamining the guidelines. Report Brief 2009.

less attention paid to diet, weight gain, and overall fetal growth patterns.[43] Given that studies of treatment of even mild forms of gestational diabetes demonstrate a favorable effect on such adverse outcomes as birth weight greater than the 90th percentile, primary cesarean delivery, neonatal hypoglycemia, preterm delivery before 37 weeks' gestation, preeclampsia, and shoulder dystocia,[29] international experts are calling for revision of diagnostic criteria for gestational diabetes based on the 2-hour 75-g GTT, using cutoffs of 92 mg/dL, 180 mg/dL, and 153 mg/dL for fasting, 1-hour, and 2-hour values, respectively.[43,44]

Both gestational weight gain and hyperglycemia are modifiable with a properly tailored, low glycemic index carbohydrate diet. Indeed, the quality rather than quantity of carbohydrate in the diet affects insulin sensitivity, glucose response curves,[45] gestational weight gain, and birth weight.[46] A diet composed of 55% to 60% carbohydrate but of low–glycemic index high-fiber foods is comparable to a diet with 40% complex carbohydrates; whereas a diet composed of equivalent protein and carbohydrate distribution (40% each), in which the carbohydrate component is of high glycemic index, produces greater gestational weight gain and a mean birth weight of more than 1 kg higher than low glycemic index carbohydrate consumers, with all infant birth weights falling in the LGA range.[46]

ULTRASONOGRAPHIC DETECTION OF ACCELERATED FETAL GROWTH

The accuracy of sonographic estimation of fetal weight is suboptimal, with margins of error approaching ±500 g, particularly when EFW increases beyond the 97th percentile.[47,48] Melamed and colleagues[49] recently demonstrated significant clinical consequences to both false-positive and false-negative antenatal ultrasonographic diagnosis of fetal macrosomia based on EFW of more than 4 kg. Among infants actually weighing less than 4 kg at birth, those with prenatal EFW greater than 4 kg (false-positive) were significantly more likely to undergo cesarean birth than similar-weight infants with true-negative antenatal ultrasonographic EFW. On the other hand, those infants with nonmacrosomic antenatal EFW who actually weighed more than 4 kg at birth were more likely to have undergone operative vaginal birth, with higher incidence of neonatal trauma, than those whose antenatal ultrasonographic results predicted macrosomia (true-positive). Shoulder dystocia incidence, however, did not differ across any of the true-negative, false-positive, true-positive, or false-negative groups.

Thus, specifically for shoulder dystocia risk assessment, ultrasonographic evaluation may be of some utility. In a retrospective study of infants weighing more than 4 kg at birth, Jazayeri and colleagues[50] found an OR of 2.97 for shoulder dystocia when abdominal circumference (AC) was greater than 35 cm within 2 weeks before delivery. Bailis and colleagues[51] recently determined that even among fetuses with EFW in the AGA percentiles (between 10% and 90%), those with AC greater than the 75th percentile (ie, with sonographic evidence of accelerated somatic growth compared with overall growth) within 3 weeks of delivery were 4 times as likely to experience shoulder dystocia compared with the general population.

Considered from a public health perspective, detection of fetuses with accelerated fetal growth toward the end of pregnancy has limited effect on shoulder dystocia incidence owing to insufficient time to intervene and affect fetal growth patterns. However, midthird trimester ultrasonographic detection of accelerated fetal AC growth is amenable to intervention that reduces both macrosomia and shoulder dystocia at the time of birth.[52–54] In randomized controlled trials, empiric treatment with exogenous insulin, tightening of glycemic targets (if diabetic), or further dietary modification (in both those with diabetes and mild hyperglycemia) on detection of AC greater than 75th percentile has a positive effect in slowing the rate of fetal growth.[52–54]

Two antenatal risk factors remain significant for shoulder dystocia independent of birth weight alone: diabetes and prior history of shoulder dystocia.[2]

Maternal Diabetes

Both maternal and neonatal delivery complications are 2 to 3 times more common among diabetic mothers than among nondiabetic mothers,[55] especially when carrying a fetus exhibiting accelerated growth.[56] Among LGA infants, a characteristic asymmetry in somatic growth ahead of overall growth renders the macrosomic infant of a diabetic mother at increased risk specifically for shoulder dystocia.[57]

Meticulous control of maternal glucose levels in diabetic pregnancy improves multiple obstetric outcomes, including a reduction in shoulder dystocia incidence.[29,55] Moses and colleagues[58] demonstrated that a low glycemic index carbohydrate diet can reduce the need for insulin among gestational diabetic patients by 50%. However, instances of demonstrable accelerated fetal growth (ie, AC$\geq$35 cm or $\geq$75% for gestational age) in spite of apparently optimal blood sugar levels still occur. As compared with nondiabetic hyperglycemic women, empiric medical treatment, tightened blood sugar targets, and dietary adjustment reduce macrosomia in such women.[52–54]

Prior Shoulder Dystocia

Recurrence of shoulder dystocia in a subsequent pregnancy varies from 6% to 20%.[21,23,24,59–62] Because prior shoulder dystocia is at times not noted in the index pregnancy, the actual recurrence rate is likely higher. Indeed, the recurrence of shoulder dystocia in women with vaginal delivery is approximately 10 times the incidence of shoulder dystocia in the general population.[62] This finding emphasizes the importance of counseling a patient about the occurrence of shoulder dystocia at the time of that delivery, even if mild and uneventful.

Because the recurrence risk is high, but the concern is for untoward outcome from subsequent recurrence rather than simply for recurrence, choice of mode of delivery in a subsequent pregnancy should be based on the risk of injury. The most consistent predictors of injury at any shoulder dystocia, including recurrent shoulder dystocia, are the birth weight of the infant[16,63–66] and the severity of the shoulder dystocia.[16,67–69]

Each of these factors should guide delivery planning in subsequent pregnancies. If the prior event resolved easily and without injury, decision regarding subsequent trial of labor may await estimation of fetal weight near term. If the EFW does not exceed the birth weight of the previous affected child, the rate of recurrence is lower. If, however, shoulder dystocia resulted in long-term or permanent injury in a prior pregnancy, then, as with the rare patient who reaches EFW above the ACOG-defined cutoffs, an elective primary cesarean delivery should be recommended for any subsequent delivery of term fetuses.[2]

Based on the earlier review of the evidence concerning the major antenatal correlates of shoulder dystocia, a rubric for the monitoring and management of the at-risk mother-infant pair is presented in **Fig. 2**. Because the identification and management of antepartum risk factors for shoulder dystocia is a chronologic one, it is amenable to prospective clinical management. Prior pregnancy history data and baseline maternal obesity are used to preselect those women who should be screened early for impaired carbohydrate metabolism. Universal glucose screening at 24 to 28 weeks' gestation, whether by current methods (as included in **Fig. 2**) or by newly adopted diagnostic criteria, provides the remainder of women with clinically significant hyperglycemia and/or overt gestational diabetes an opportunity to intervene (via dietary modification and exercise). Borderline or abnormal test results, as well as detection of gestational weight gain beyond target range and/or increased fundal height, identify women at increased risk who should undergo ultrasonographic evaluation of fetal growth and repeat GTT as indicated. Modification of delivery planning at term is reserved for those at highest risk.

INTRAPARTUM RISK FACTORS FOR SHOULDER DYSTOCIA

Once a trial of labor is undertaken, additional risk factors for shoulder dystocia can accrue, which independently increase the likelihood of the condition's occurrence. Induction of labor and use of epidural analgesia, although variably associated with

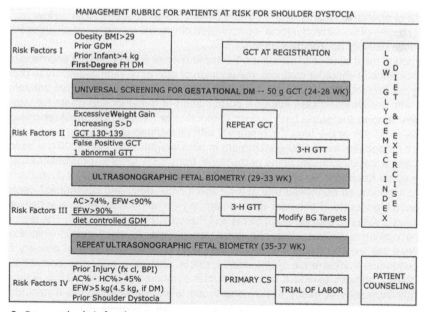

Fig. 2. Proposed rubric for the management of patients at risk for shoulder dystocia. A chronologic algorithm for the identification and management of antepartum risk factors for shoulder dystocia is presented. BG, blood glucose; BMI, body mass index; BPI, brachial plexus injury; CS, cesarean section; DM, diabetes mellitus; FH DM, family history of diabetes mellitus; fx cl, fractured clavicle; GDM, gestational diabetes mellitus; HC, head circumference; S>D, size greater than dates.

increased risk of shoulder dystocia, are also exceedingly common, multipurposeful, and most often clinically indicated. Thus, curtailing their use specifically for avoiding shoulder dystocia is perhaps only justified in the circumstance in which induction of labor is undertaken solely for impending or suspected macrosomia. This latter strategy is ineffective in reducing shoulder dystocia incidence.[2] By contrast, postdates induction of labor at 41 rather than at 42 weeks' gestation has been shown to reduce multiple perinatal morbidities, including shoulder dystocia.[70]

Precipitous second stage of labor and operative vaginal delivery are intrapartum events most strongly associated with shoulder dystocia.[25,71] Pathophysiologically, the interval between emergence of the head and subsequent restitution with simultaneous shoulder rotation is shortened with either a precipitous second stage or an operative vaginal delivery. Whether the birth attendant expedites completion of fetal expulsion operatively or whether fetal expulsion occurs spontaneously, there may not be sufficient time for the shoulders to rotate and occupy the oblique dimensions of the pelvis before complete descent, culminating in shoulder impingement behind the bony prominences of the pelvis. Precipitous second stage precedes 30% of shoulder dystocia deliveries and is the most prevalent intrapartum risk factor for shoulder dystocia.[71] In these settings, patience and/or a noninterventionist approach to allow time for spontaneous restitution can avert or mitigate the likelihood of fetal injury.[72–74] Awaiting the next contraction after the head delivers also allows time for proper suctioning of the oropharynx and nasopharynx, assessment for presence of a nuchal cord, and palpation for (and even manual adjustment to) oblique positioning of the shoulders and reduces the incidence of shoulder dystocia.[72,74,75]

Although spontaneous precipitous second stage is beyond the control of a clinician, operative intervention via forceps or vacuum is a modifiable choice. The overall incidence of operative vaginal delivery in the United States is about 15%.[14] However, in most studies of shoulder dystocia–complicated births, the incidence of an antecedent operative delivery approaches 35%.[71,76,77]

Although the presence of more than 1 antepartum risk factor does not seem to affect the incidence of shoulder dystocia, the addition of operative vaginal delivery to preexisting risk factors exhibits a cumulative effect, especially when risk factors are coincident with a suspected LGA infant. A combination of diabetes and operative vaginal delivery among the same birth-weight categories is followed by shoulder dystocia 12.2% to 34.8% of the time.[56] Compared with unassisted deliveries of similar–birth-weight categories, every 250-g increment in birth weight more than 4000 g is associated with a steady increase in the percentage, from 8.6% to 29%, of infants delivered using either forceps or vacuum who subsequently experience shoulder dystocia.[8,56]

In a randomized controlled trial of instrument type, Bofill and colleagues[8] demonstrated a higher rate of shoulder dystocia among vacuum deliveries than in deliveries completed with the assistance of forceps (4.7% vs 1.9%, respectively). The difficulty of the operative delivery also has important effects. A direct relationship exists between the length of time needed to complete an operative vaginal delivery and the subsequent occurrence of shoulder dystocia. Operative deliveries completed in less than 2 minutes exhibit a rate of shoulder dystocia of less than 0.5%, whereas the rate increases to nearly 4% among those taking between 2 and 6 minutes to complete and nearly twice (7.9%) among operative deliveries lasting longer than 6 minutes.[8,77] Although the incidence of shoulder dystocia is higher among operative deliveries, associated permanent injuries are not any more common or severe than among spontaneous vaginal deliveries.[78]

Thus, a prospective decision to use an instrument in a particular delivery should be made with the knowledge that doing so at least doubles the risk of shoulder dystocia.

In the presence of other antenatal risk factors, such as high EFW, diabetes, or prior shoulder dystocia, the decision to use operative delivery, and which instrument to use, should be made only with informed discussion with the patient about the additional risk of shoulder dystocia and neonatal injury.

MECHANISMS OF NEONATAL INJURY

Four main neonatal complications are associated with shoulder dystocia. These are clavicle fracture, humeral fracture, brachial plexus injury, and anoxic injury. Humeral fractures may occur, albeit infrequently, in the course of delivery of the posterior arm. Fractured clavicles occur by the passage of anterior shoulder beneath the pubis during vaginal deliveries with and without shoulder dystocia.[79] Although disconcerting at the time of birth, these injuries are often unavoidable and always heal without sequelae during the neonatal period.

Anoxic and brachial plexus injuries, although infrequent and often unavoidable, can be devastating to the patient and the provider. In this section, the authors present the mechanism of injury and potential ways to lower the risk to the patient.

Anoxic Injury

Central nervous system injury resulting from shoulder dystocia involves the interruption of cord blood flow during the head-to-body interval. Mechanical obstruction to blood flow can occur in 2 ways: either by external compression via entrapment of a segment of cord between the fetal upper torso or neck and the soft tissues of the birth canal or via stretching of the cord, which constricts the elastic intima of the blood vessels. The vulnerability of the cord to compression during shoulder dystocia is thus variable and inconsistent. As in all intrapartum occurrences of cord compression, the severity and duration of fetal circulatory effect depend on the presence, frequency, and intensity of uterine contractions. Rarely, complete obstruction to blood flow occurs, unless the umbilical cord is severed (iatrogenically) before delivery is complete. Nuchal cord management in any delivery, and especially in those already recognized as being complicated by shoulder dystocia, requires assurance of freedom of motion of the anterior shoulder before cutting the cord.[80,81]

Unequal compression of the umbilical vein greater than that of the artery during shoulder dystocia leads to preferential transfusion of blood from the fetus to the placenta with resultant fetal hypovolemia.[82] During the shoulder dystocia episode, the natural effect of vaginal wall pressure on the fetus is protective in maintaining central circulation; however, immediately on resolution of the shoulder dystocia, the release of this pressure and return of peripheral circulation can produce cardiovascular collapse and asystole even moments after a normal fetal heart rate had been detected.[82] Delaying clamping of the cord after a long shoulder dystocia episode may allow reperfusion from the placenta once the pressure on the umbilical veins has been released.[82]

Erratic or incomplete circulatory effects render the relationship between head-to-body interval and hypoxic ischemic encephalopathy or fatality resulting from shoulder dystocia fairly complex.[83] Yet it seems that having to manage shoulder dystocia within the commonly used 4-minute rule is conservative because the rule is based only on extrapolated data from nonshoulder dystocia deliveries; a decline in cord pH of 0.14 per minute during the head-to-body delivery interval was retroactively calculated.[84] A recent study found a decline in arterial pH in 200 shoulder dystocia deliveries to be only 0.011 per minute.[85] Four studies specifically examining the effect of the head-to-body interval during shoulder dystocia found no clinically significant decrease in cord pH or increase in occurrence of 5-minute Apgar scores less than 7 for up to a 6 minutes' head-to-body interval.[10,67,86,87] Together, these 5 studies demonstrate that cord arterial pH drops with head-to-body interval during shoulder dystocia but does so slowly, and the risk of acidosis or hypoxic ischemic encephalopathy is very low with an otherwise healthy fetus when the head-to-body interval is less than 6 minutes. Actively measuring head-to-body interval during shoulder dystocia delivery by marking the time of emergence of the fetal head and recognizing that at least 6 minutes is available should help clinicians in shoulder dystocia management.

Brachial Plexus Injury

Although, there are many etiologies for neonatal BP impairment,[88,89] obstetric brachial plexus injuries that are permanent and require neurosurgical treatment universally demonstrate (at the time of surgery) evidence of having undergone forceful stretch.[90–94] Most mechanical brachial plexus injuries evident at birth are upper praxis injuries, are temporary, and resolve any time from while still in the delivery room to up to as long as 18 months postnatally. However, if any of the nerves are mechanically ruptured or avulsed, then the result is an injury that does not recover fully even with surgical intervention. There are 3 types of permanent mechanical nerve stretch injuries: neuroma, rupture, or avulsion; examples are shown in **Fig. 3**. Mechanical stretch injury of the brachial plexus occurs as a result of hyperextension of one side of the neck, thereby elongating the 5 brachial plexus nerves (C5-T1) beyond their injury threshold. The pattern of mechanical stretch injury consistently noted in neurosurgically treated obstetric brachial plexus palsy is that the upper roots (C5-C6) are always injured first. If limited to C5-C6, this is an upper injury, referred to as Erb-Duchenne

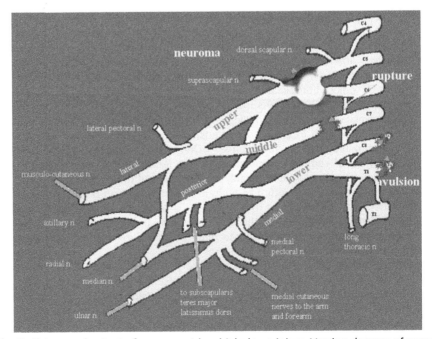

Fig. 3. Nature and extent of permanent brachial plexus injury. Varying degrees of axonal and surrounding nerve sheath disruption results in a range of nerve stretch injuries. From least to most severe, these injuries are (1) neuroma in continuity (axonotmesis) (illustrated at C5-C6;), (2) rupture (neurotmesis) (illustrated at C7), and (3) avulsion (illustrated at C8-T1).

palsy. Clinically, this injury affects the shoulder and elbow only. With increasing stretch, C7 may also be injured (middle injury); this manifests with symptoms involving wrist and finger extension. With even more stretch and/or twist, the lower roots C8-T1 may also be affected (complete injury). With a complete injury, the hand and fingers are also affected.[95] If the lower roots are involved and the sympathetic nervous system (T1) is affected, there may be concomitant Horner syndrome.[89]

Neonatal brachial plexus injuries occur in nonshoulder dystocia–complicated births.[2,18,96,97] The reported rates (depending on the definition of shoulder dystocia) vary from 100% of injuries being associated with shoulder dystocia to an average of 47%, with a peak of 77% of injuries not associated with shoulder dystocia.[98–101] However, the most consistent risk factor for either transient or permanent neonatal brachial plexus injury is antecedent shoulder dystocia.[63,87,98,99,102–105] During shoulder dystocia, neonatal brachial plexus injury occurs as a result of increased lateral traction to and/or twist of the head in an attempt to deliver the trunk.[4,103,106–112]

Based on retrospective studies and limited computer modeling, many investigators have proposed alternative theories about permanent mechanical brachial plexus injury causation. These theories include intrauterine forces, precipitous second stage, and shoulder dystocia itself.[100,113,114] However, none of these theories have been proved prospectively, by experimental evidence, or with rigorous computer modeling. Several retrospective and experimental studies exist that counter these theories.[98,99,103,110,115–117] The merits and demerits of this literature have been presented elsewhere[118] and are beyond the scope of this article.

Randomized prospective intentional in vivo measurement of the traction limits for neonatal injury causation is, of course, unethical. Until recently, the only study measuring the lateral force needed to cause permanent injury has been experimental. Cadaveric work by Metaizeau and colleagues[112] demonstrated that mechanical injury (rupture of the upper roots) only became observable with laterally applied traction of 44 pounds; to rupture and/or avulse the middle and lower roots, up to 88 pounds of lateral traction is needed. However, the strongest evidence derives from the only multicenter prospective study on permanent brachial plexus injuries in history, which has recently been completed in Sweden by Mollberg and colleagues.[77,90,91,119]

Using a visual analog scale (VAS) for quantifying traction and a detailed protocol for documenting manual assistance, clinician-applied traction was assessed in more than 31,000 vaginal deliveries in which 18 permanent brachial plexopathies occurred. In all the 18 plexopathies, Mollberg and colleagues[91] found that "downward traction of the head had been applied more often and with greater force (VAS >77) in the group with persistent damage and there was a significant correlation between the force used and the number of affected nerve roots" (Mollberg, Personal communication, 2011). This is the most compelling evidence, especially because it confirms the experimental and cadaveric studies, and graphical evidence in videotaped deliveries-that mechanical permanent brachial plexus injuries during vaginal deliveries in otherwise normal patients do not occur without strong lateral traction.

Thus, the single greatest correlate with neonatal brachial plexus injury after shoulder dystocia is degree of clinician-applied traction. Nonetheless, iatrogenic temporary and permanent injuries may be unavoidable in certain circumstances and does not necessarily imply negligence or malpractice on the part of the provider.[27,118] Whether an injury is temporary or permanent, and if permanent, whether the injury is to the upper nerves or to the upper and middle nerves or whether it is a pan-plexus injury, is dependent on the fetus (its size, head position, muscle tone, and innate biological variability) and the delivering clinician's manipulation (traction magnitude, direction, and rate, as well as head rotation). Although fetal determinants of injury cannot be controlled once shoulder dystocia is underway, at least the traction applied at delivery is a modifiable determinant of injury permanence and severity. Although it is not possible to predict at what specific traction magnitude an injury occurs in a specific delivery, based on the clinical, experimental, and cadaveric data reviewed earlier, it is possible to relate the ranges of traction and their concomitant brachial plexus stretch to the risk and type of injury they may produce, as shown in **Fig. 4**.[4,90,91,120–123] This provides an objective metric by which to assess provider acquisition and retention of competency in simulation-based training[124–126] (discussed further later). As a result, with attention to traction-reducing strategies, many injuries are likely amenable to prevention or mitigation.

Although sometimes unavoidable, many injuries can be averted by using at most moderate traction (up to 20 pounds).[4,73,74,121,127,128] Beyond magnitude, clinician-applied traction during shoulder dystocia should, to the extent possible, be directed axially and not laterally relative to the fetal spine to reduce the risk of injury.[90,111,121,129] With the direction of the traction as much in line with the fetal spine as possible, the least amount of brachial plexus stretch is produced and protects against injury.[111,130] Before applying traction to the head, checking the orientation of the shoulders is important to limit inadvertent excessive rotational manipulation of the head, as shown in **Fig. 5**. If performed as an initial step in every shoulder dystocia management algorithm, confirming the position of the shoulders and adjusting them to the oblique diameter of the pelvis has been shown to reduce injuries in clinical practice.[75]

MANAGEMENT OF SHOULDER DYSTOCIA

Only after the fetal head has emerged can diagnosis of shoulder dystocia be made. Simply awaiting the next contraction, even in deliveries exhibiting a turtle sign, actually

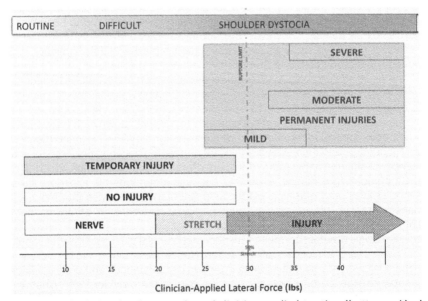

Fig. 4. Graph of relationship between lateral clinician-applied traction (*bottom axis*), characterization of delivery difficulty (*top axis*), and nature and extent of potential-associated neonatal brachial plexus injury (*boxes*). The elastic property of nerve is superimposed on the force graph with the elastic limit (*broken vertical line*) demarcated. This assumes no additional rotation of the head.

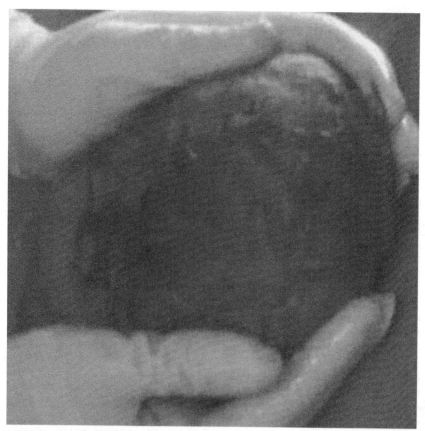

Fig. 5. In this shoulder dystocia delivery, head appears to be in LOA position, implying that the right shoulder is anterior. In fact, the left shoulder was the anterior and the head is twisted nearly 180° by the delivering clinician. No maneuvers were done, and the head-to-body interval was about 70 seconds, most of which the clinician was applying traction to the head and twisting it. However, the resulting injury to this infant involved multiple avulsions.

lowers the incidence of shoulder dystocia.[72,73,131,132] In a prospective study of head-to-body interval in 789 vaginal deliveries, use of a 2-step approach (pausing after the head delivers and waiting for a contraction) reduced the shoulder dystocia rate to 0.25%.[72] Nonetheless, even when these principles are strictly observed, a delivery obstructed by true shoulder dystocia often is not overcome by either patience or gentle or even moderate traction alone. To successfully deliver the infant, attempting to avoid injury, specialized maneuvers have to be used. A review of the techniques of individual shoulder dystocia maneuvers and how to perform them have appeared multiple times in book chapters, review articles, and online[7,67,76,89] and are not presented here. However, despite views to the contrary,[133] evidence does exist regarding the comparative effectiveness of different shoulder dystocia maneuvers in reducing the risk of injury by reducing clinician-applied traction to the head. Those maneuvers that use direct manipulation of the fetus within the birth canal (eg, Rubin maneuver, Woods screw, or posterior arm delivery) ultimately require less traction to the fetal head compared with shoulder dystocia maneuvers that involve manipulation of the mother by assistants (eg, McRoberts positioning and application of suprapubic pressure) while the delivering clinician applies usual delivery traction to the head. The evidence is as follows:

1. A 400% decrease in neonatal brachial plexus injury rate (from 1.6–0.38 per 1000 deliveries) occurred over 23 years (1939–1962) at the New York Hospital.[117] During that time, the Woods screw and delivery of the posterior arm maneuvers were introduced and practiced in the New York area.[115,134,135]
2. A simulation experiment demonstrated that for milder shoulder dystocia deliveries, McRoberts maneuver, compared with lithotomy position, reduced delivery force, brachial plexus stretch, and incidence of clavicle fracture. However, as shoulder dystocia deliveries became more severe, there was no benefit of McRoberts maneuver compared with lithotomy in reducing injury.[121]
3. Although few in number, when shoulder dystocia is initially managed with shoulder rotation, Woods maneuver, or delivery of the posterior arm, the injury rate is significantly lower than when initially managed with McRoberts maneuver and traction.[75,103,136,137]
4. In a shoulder dystocia delivery measuring clinician traction during the delivery, delivery of the posterior arm resolved the shoulder dystocia with half the force used during an earlier unsuccessful attempt using McRoberts maneuver.[5]
5. In a shoulder dystocia case report comparing McRoberts maneuver with posterior arm delivery, the clearance provided by the fetal maneuver is more than twice (20 mm) that of McRoberts maneuver (9 mm).[36]
6. In a simulation study comparing McRoberts positioning with Rubin rotation as the initial maneuver, delivery traction, brachial plexus stretch, and head rotation were significantly lower using Rubin maneuver.[138]
7. A rigid body computer simulation study found that brachial plexus stretch was significantly lower with fetal maneuvers than with maternal maneuvers.[139]
8. By creating a protocol to check and adjust shoulder position before attempting other shoulder dystocia maneuvers, injury rate decreased significantly in clinical practice.[75]

The effective difference between maternal and fetal maneuvers is in the locus and timing of application of traction by the clinician. During McRoberts maneuver, suprapubic pressure, or both, traction force is applied to the fetal head while the shoulder is still impacted in an attempt to overcome the obstruction, whereas in Rubin maneuver, Woods maneuver, and delivery of the posterior arm, finesse is used to release the obstruction and traction is mainly applied directly to the fetal trunk to deliver it. Although there is enough evidence to change the current management guidelines regarding order of maneuvers, a multicenter randomized trial is the best way to evaluate different shoulder dystocia maneuvers in the clinical environment in sizable numbers.

SIMULATION-BASED INSTRUCTION AND REHEARSAL OF SHOULDER DYSTOCIA MANEUVERS

Because shoulder dystocia is relatively infrequent and certainly unplanned, any clinician's experience in managing shoulder dystocia is limited. Because most shoulder dystocia events are resolved by McRoberts maneuver, with or without suprapubic pressure, and moderate traction[140] and most clinicians are unwilling to practice fetal maneuvers during routine deliveries, developing proficiency and competency in fetal manipulation techniques for atraumatic resolution of shoulder dystocia is challenging.

Medical simulation in obstetrics is a rapidly growing training and retraining tool,[143] and success has already been reported in improving shoulder dystocia management using birth simulators.[116,138,141–146] During the last 20 years, in more than a dozen quantitative research and simulation studies, clinician-applied forces have been measured in more than 1000 clinical and simulated deliveries,[4,5,121,127,138,147–153] including routine, difficult, and shoulder dystocia deliveries in the simulated and clinical environment. The principal findings are as follows: (1) In the simulated environment, clinicians can generally distinguish between 3 levels of delivery traction magnitude, routine, difficult, and shoulder dystocia,[4,154,155] and thus can be prospectively aware of degrees of applied traction. (2) The typical traction applied during a routine delivery varies from 0 to 10 pounds; this increases to 20 pounds or more during shoulder dystocia delivery.[4,5,147,149–151] Beyond this range, most clinicians can recognize the need to progress to shoulder dystocia maneuvers to complete delivery without increasing traction force further. (3) In more difficult deliveries in which traction attempts are repeated, increasing traction is always applied during successive delivery attempts if using McRoberts maneuver, suprapubic pressure, or both.[4,5,127] This requires conscious effort and training to avoid. (4) Simulation-based training in shoulder dystocia delivery management reduces clinician traction in subsequent simulated deliveries by the same provider.[142,151–153] Most importantly, training of obstetric staff has led to improved neonatal outcome.[75,152]

SUMMARY

The major findings of this review are as follows:

- In contrast to the lower incidences in retrospective studies, prospective studies reveal that the incidence of shoulder dystocia among term vaginal deliveries is between 3% and 7%. Because definitions and patient populations vary, the true incidence of shoulder dystocia is unknowable, but it occurs more frequently than previously thought.
- Despite the existence of risk factors, nearly half of shoulder dystocia deliveries occur in the absence of risk factors; thus, shoulder dystocia is unpredictable in any given patient.
- History of shoulder dystocia in a prior pregnancy, fetal macrosomia, and maternal diabetes are the major antepartum risk factors for shoulder dystocia; other risk factors such as obesity, excessive gestational weight gain, and postdatism relate to the tendency to produce LGA infants.
- False-positive and false-negative ultrasonographic diagnoses of fetal macrosomia (>4 kg) near delivery increase primary cesarean and traumatic operative vaginal delivery, respectively, but do not affect shoulder dystocia incidence; mid-third trimester ultrasonographic detection of accelerated fetal AC growth is amenable to intervention that reduces both macrosomia and shoulder dystocia at the time of birth.
- Shoulder dystocia incidence can be lowered by maintaining within-target gestational weight gain antenatally, controlling maternal glycemia through properly configured low glycemic index diet and exercise and monitoring fetal growth throughout the prenatal period.
- Elective induction for impending macrosomia before 41 weeks' gestation does not reduce the incidence of shoulder dystocia but is effective at 41 weeks' gestation compared with 42 weeks' gestation.
- Operative vaginal delivery and precipitous second stage are the major intrapartum risk factors for shoulder dystocia owing to insufficient time for the fetal

shoulder girdle to rotate into the oblique diameter of the maternal pelvis. Operative delivery increases the risk of shoulder dystocia by at least a factor of 2; thus, instrumented delivery is the most significant modifiable intrapartum risk factor for subsequent shoulder dystocia and associated injury, especially among LGA infants.

- Neonatal brachial plexus stretch injury is produced by forcible hyperextension of one side of the fetal neck; although several etiologies exist, the single greatest risk factor for permanent neonatal brachial plexus injury is clinician-applied lateral traction during antecedent shoulder dystocia.
- The degree and extent of neonatal brachial plexus injury after shoulder dystocia correlates with magnitude, direction, and rate of clinician-applied traction. The best way to prevent an injury is by minimizing lateral traction and head rotation.
- Iatrogenic temporary and permanent injuries may be unavoidable in certain circumstances and does not necessarily imply negligence or malpractice on the part of the provider.
- Waiting for a contraction after the head delivers reduces the incidence of shoulder dystocia and mechanical injury with no increase in incidence of neonatal depression or acidosis.
- Checking for the shoulders before managing shoulder dystocia reduces the risk of brachial plexus injury.
- Using shoulder dystocia maneuvers that minimize or eliminate direct application of traction to the fetal head reduces the risk of neonatal brachial plexus injury. Compared with those maneuvers that still use such traction, direct fetal manipulation confers greater mechanical advantage in resolving shoulder dystocia and should be prioritized in management algorithms.
- The safe environment of medical simulation is best for training in and rehearsal of fetal maneuvers for the management of shoulder dystocia; competency assessment can be achieved by simulator-derived objective metrics correlating clinician-applied force with resultant fetal mechanical response.

REFERENCES

1. Royal College of Obstetricians and Gynaecologists. Shoulder dystocia. London: RCOG Guideline; 2005. No. 42.
2. American College of Obstetricians and Gynecologists. Practice Bulletin No. 40. Shoulder dystocia, 100. Washington, DC: ACOG; 2002. p. 1045–50.
3. Christoffersson M, Rydhstroem H. Shoulder dystocia and brachial plexus injury: a population-based study. Gynecol Obstet Invest 2002;53:42–7.
4. Allen R, Sorab J, Gonik B. Risk factors for shoulder dystocia: an engineering study of clinician-applied forces. Obstet Gynecol 1991;77:352–5.
5. Poggi SH, Allen RH, Patel CR, et al. Randomized trial of McRoberts' versus lithotomy positioning to decrease the force that is applied to the fetus during delivery. Obstet Gynecol 2004;191:874–8.
6. Young WW. Shoulder dystocia [educational video recording]. American College of Obstetricians & Gynecologist. Washington, DC; 1993.
7. Allen RH, Gurewitsch ED. Shoulder dystocia. eMedicine from WebMD. Available at: http://emedicine.medscape.com/article/1602970-overview. Accessed October 12, 2010.
8. Bofill JA, Rust OA, Devidas M, et al. Shoulder dystocia and operative vaginal delivery. J Matern Fetal Med 1997;6:220–4.

9. Beall MH, Spong C, McKay J, et al. Objective definition of shoulder dystocia: a prospective evaluation. Obstet Gynecol 1998;179:934–7.

10. Spong CY, Beall M, Rodrigues D, et al. An objective definition of shoulder dystocia: prolonged head to body delivery intervals and/or the use of ancillary obstetric maneuvers. Obstet Gynecol 1995;86:433–6.

11. Hankins GD, Clark SM, Munn MB. Cesarean section on request at 39 weeks: impact on shoulder dystocia, fetal trauma, neonatal encephalopathy, and intra-uterine fetal demise. Semin Perinatol 2006;30:276–87.

12. Lee YM, D'Alton ME. Cesarean delivery on maternal request: maternal and neonatal complications. Curr Opin Obstet Gynecol 2008;20:597–601.

13. Rouse DJ, Owen J, Goldenberg RL, et al. The effectiveness and costs of elective cesarean delivery for fetal macrosomia diagnosed by ultrasound. J Am Med Assoc 1996;276:1480–6.

14. Towner D, Castro MA, Eby-Wilkens E, et al. Effect of mode of delivery in nulliparous women on neonatal intracranial injury. N Engl J Med 1999;341:1709–14.

15. Gherman RB, Goodwin TM, Ouzounian JG, et al. Brachial plexus palsy associated with cesarean section: an in utero injury? Obstet Gynecol 1997;177:1162–4.

16. McFarland LV, Raskin M, Daling J, et al. Erb-Duchenne's palsy: a consequence of fetal macrosomia and method of delivery. Obstet Gynecol 1986;68:784–8.

17. Gilbert WM, Nesbitt TS, Danielsen B. Associated factors in 1611 cases of brachial plexus injury. Obstet Gynecol 1999;93:536–40.

18. Acker DB, Sachs BP, Friedman EA. Risk factors for shoulder dystocia in the average-weight infant. Obstet Gynecol 1986;67:614–8.

19. Ruis K, Allen R, Gurewitsch E. Severe shoulder dystocia with small-for-gestational age infant. J Reprod Med 2011;56:178–80.

20. Rouse DJ, Owen J. Prophylactic cesarean delivery for fetal macrosomia diagnosed by means of ultrasonography—a Faustian bargain. Obstet Gynecol 1999;181:332–8.

21. Lewis D, Raymond RC, Perkins MB, et al. Recurrence rate of shoulder dystocia. Obstet Gynecol 1995;172:1369–71.

22. Gurewitsch ED. Optimizing shoulder dystocia management to prevent birth injury. Clin Obstet Gynecol 2007;50:592–606.

23. Smith RB, Lane C, Pearson JF. Shoulder dystocia: what happens at the next delivery? Br J Obstet Gynaecol 1994;101:713–5.

24. Gurewitsch ED, Johnson TL, Allen RH. After shoulder dystocia: managing the subsequent pregnancy and delivery. Semin Perinatol 2007;31:185–95.

25. Dodds SD, Wolfe SW. Perinatal brachial plexus palsy. Curr Opin Pediatr 2000; 12:40–7.

26. Acker DB, Sachs BP, Friedman EA. Risk factors for shoulder dystocia. Obstet Gynecol 1985;66:762–8.

27. Gonik B, Hollyer VL, Allen R. Shoulder dystocia recognition: differences in neonatal risks for injury. Am J Perinatol 1991;8:31–4.

28. Sheiner E, Levy A, Hershkovitz R, et al. Determining factors associated with shoulder dystocia: a population-based study. Eur J Obstet Gynecol Reprod Biol 2006;126:11–5.

29. Landon MB, Spong CY, Thom E, et al. A multicenter, randomized trial of treatment for mild gestational diabetes. N Engl J Med 2009;361:1339–48.

30. Barker DJ. Fetal and infant origins of adult disease. BMJ 1990;301:1111.

31. Oken E, Gillman MW. Fetal origins of obesity. Obes Res 2003;11:496–506.

32. Yogev Y, Langer O. Pregnancy outcome in obese and morbidly obese gestational diabetic women. Eur J Obstet Gynecol Reprod Biol 2008;137:21–6.

33. Jensen DM, Damm P, Sorensen B, et al. Pregnancy outcome and prepregnancy body mass index in 2459 glucose-tolerant Danish women. Obstet Gynecol 2003;189:239–44.

34. Cedergren MI. Maternal morbid obesity and the risk of adverse pregnancy outcome. Obstet Gynecol 2004;103:219–24.

35. Allen R, Petersen S, Moore P, et al. Do antepartum and intrapartum risk factors differ between mild and severe shoulder dystocia? Obstet Gynecol 2003;189:S208.

36. Poggi SH, Spong CY, Allen RH. Prioritizing posterior arm delivery during severe shoulder dystocia. Obstet Gynecol 2003;101:1068–72.

37. Ray JG, Vermeulen MJ, Shapiro JL, et al. Maternal and neonatal outcomes in pregestational and gestational diabetes mellitus, and the influence of maternal obesity and weight gain: the DEPOSIT study. Diabetes Endocrine Pregnancy Outcome Study in Toronto. QJM 2001;94:347–56.

38. Spellacy WN. Obstetric practice in the United States of America may contribute to the obesity epidemic. J Reprod Med 2008;53:955–6.

39. Stotland NE, Hopkins LM, Caughey AB. Gestational weight gain, macrosomia, and risk of cesarean birth in nondiabetic nulliparas. Obstet Gynecol 2004;104:671–7.

40. Hinkle SN, Sharma AJ, Dietz PM. Gestational weight gain in obese mothers and associations with fetal growth. Am J Clin Nutr 2010;92:644–51.

41. Grotegut CA, Tatineni H, Dandolu V, et al. Obstetric outcomes with a false-positive one-hour glucose challenge test by the Carpenter-Coustan criteria. J Matern Fetal Neonatal Med 2008;21:315–20.

42. Stamilio DM, Olsen T, Ratcliffe S, et al. False-positive 1-hour glucose challenge test and adverse perinatal outcomes. Obstet Gynecol 2004;103:148–56.

43. Coustan DR, Lowe LP, Metzger BE, et al. International Association of Diabetes and Pregnancy Study Groups. The Hyperglycemia and Adverse Pregnancy Outcome (HAPO) study: paving the way for new diagnostic criteria for gestational diabetes mellitus. Am J Obstet Gynecol 2010;202:654. e1–654. e6.

44. Hadar E, Hod M. Establishing consensus criteria for the diagnosis of diabetes in pregnancy following the HAPO study. Ann N Y Acad Sci 2010;1205:86–93.

45. Fraser RB, Ford FA, Lawrence GF. Insulin sensitivity in third trimester pregnancy. A randomized study of dietary effects. Br J Obstet Gynaecol 1988;95:223–9.

46. Clapp JF. Effects of diet and exercise on insulin resistance during pregnancy. Metab Syndr Relat Disord 2006;4:84–90.

47. Chauhan SP, Hendrix NW, Magann EF, et al. Limitations of clinical sonographic estimates of birth weight: experience with 1034 parturients. Obstet Gynecol 1998;91:72–7.

48. Weiner Z, Ben-Shlomo I, Beck-Fruchter R, et al. Clinical and ultrasonographic weight estimation in large for gestational age fetus. Eur J Obstet Gynecol Reprod Biol 2002;105:20–4.

49. Melamed N, Yogev Y, Meizner I, et al. Sonographic prediction of fetal macrosomia: the consequences of false diagnosis. J Ultrasound Med 2010;29:225–30.

50. Jazayeri A, Heffron JA, Phillips R, et al. Macrosomia prediction using ultrasound fetal abdominal circumference of 35 centimeters or more. Obstet Gynecol 1999;93:523–6.

51. Bailis A, Syzmanski L, Ibrahim S, et al. Accelerated abdominal circumference growth (>75th%ile) in average gestational age fetuses increases risk of shoulder dystocia. Reprod Sci 2010;17:S187A.

52. Bonomo M, Cetin I, Pisoni MP, et al. Flexible treatment of gestational diabetes modulated on ultrasound evaluation of intrauterine growth: a controlled randomized clinical trial. Diabetes Metab 2004;30:237–44.

53. Kjos SL, Schaefer-Graf U, Sardesi S, et al. A randomized controlled trial using glycemic plus fetal ultrasound parameters versus glycemic parameters to determine insulin therapy in gestational diabetes with fasting hyperglycemia. Diabetes Care 2001;24:1904–10.

54. Schaefer-Graf UM, Kjos SL, Fauzan OH, et al. A randomized trial evaluating a predominantly fetal growth-based strategy to guide management of gestational diabetes in Caucasian women. Diabetes Care 2004;27:297–302.

55. Langer O, Berkus MD, Huff RW, et al. Shoulder dystocia: should the fetus weighing ≥ 4000 grams be delivered by cesarean section? Obstet Gynecol 1991;165:831–7.

56. Nesbitt T, Gilbert W, Herrchen B. Shoulder dystocia and associated risk factors with macrosomic infants born in California. Obstet Gynecol 1998;179:476–80.

57. McFarland MB, Tshibangu KC, Langer O. Anthropometric differences in macrosomic infants of diabetic and nondiabetic mothers. J Matern Fetal Med 1998;7:292–5.

58. Moses RG, Barker M, Winter M, et al. Can a low-glycemic index diet reduce the need for insulin in gestational diabetes mellitus? A randomized trial. Diabetes Care 2009;32:996–1000.

59. Baskett TF, O'Connell CM, Allen A. Antecedents, prevalence, and recurrence of shoulder dystocia and brachial plexus injury. Obstet Gynecol 2006;107:63S.

60. Ginsberg NA, Moisidis C. How to predict recurrent shoulder dystocia. Obstet Gynecol 2001;184:1427–30.

61. Johnstone FD, Myerscough PR. Shoulder dystocia. Br J Obstet Gynaecol 1998;105:811–5.

62. Mehta SH, Blackwell SC, Chadha R, et al. Shoulder dystocia and the next delivery: outcomes and management. J Matern Fetal Neonatal Med 2007;20:729–33.

63. Acker DB, Gregory KD, Sachs BP, et al. Risk factors for Erb-Duchenne palsy. Obstet Gynecol 1988;71:389–92.

64. Christoffersson M, Kannisto P, Rydhstroem H, et al. Shoulder dystocia and brachial plexus injury: a case-control study. Acta Obstet Gynecol Scand 2003;82:147–51.

65. Iffy L, Varadi V, Jakobovits A. Common intrapartum denominators of shoulder dystocia related birth injuries. Zentralbl Gynakol 1994;116:33–7.

66. Iffy L, Brimacombe M, Apuzzio JJ, et al. The risk of shoulder dystocia related permanent fetal injury in relation to birth weight. Eur J Obstet Gynecol Reprod Biol 2008;136:53–60.

67. Gurewitsch ED, Allen RH. Fetal manipulation for management of shoulder dystocia. Fet Mat Med Rev 2006;17:185–204.

68. McFarland MB, Langer O, Piper JM, et al. Perinatal outcome and the type and number of maneuvers in shoulder dystocia. Int J Gynaecol Obstet 1996;55:219–24.

69. Moore HM, Reed SD, Batra M, et al. Risk factors for recurrent shoulder dystocia, Washington State, 1987–2004. Am J Obstet Gynecol 2008;198:e16–24.

70. Kaimal AJ, Little SE, Odibo AO, et al. Cost-effectiveness of elective induction of labor at 41 weeks in nulliparous women. Am J Obstet Gynecol 2011;204:137. e1–137, e9.

71. Poggi SH, Stallings SP, Ghidini A, et al. Intrapartum risk factors for permanent brachial plexus injury. Obstet Gynecol 2003;189:725–9.

72. Strobelt N, Locatelli A, Casarico G, et al. Head-to-body interval time: what's the normal range? Obstet Gynecol 2006;195:S110.

73. Hart G. Waiting for shoulders. Midwifery Today 1997;42:32–4.

74. Bottoms SF, Sokol RJ. Mechanisms and conduct of labor. In: Iffy L, Kaminetzky HA, editors. Principles and practice of obstetrics & perinatology. New York: John Wiley & Sons; 1981. p. 815–37.

75. Inglis SR, Feier N, Chetiyaar J, et al. Effects of a shoulder dystocia management protocol on the incidence of brachial plexus injury. Am J Obstet Gynecol 2011; 204:322, e1–6.

76. Dildy GA, Clark SL. Shoulder dystocia: risk identification. Clin Obstet Gynecol 2000;43:265–82.

77. Mollberg M, Hagberg H, Bager B, et al. Risk factors for obstetric brachial plexus palsy among neonates delivered by vacuum extraction. Obstet Gynecol 2005; 106:913–8.

78. Poggi SH, Ghidini A, Allen RH, et al. Effect of operative vaginal delivery on the outcome of permanent brachial plexus injury. J Reprod Med 2003;48:692–6.

79. Cohen AW, Otto SR. Obstetric clavicular fractures: a three-year analysis. J Reprod Med 1980;25:119–22.

80. Iffy L, Gittens-Williams LN. Shoulder dystocia and nuchal cord. Acta Obstet Gynecol Scand 2007;86:253.

81. Cunningham FG, MacDonald PC, Grant NF, et al. Williams obstetrics. 20th edition. Norwalk (CT): Appleton & Lange; 1997.

82. Mercer J, Erickson-Owens D, Skovgaard R. Cardiac asystole at birth: is hypovolemic shock the cause? Med Hypotheses 2008;72:458–63.

83. Hope P, Breslin S, Lamont L, et al. Fatal shoulder dystocia: a review of 56 cases reported to the Confidential Enquiry into Stillbirths and Deaths in Infancy. Br J Obstet Gynaecol 1998;105:1256–61.

84. Wood C, Ng KH, Hounslow D. Time—an important variable in normal delivery. J Obstet Gynaecol Br Commonw 1973;80:295–300.

85. Leung T, Stuart O, Sahota D, et al. Head-to-body delivery interval and risk of fetal acidosis and hypoxic ischaemic encephalopathy in shoulder dystocia: a retrospective review. BJOG 2011;118(4):474–9. DOI: 10.1111/j.1471-0528.2010.02834.x.

86. Stallings SP, Edwards RK, Johnson JW. Correlation of head-to-body delivery intervals in shoulder dystocia and umbilical artery acidosis. Am J Obstet Gynecol 2001;185:268–74.

87. Allen RH, Rosenbaum TC, Ghidini A, et al. Correlating head-to-body delivery intervals with neonatal depression in vaginal births that result in permanent brachial plexus injury. Obstet Gynecol 2002;187:839–42.

88. Alfonso I, Diaz-Arca G, Alfonso DT, et al. Fetal deformations: a risk factor for obstetrical brachial plexus palsy? Pediatr Neurol 2006;35:246–9.

89. Gurewitsch ED, Allen RH. Epidemiology of shoulder dystocia and its associated neonatal complications. In: Sheiner E, editor. Textbook of perinatal epidemiology. Hauppauge (NY): Nova Scientific Publishers; 2010. p. 453–98.

90. Mollberg M, Wennergren M, Bager B, et al. Obstetric brachial plexus palsy: a prospective study on risk factors related to manual assistance during the second stage of labor. Acta Obstet Gynecol Scand 2007;86:198–204.

91. Mollberg M, Lagerkvist AL, Johansson U, et al. Comparison in obstetric management on infants with transient and persistent obstetric brachial plexus palsy. J Child Neurol 2008;23:1424–32.

92. Alfonso I, Alfonso DT, Papazian O. Focal upper extremity neuropathy in neonates. Semin Pediatr Neurol 2000;7:4–14.

93. Belzberg AJ, Dorsi MJ, Storm PB, et al. Surgical repair of brachial plexus injury: a multinational survey of experienced peripheral nerve surgeons. J Neurosurg 2004;101:365–76.

94. Sunderland S, Bradley KC. Stress-strain phenomena in human peripheral nerve trunks. Brain 1961;84:102–19.
95. Pondaag W, Allen RH, Malessy MJ. Correlating birth weight with neurological severity of obstetric brachial plexus lesions. Br J Obstet Gynaecol, in press.
96. Graham EM, Forouzan I, Morgan MA. A retrospective analysis of Erb's palsy cases and their relation to birth weight and trauma at delivery. J Matern Fetal Med 1997;6:1–5.
97. Allen RH, Gurewitsch ED. Temporary Erb-Duchenne palsy without shoulder dystocia or traction to the fetal head. Obstet Gynecol 2005;105:1210–2.
98. Morrison JC, Sanders JR, Magann EF, et al. The diagnosis and management of dystocia of the shoulder. Surg Gynecol Obstet 1992;175:515–22.
99. Ubachs JM, Slooff AC, Peeters LL. Obstetric antecedents of surgically treated obstetric brachial-plexus injuries. Br J Obstet Gynaecol 1995;102:813–7.
100. Gherman RB, Ouzounian JG, Miller DA, et al. Spontaneous vaginal delivery: a risk factor for Erb's palsy? Obstet Gynecol 1998;178:423–7.
101. Levine MG, Holroyde J, Woods JR, et al. Birth trauma: incidence and predisposing factors. Obstet Gynecol 1984;63:792–5.
102. Nocon JJ, McKenzie DK, Thomas LJ, et al. Shoulder dystocia: an analysis of risks and obstetric maneuvers. Obstet Gynecol 1993;168:1732–9.
103. Baskett TF, Allen AC. Perinatal implications of shoulder dystocia. Obstet Gynecol 1995;86:14–7.
104. Allen RH, Edelberg SC. Brachial plexus palsy causation [letter]. Birth 2003;30: 141–3 [author reply: 143–5].
105. Ouzounian JG, Korst L, Phelan J. Permanent Erb's palsy: a lack of a relationship with obstetrical risk factors. Am J Perinatol 1998;15:221–3.
106. Fieux G. Pathogenesis of brachial paralyses in the neonate. Obstetrical paralyses. Ann Gynecol Obstet 1897;47:52–64.
107. Thorburn W. Obstetrical paralysis. J Obstet Gynecol Br Empire 1903;3:454–8.
108. Clark LP, Taylor AS, Prout TP. A study on brachial birth palsy. Am J Med Sci 1905;130:670–707.
109. Sever JW. Obstetric paralysis: its etiology, pathology, clinical aspects and treatment, with a report of four hundred and seventy cases. Am J Dis Child 1916;12: 541–78.
110. Stander HJ, editor. Williams textbook of obstetrics. 9th edition. New York: Appleton-Century; 1945.
111. Morris WI. Shoulder dystocia. J Obstet Gynecol Br Empire 1955;62:302–6.
112. Metaizeau JP, Gayet C, Plenat F. Brachial plexus injuries: an experimental study. Chir Pediatr 1979;20:159–63 [in French].
113. Gonik B, Zhang N, Grimm MJ. Prediction of brachial plexus stretching during shoulder dystocia using a computer simulation model. Obstet Gynecol 2003; 1989:1168–72.
114. Ouzounian JG, Korst L, Phelan J. Permanent Erb's palsy- a traction related injury? Obstet Gynecol 1997;89:139–41.
115. Adler J, Patterson RL. Erb's palsy: long term results of treatment in eighty-eight cases. J Bone Joint Surg Am 1967;49:1052–64.
116. Allen RH, Cha SL, Kranker LM, et al. Comparing mechanical fetal response during descent, crowning and restitution among deliveries with and without shoulder dystocia. Am J Obstet Gynecol 2007;196:e1–5.
117. Foad SC, Mehlman CT, Ying J. The epidemiology of neonatal brachial plexus injury. J Bone Joint Surg Am 2008;90:1258–64.

118. Gurewitsch ED, Allen RH. Shoulder dystocia. Clin Perinatol 2007;34:365–85.
119. Mollberg M. Obstetric brachial plexus palsy. Sweden: Department of Obstetrics and Gynaecology, The Institute of Clinical Sciences, Sahlgrenska Academy at Göteborg University; 2007.
120. American College of Obstetricians and Gynecologists. Shoulder dystocia. Practice patterns No. 7. Washington, DC: ACOG; 1997.
121. Gonik B, Allen R, Sorab J. Objective evaluation of the shoulder dystocia phenomenon: effect of maternal pelvic orientation on force reduction. Obstet Gynecol 1989;74:44–8.
122. American College of Obstetricians and Gynecologist. Shoulder dystocia. Int J Gynaecol Obstet 1998;60:306–13.
123. Kalmin OV. Structural based for tensile strength properties of nerves. Morfologiia 1997;111:39–43 [in Russian].
124. Gurewitsch ED, Johnson TL, Narayan AK, et al. Clinician-educators traction estimation and injury prediction during simulated shoulder dystocia. Reprod Sci 2009;16:308A.
125. Gurewitsch ED, Johnson TL, Narayan AK, et al. Subjective debriefing following shoulder dystocia: how good is it? Reprod Sci 2009;16:308A.
126. Johnson TL, Allen RH, Narayan AK, et al. Clinician-educators ranking of factors contributing to injury following shoulder dystocia. Reprod Sci 2009; 16:311A.
127. Tam W, Hoe YS, Huang S, et al. Measuring hand-applied forces during vaginal delivery without instrumenting the fetus or interfering with grasping function. J Soc Gynecol Investig 2004;11:205A.
128. Crofts JF, Bartlett C, Ellis D, et al. Training for shoulder dystocia—a trial of simulation using low-fidelity and high-fidelity mannequins. Obstet Gynecol 2006;108: 1477–85.
129. Gonik B, Zhang N, Grimm MJ. Defining forces that are associated with shoulder dystocia: the use of a mathematic dynamic computer model. Obstet Gynecol 2003;188:1068–72.
130. Allen RH. On the mechanical aspects of shoulder dystocia and birth injury. Clin Obstet Gynecol 2007;50:607–23.
131. Iffy L, Ganesh V, Gittens L. Obstetric maneuvers for shoulder dystocia [letter]. Obstet Gynecol 1998;179:1379–80.
132. Andersen J, Watt J, Olson J, et al. Perinatal brachial plexus palsy. Paediat Child Health 2006;11:93–100.
133. Gherman RB, Chauhan S, Ouzounian JG, et al. Shoulder dystocia: the unpreventable obstetric emergency with empiric management guidelines. Am J Obstet Gynecol 2006;195:657–72.
134. Woods CE. A principle of physics as applicable to shoulder dystocia. Obstet Gynecol 1943;45:796–804.
135. Barnum CG. Dystocia due to the shoulders. Obstet Gynecol 1945;50:439–42.
136. Gross SJ, Shime J, Farine D. Shoulder dystocia: predictors and outcome. Obstet Gynecol 1987;156:334–6.
137. Schwartz BC, Dixon DM. Shoulder dystocia. Obstet Gynecol 1958;11:468–71.
138. Gurewitsch ED, Kim EJ, Yang JH, et al. Comparing McRoberts' and Rubin's maneuvers for initial management of shoulder dystocia: an objective evaluation. Am J Obstet Gynecol 2005;192:153–60.
139. Grimm MJ, Costello RE, Gonik B. Effect of clinician-applied maneuvers on brachial plexus stretch during a shoulder dystocia event: investigation using a computer simulation model. Am J Obstet Gynecol 2010;203:e1–5.

140. Gherman RB, Ouzounian JG, Goodwin TM. Obstetric maneuvers for shoulder dystocia and associated fetal morbidity. Am J Obstet Gynecol 1998;178: 1126–30.

141. Gardner R, Walzer TB. Obstetric simulation: state of the art in 2005. Cont Obstet Gynecol 2005. Available at: http://contemporaryobgyn.net/obgyn/content/printcontentpopup.jsp?id=18115. Accessed August 28, 2006.

142. Crofts JF, Bartlett C, Ellis D, et al. Management of shoulder dystocia—skill retention 6 and 12 months after training. Obstet Gynecol 2007;110:1069–74.

143. Crofts JF, Attilakos G, Read M, et al. Shoulder dystocia training using a new birth training mannequin. BJOG 2005;112:997–9.

144. Macedonia CR, Gherman RB, Satin AJ. Simulation laboratories for training in obstetrics and gynecology. Obstet Gynecol 2003;102:388–92.

145. Deering S, Poggi S, Macedonia C, et al. Improving resident competency in the management of shoulder dystocia with simulation training. Obstet Gynecol 2004;103:1224–8.

146. Goffman D, Heo H, Pardanani S, et al. Improving shoulder dystocia management among resident and attending physicians using simulations. Obstet Gynecol 2007;197:S185.

147. Poggi SH, Allen RH, Patel C, et al. Effect of epidural anaesthesia on clinician-applied force during vaginal delivery. Obstet Gynecol 2004;191:903–6.

148. Bankoski BR, Allen RH, Nagey DA, et al. Measuring clavicle strength and modeling birth: towards understanding birth injury. In: Vossoughi J, editor. Proc 13th Southern Biomedical Engineering Conference. Washington, DC, April 1994. p. 586–9.

149. Sorab J, Allen RH, Gonik B. Tactile sensory monitoring of clinician-applied forces during delivery of newborns. IEEE Trans Biomed Eng 1988;35:1090–3.

150. Crofts JF, Ellis D, James M, et al. Pattern and degree of forces applied during simulation of shoulder dystocia. Obstet Gynecol 2007;197:156.

151. Deering SH, Weeks L, Benedetti T. Evaluation of force applied during deliveries complicated by shoulder dystocia using simulation. Am J Obstet Gynecol 2011; 204:234, e1–5.

152. Draycott TJ, Crofts JF, Ash JP, et al. Improving neonatal outcome through practical shoulder dystocia training. Obstet Gynecol 2008;112:14–20.

153. Kelly J, Guise JM, Osterweil P, et al. 211: determining the value of force-feedback simulation training for shoulder dystocia. Obstet Gynecol 2008;199: S70.

154. Allen RH, Bankoski BR, Nagey DA. Simulating birth to investigate clinician-applied loads on newborns. Med Eng Phys 1995;17:380–4.

155. Allen RH, Bankoski BR, Butzin CA, et al. Comparing clinician-applied loads for routine, difficult, and shoulder dystocia deliveries. Obstet Gynecol 1994;171: 1621–7.

Acquired and Inherited Thrombophilia Disorders in Pregnancy

Silvia S. Pierangeli, PhD[a],*, Benjamin Leader, MD, PhD[b],
Giuseppe Barilaro, MD[a], Rohan Willis, MD[a],
D. Ware Branch, MD[c]

KEYWORDS

- Thrombosis in pregnancy • Antiphospholipid syndrome
- Antiphospholipid antibodies • Pregnancy loss

ACQUIRED THROMBOPHILIAS AND PREGNANCY MORBIDITY

The most common acquired thrombophilia is the antiphospholipid syndrome (APS). Nigel Harris first used the term antiphospholipid syndrome in 1986[1] to refer to what is now a well-known clinical condition of thrombosis and/or pregnancy morbidity associated with repeatedly positive tests for antiphospholipid (aPL) antibodies. Obstetrics and gynecology quickly embraced APS as one of the few, if any, treatable causes of fetal loss. It was not long before numerous other reproductive and medical maladies were linked to aPL antibodies, although with debatable certainty. The curious association of thrombosis with fetal loss ushered in an era of collaborative research between reproductive specialists, hematologists, and rheumatologists, as well as a new area of basic science investigation involving autoantibodies, coagulation, and inflammation. This work, along with more than a dozen international congresses, has led to 2 published sets of International Criteria for the diagnosis of APS, numerous attempts to standardize clinical testing, and exciting laboratory findings in vitro and in animal models that await corroboration in humans. Controversies still thrive, especially in terms of how best to define APS and in particular with regard to autoantibody testing.

Disclosures of interest: SP is the owner and technical director of Louisville APL Diagnostics Inc (manufacturer of the APhL enzyme-linked immunoassay mentioned in this paper). BL is the CEO of Reprosource Inc.

[a] Antiphospholipid Standardization Laboratory, Division of Rheumatology, Department of Internal Medicine, University of Texas Medical Branch, 301 University Boulevard, Galveston, TX 77555-0883, USA
[b] Clinical Research Division, Reprosource, Inc, 300 Trade Center, Suite 6540, Woburn, MA 01801, USA
[c] Department of Obstetrics and Gynecology, University of Utah Health Sciences Center and Intermountain Healthcare, 30 North 1900 East, Room 2B200 SOM, Salt Lake City, UT 84132, USA
* Corresponding author.
E-mail address: sspieran@utmb.edu

Obstet Gynecol Clin N Am 38 (2011) 271–295
doi:10.1016/j.ogc.2011.02.016
0889-8545/11/$ – see front matter © 2011 Elsevier Inc. All rights reserved.

obgyn.theclinics.com

Clinical Features of APS

APS is a clinical diagnosis (**Box 1**). The accepted clinical features are (1) 1 or more episodes of thrombosis, (2) recurrent ($\geq$3) early miscarriage (<10 weeks' gestation), (3) 1 or more fetal deaths ($\geq$10 weeks' gestation), or (4) preterm delivery of less than 34 weeks' gestation for severe preeclampsia or placental insufficiency.[2] Thromboses may be arterial, venous, or small vessel in nature, in any tissue or organ, and should be objectively shown (ie, by unequivocal findings of appropriate imaging studies or histopathology). For histopathologic support, thrombosis should be present without substantial evidence of inflammation in the vessel wall. The most common presenting

---

Box 1
Classification criteria for APS

Clinical criteria

Vascular thrombosis

- One or more clinical episodes of arterial, venous, or small-vessel thrombosis, in any tissue or organ.
  - Thrombosis should be supported by objective validated criteria (ie, unequivocal findings of appropriate imaging studies or histopathology). For histopathologic support, thrombosis should be present without substantial evidence of inflammation in the vessel wall.

Pregnancy morbidity, defined by 1 of the following criteria:

- One or more unexplained deaths of a morphologically healthy fetus at or beyond the 10th week of gestation, with healthy fetal morphology documented by ultrasound or by direct examination of the fetus

- One or more premature births of a morphologically healthy newborn baby before the 34th week of gestation because of: eclampsia or severe preeclampsia defined according to standard definitions or recognized features of placental failure

- Three or more unexplained consecutive spontaneous abortions before the 10th week of gestation, with maternal anatomic or hormonal abnormalities and paternal and maternal chromosomal causes excluded

  - In studies of populations of patients who have more than 1 type of pregnancy morbidity, investigators are strongly encouraged to stratify groups of patients according to 1 of the 3 criteria

Laboratory criteria

- Lupus anticoagulant (LAC) present in plasma, on 2 or more occasions at least 12 weeks apart, detected according to the guidelines of the International Society on Thrombosis and Hemostasis (Scientific Subcommittee on LAC/phospholipid-dependent antibodies)

- Anticardiolipin (aCL) antibody of IgG or IgM isotype, or both, in serum or plasma, present in medium or high titers (ie, >40 GPL or MPL, or greater than the 99th percentile) on 2 or more occasions, at least 12 weeks apart, measured by a standardized enzyme-linked immunoassay (ELISA)

- Anti-β_2-glycoprotein I (anti-β_2GPI) antibody of IgG or IgM isotype, or both, in serum or plasma (in titers greater than the 99th percentile), present on 2 or more occasions, at least 12 weeks apart, measured by a standardized ELISA, according to recommended procedures

Abbreviations: GPL, G phospholipid units; MPL, M phospholipid units.
Adapted from Miyakis S, Lockshin MD, Atsumi T, et al. International consensus statement on an update of the classification criteria for definite antiphospholipid syndrome (APS). J Thromb Haemost 2006;4:295–306; with permission.

thrombotic event is venous thrombosis (or embolism), most often in typical locations such as the left lower extremity. However, APS should be considered with more unusual thrombotic events such as mesenteric, renal, or intracranial thromboses.

With regard to the pregnancy-related clinical criteria, both recurrent early miscarriage (REM) and fetal death should be otherwise unexplained. For REM, international consensus[2] calls for excluding maternal anatomic or hormonal abnormalities and paternal and maternal chromosomal causes. For fetal death, the consensus calls for normal fetal morphology by ultrasound or physical examination. Severe preeclampsia is diagnosed by standard criteria (American College of Obstetricians and Gynecologists [ACOG] Practice bulletin) and placental insufficiency is defined as (1) abnormal or nonreassuring fetal surveillance test(s) (eg, a nonreactive nonstress test), suggestive of fetal hypoxemia, (2) abnormal Doppler flow velocimetry waveform analysis suggestive of fetal hypoxemia (eg, absent end-diastolic flow in the umbilical artery), (3) oligohydramnios (eg, an amniotic fluid index of 5 cm or less), or (4) a postnatal birth weight less than the 10th percentile for the gestational age.[2]

Experts debate two related major issues regarding the obstetric criteria for APS. The first is that of the frequency with which a given clinical presentation is attributable to APS (ie, the frequency of cases in which repeatedly positive, significant levels of aPL antibodies are found). Recurrent miscarriage occurs in about 1% of the general population attempting to have children.[3] About 10% to 15% of women with recurrent miscarriage are diagnosed with APS.[4,5] Branch and colleagues[6] have challenged this high frequency, noting that although they see about 100 new patients with REM per year, only a rare case meets the current criteria for APS by having LAC or more than 40 GPL or MPL units of aCL or titre greater than 99th percentile of anti-β_2GPI antibodies, much less have repeatedly positive results.[6] This finding, coupled with results from recent trials in which women with recurrent miscarriage and aPL antibodies were found to have benign pregnancy outcomes without heparin treatment,[7,8] strongly suggests the need for more research in this area of obstetric APS. A recently convened expert task force concluded that such research into the relationship of aPL antibodies and recurrent miscarriage is warranted.[9]

Fetal death in the second or third trimesters of pregnancy occurs in up to 5% of unselected pregnancies progressing beyond the early second trimester,[10] but is less likely as pregnancy advances.[11] Although fetal death is linked to APS,[12] the overall contribution of this syndrome is uncertain, partly because of the effect of other possible contributing factors such as underlying hypertension or preexisting comorbidities such as systemic lupus erythematosus (SLE) or renal disease. Results of a population-based study of fetal deaths at more than 20 weeks' gestation (the Stillbirth Collaborative Research Network sponsored by the National Institutes of Health) should prove relevant to better understanding of the frequency of APS as a cause of fetal death. However, fetal deaths occurring between 10 and 20 weeks are poorly studied with regard to cause, including with regard to aPL antibodies. Further work in this area is required.[6]

About 5% to 10% of all pregnancies are complicated by preeclampsia or placental insufficiency (as manifested by fetal growth restriction), or both, and severe manifestations of these disorders account for about 75% of indicated preterm deliveries.[13] Pregnant women with a previous diagnosis of APS syndrome are at increased risk for developing preeclampsia or placental insufficiency, but the association between aPL antibodies and these disorders in the absence of preexisting APS is less certain.[14] Results of case-control studies show that aPL antibodies are detected in 11% to 29% of women with preeclampsia, compared with 7% or less in controls. A recent meta-analysis found that moderate to high levels of aCL antibodies are associated with preeclampsia, but there is insufficient evidence to use aCL antibodies as predictors of preeclampsia in clinical practice.[15] Findings from one study showed that 25% of women delivering growth-restricted fetuses had aPL antibodies, but results from others do not show an association.[14] Results from prospective cohort studies indicate that of pregnant women with high titers of aPL antibodies, 10% to 50% develop preeclampsia, and more than 10% of these women deliver infants who are small for gestational age.[14] Taken together, the available evidence regarding the frequency and magnitude of the association between aPL antibodies and second-trimester or third-trimester adverse outcomes in the absence of APS is weak at best. The Obstetric Task Force has called for additional studies to firmly establish the significance and magnitude of the association between aPL antibodies and preterm birth caused by severe preeclampsia and placental insufficiency.[6,7]

The second major area of debate is the specificity of the clinical presentations for APS; this is a topic directly related to the earlier discussion of the frequency and magnitude of the association between aPL antibodies and the obstetric criteria. Each of the clinical criteria for APS (including thrombosis) is a common presentation, and each is of heterogeneous cause. Couple this with the reality that moderately positive aPL tests may occur in 1% to 5% of the normal population, and the distinct possibility of a false diagnosis of APS becomes apparent. In contrast to SLE, only 1 clinical criterion is required to make a diagnosis of APS. The international community has yet to struggle with the issue of clinical criteria specificity; however, the current International Criteria call for excluding other causes of either recurrent miscarriage or fetal death before attributing these to APS.

Mechanisms of APS-related Obstetric Disease

Thrombotic mechanisms in obstetric APS

Given that aPL antibodies were linked to thrombosis, impairment of maternal-fetal blood exchange as a result of thrombus formation in the uteroplacental vasculature was believed to be the main mechanism underlying APS pregnancy morbidity,[16] and was supported by findings of placental thrombosis in patients with APS with first-trimester and second-trimester abortions by some investigators.[17,18] However, such a histologic finding is not specific for APS, being also present in other conditions. IgG fractions from LAC-positive patients with APS are able to induce a procoagulant phenotype, with significant increases in thromboxane synthesis in placental explants from normal human pregnancies.[19] In favor of the pathogenic role of thrombotic events in aPL-associated pregnancy loss there is evidence from in vitro studies that aPL may induce a procoagulant state.[20] A further thrombophilic mechanism mediated by aPL antibodies involves the relationship between the autoantibodies and annexin A5. In physiologic conditions, a crystal shield of annexin A5 is suggested to cover thrombogenic anionic surfaces and prevent the activation of the coagulation cascade by inhibiting the binding of activated factor X and prothrombin. In vitro studies showed that aPL/anti-β_2GPI might disrupt the anticoagulant annexin A5 crystal shield; such an effect was reproduced also on trophoblast and endothelial cell monolayers.[21–23] According to the hypothesis that a loss of the annexin A5 shield may play a pathogenic role, the same group reported a significantly lower amount of annexin A5 covering the intervillous surfaces in the placentas of aPL-positive women.[21–23] A new mechanistic test that measures the decrease of the anticoagulant effect of annexin A5 by aPL antibodies in plasma has been recently developed. Studies using this test have shown that the assay correctly identifies aPL-antibodies associated thrombosis and pregnancy losses and it is positive in approximately 50% of the patients with APS.[21–23]

Nonthrombotic mechanisms in obstetric APS

Despite experimental models providing evidence for a role of thrombosis in APS-related pregnancy losses, histologic evidence of thrombosis in the uteroplacental circulation cannot be shown in many placentas from patients with APS.[24]

Other theories have thus been put forward to explain APS-related pregnancy morbidity such as defective trophoblast invasion and decidual transformation in early pregnancy and placental injury as a result of local inflammatory events.[25] It is likely that abnormalities of early trophoblast invasion and defective placentation rather than thrombosis may be the primary pathologic mechanism involved in first-trimester losses in these patients,[26] and more recent investigators focus on cellular dysfunction and inflammation as primary mediators of APS-related obstetric disease.

Cellular dysfunction Investigators have sought evidence for a direct effect of aPL on trophoblast function, hypothesizing that aPL may increase trophoblast apoptosis and abnormal proliferation, decrease human chorionic gonadotropin (hCG) release, diminish trophoblast invasiveness, alter adhesion molecule expression, and alter maternal spiral artery transformation and the maturation and differentiation of maternal decidual endometrial cells.[25] Murine and human monoclonal aPL and polyclonal IgG antibodies from patients with APS show β_2GPI-dependent binding to trophoblast monolayers.[27,28] Bound murine monoclonal aPLs have been shown to react with syncytiotrophoblast and to prevent intertrophoblast fusion, trophoblast invasiveness, and hCG secretion.[27,29,30] APL may also act by decreasing expression of heparin-binding epidermal growth factor-like growth factor (EGF-like GF), an important factor in blastocyst implantation.[31] Increased apoptosis has been shown in rat embryos and placental explant cultures incubated with polyclonal IgG from women with APS and associated pregnancy loss, as well as in rat embryos incubated with monoclonal anti-phosphatidylserine antibodies.[32,33]

It has been shown that aPLs, particularly anti-β_2GPI, also react with human stromal decidual cells, thus potentially affecting the maternal side of the placenta. Polyclonal and monoclonal β_2GPI-dependent aPL can bind stromal decidual cell monolayers and induce a proinflammatory phenotype characterized by increased intercellular adhesion molecule 1 (ICAM-1) expression and tumor necrosis factor α (TNF-α) secretion.[34] Impaired endometrial differentiation, as well as diminished expression of the complement regulatory protein decay accelerating factor (DAF), have been shown in endometrial biopsy samples from patients with APS with recurrent pregnancy loss (RPL).[35] Using in vitro human endometrial endothelial angiogenesis or an in vivo angiogenesis murine model, aPL can be shown to significantly decrease the number and total length of tubule formation, vascular endothelial growth factor (VEGF) and matrix metalloproteinase (MMP) production and nuclear factor κB DNA-binding activity by endometrial endothelial cells.[36] Newly formed vessels also were significantly reduced in aPL-inoculated mice, suggesting that inhibition of angiogenesis is a potential mechanism of defective placentation in patients with APS.[36]

Immune injury Experimental models have shown a role for complement, tissue factor (TF), TNF-α, and chemotactic chemokines in aPL-mediated fetal loss.[37,38] Initial murine models used to evaluate the role of complement activation in aPL-induced fetal loss had focused on complement components C3 and C5. Passive transfer of large amounts of human IgG-aPL from patients with APS to pregnant naive mice induced extensive placental damage, increased fetal resorption, and fetal growth retardation at day 15 of pregnancy.[37] Placental inflammation in these mice was characterized by recruitment of neutrophils, upregulated TF and TNF-α secretion, focal decidual necrosis and apoptosis, and complement deposition. Complement receptor

1 related gene/protein y (Crry)-Ig, an inhibitor of classic and alternative pathway complement C3 convertases, was shown to reduce the frequency of fetal resorption, prevent growth restriction in surviving fetuses, and limit the development of placental lesions.[39] Additional murine studies have shown the key role that complement component C5 plays in aPL-induced placental injury. Induced by aPL pregnancy complications were reduced in C5 or C5a receptor (C5aR)-deficient mice and in mice treated with monoclonal anti-C5 antibodies or a highly specific peptide antagonist of C5aR (C5aR-AP).[40] These findings highlight the critical importance of C5a-C5aR interaction in inducing aPL-mediated placental injury. On the other hand, C6-deficient mice are not protected from aPL-mediated fetal loss, indicating that the membrane attack complex (C5b-9) is unlikely to play an essential role in this process.[41] Deciduas from $C5^{-/-}$ mice treated with aPL had normal morphology with absent neutrophil infiltration, and in similar experiments mice depleted of neutrophils did not have pregnancy loss, fetal growth restriction, or inflammatory infiltrates.[41] Studies also suggest a possible role for C5a activation of monocytes resulting in soluble VEGF receptor-1 (sVEGFR-1) expression and subsequently diminished VEGF levels in conditions associated with fetal loss.[42,43] Taken together, the available data indicate a mechanism in which aPLs bind trophoblast and induce complement activation, generating C5a and subsequent C5a-C5aR interactions, including those on neutrophils and monocytes. C5a induces TF expression and superoxide production in neutrophils, causing oxidative damage, and possibly sVEGFR-1 secretion by monocytes, causing diminished VEGF levels and inadequate placental development and perfusion. This situation results in placental injury, fetal growth restriction, or resorption. The efficacy of heparin in preventing obstetric complications in women with APS has been shown not to be a function of its ability to inhibit thrombosis, as was once believed, but rather a function of its ability to limit aPL-induced complement activation and subsequent placental inflammation.[44] Although complement deposition in abortive specimens from patients with APS has been reported in some case series, others were unable to show this pathologic finding.[45,46] Thus, conclusive immunohistologic evidence of complement activation in abortive material and placentas from women with APS is still lacking. One possibility is that the inflammation leading to placental damage occurs early in pregnancy and is no longer apparent at the time of pregnancy outcome. Further analysis of the applicability of murine models to aPL-induced obstetric complications in patients with APS is thus required to translate these findings into the development of targeted therapies for these patients. A prospective, multicenter, observational study entitled PROMISSE (Predictors of Pregnancy Outcome: Biomarkers in Antiphospholipid Antibody Syndrome and SLE–NCT00198068) to examine the role of complement as a potential surrogate marker that predicts poor pregnancy outcomes in patients with APS is under way and scheduled for completion in 2013 (**Fig. 1**).[47]

Laboratory Diagnosis of APS

Criteria aPL tests

Since the APS was first identified, more than 25 years ago, the attention of physicians has been focused on patients with the clinical features of the disease, identified as vascular thrombosis and pregnancy morbidity, which includes both miscarriages and fetal losses.[1] Some of these symptoms, such as deep vein thrombosis (DVT) or recurrent miscarriages, are common in the general population. Therefore, the need for a correct classification of patients with APS was felt from the beginning. To be classified as APS, patients with suspected clinical features should carry confirmed and persistent positivity for aPL antibodies.[2] This is a task that brings along some

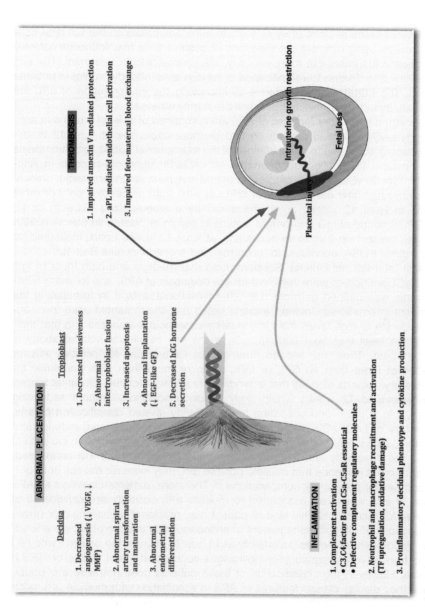

Fig. 1. Pathogenic mechanisms leading to obstetric complications in APS. (*From* Willis R, Pierangeli S. Pathophysiology of the antiphospholipid antibody syndrome. Autoimmun Highlights. online March 24, 2011. doi: 10.1007/s13317-011-0017-9; with permission.)

The figure contains the following labels:

ABNORMAL PLACENTATION

Decidua
1. Decreased angiogenesis (↓ VEGF, ↓ MMP)
2. Abnormal spiral artery transformation and maturation
3. Abnormal endometrial differentiation

Trophoblast
1. Decreased invasiveness
2. Abnormal intertrophoblast fusion
3. Increased apoptosis
4. Abnormal implantation (↓ EGF-like GF)
5. Decreased hCG hormone secretion

THROMBOSIS
1. Impaired annexin V mediated protection
2. aPL mediated endothelial cell activation
3. Impaired feto-maternal blood exchange

INFLAMMATION
1. Complement activation
 • C3,C4,factor B and C5a-C5aR essential
 • Defective complement regulatory molecules
2. Neutrophil and macrophage recruitment and activation (TF upregulation, oxidative damage)
3. Proinflammatory decidual phenotype and cytokine production

Intrauterine growth restriction

Placental injury

Fetal loss

difficulties. All three tests formally included in the classification criteria (LAC, aCL, and anti-β_2GPI) display some technical problems, making the results sometimes difficult to interpret. According to the revised classification criteria, the stable positivity of a single test is sufficient to classify a patient as APS.[2] As a consequence, clinicians have been wondering whether patients with similar clinical features but with different positivity pattern (profile) in the three aPL tests should be considered completely comparable or not. From a practical point of view, such an approach based on the subclassification of patients using different combinations of positive tests may influence not only the prognostic judgment but more critically, the pharmacologic treatment. The aim of this review is to discuss the significance of various autoantibody profiles in patients with APS. The hottest issues in terms of improving the interpretation of aPL are pointed out, including promising novel tests that may emerge.

The accepted laboratory features of APS are comprised of at least 1 of 3 autoantibodies: (1) LAC present in plasma on two or more occasions at least 12 weeks apart, detected according to the guidelines of the International Society on Thrombosis and Hemostasis (Scientific Subcommittee on LACs/Phospholipid-dependent Antibodies)[48,49]; or (2) aCL antibody of IgG and/or IgM isotype in serum or plasma, present in medium or high titer (ie, >40 GPL or MPL, or >the 99th percentile), on 2 or more occasion at least 12 weeks apart, measured by a standardized ELISA[50]; or (3) anti-β_2GPI antibody of IgG and/or IgM isotype in serum or plasma (in titer >the 99th percentile), present on 2 or more occasions, at least 12 weeks apart, measured by a standardized ELISA, according to recommended procedures (see **Box 1**).[50]

The first International Criteria (Sapporo) held that medium and high titers of IgG and IgM aCL antibodies were sufficient for the diagnosis of APS, and for many laboratories this was defined as more than 20 international units.[51] In formulating the most recent International Criteria,[2] experts noted that the threshold used to distinguish moderate to high levels from low levels was without a standard and that definition of the level that best corresponds to the risk of clinical manifestations is difficult at best. Thus, the second International Criteria call for positive aCL or anti-β_2GPI at more than 40 GPL or MPL units, or more than 99th percentile for the laboratory. Experts also felt that extending the interval required for repeat testing from 6 weeks to 12 weeks would likely enhance specificity without sacrificing sensitivity.[2] In addition and according to the recently revised classification criteria, the positivity of LAC, aCL, and anti-β_2GPI antibodies are considered independent risk factors, so a single stable positivity is enough to classify a symptomatic patient as APS. The specificity and the predictive value of each test are still unresolved, however, there is evidence that multiple positive aPL may increase the risk of thrombosis and severe pregnancy complications.[52] Therefore, patients classified as APS because of a clinical event associated to multiple aPL positivity are considered at higher risk for recurrence. This kind of patient may represent a challenge for physicians, because of difficult management of anticoagulation in case of severe arterial/venous thrombosis as well as uncertainty as to how to counsel the patients who had suffered from severe pregnancy complications such as late fetal losses or HELLP syndrome. However, the classification of these patients does not raise any doubt, because they display classic features of APS in association with multiple aPL positivity. In contrast the picture is not clear when we deal with patients with a single positive test.

It is largely accepted that LAC better correlates with thrombosis and pregnancy morbidity than aCL or anti-β_2GPI regardless of the type of assay used. A well-known, large meta-analysis study showed that LAC is the most important risk factor for thrombosis occurrence independently from the type of assay used.[44]

Several attempts have been made to standardize the aCL and the anti-β_2GPI tests, including several international workshops, a European forum that convened for this purpose, an Australasian Anticardiolipin Working Group, the College of American Pathologists in the United States, and the National External Quality Assessment Scheme in the United Kingdom.[53–59] For example, the College of American Pathologists (CAP) enrolls certified laboratories in the proficiency testing for aCL/anti-β_2GPI assays and requires participation in the program for accreditation purposes. The interlaboratory agreement has significantly improved over the last 7 years for the aCL and the anti-β_2GPI assays. The lack of consensus was observed particularly when samples were in the low to indeterminate range.

Noncriteria aPL tests

Several other autoantibodies shown to be directed to phospholipids and/or their complexes with proteins and/or to proteins of the coagulation cascade have been proposed to be relevant to APS. However, the clinical usefulness of these newly developed assays and their diagnostic value remains elusive. The issue of the value of IgA aPL antibodies and whether this test should be part of the routine diagnostic algorithm has also been a subject of debate. The following sections include an update of issues related to these noncriteria aPL tests as well as recent recommendations from an aPL task force that gathered at the 13th International Congress on Antiphospholipid Antibodies (APLA 2010) in Galveston in April 2010.[60]

Antibodies to negatively charged phospholipids other than cardiolipin Antibodies directed against negatively charged phospholipids such as phosphatidic acid (PA), phosphatidylinositol (PI), phosphatidylserine (PS), and phosphatidylglycerol have been reported in patients with APS. These tests are frequently ordered by obstetricians and maternal fetal medicine and reproductive immunology specialists, in searching for a cause of pregnancy morbidity, particularly in patients with RPL, who may benefit from treatment.[61–64] Of the three major negatively charged aPL antibodies (anti-PA, anti-PI, and anti-PS), anti-PS has been most extensively investigated in thrombosis and pregnancy-related morbidity APS.[61–66] These antibodies, particularly anti-PS, have been shown to be more specific for APS when compared with aCL, because aCL is often seen positive in infectious diseases and other disorders.[67–69] Assays that use a mixture of negatively charged phospholipids instead of cardiolipin as an antigen (such as the APhL ELISA) have shown to have superior specificity compared with aCL due to negligible reactivity with aPL antibodies from infectious diseases sera and retain excellent sensitivity and the best positive and negative predictive values for diagnosis of APS in independent studies.[70,71] One study has shown that the APhL ELISA test is an independent risk factor of pregnancy loss.[72]

Anti-PS antibodies have been shown to inhibit trophoblast development and invasion using an in vitro model system.[28] The anti-PS antibodies retard syncytiotrophoblast formations and decrease the synthesis of hCG. Both low-molecular-weight heparin (LMWH) and unfractionated heparin (UFH) have been shown to reduce the in vitro binding of anti-PS as well as aCL.[73] Furthermore, some clinical data are available to suggest that some of these women with a diagnosis of RPL and aPL positivity may benefit from treatments that have assisted women with RPL and aCL to deliver healthy offspring.[74] However, the conditions necessary to achieve optimal clinical and analytical performance of these assays are yet to be determined. In addition, controversy has arisen as to the significance of these antibodies and whether treatment should be based on positive results of aCL only or based on positive results of any of the other aPLs. This ongoing debate of the clinical significance of aCL and other aPLs has prompted some clinicians to screen patients with RPL and identify those patients who might be missed if only aCL were considered significant. In one study by Branch and colleagues[75] the investigators found using the 99th percentile for a panel of phospholipids in 147 women with RPL, APS, and fertile controls that 26 of 147 (17.7%) of women with RPL had positive antibodies to CL and 13 of 147 (8.8%) of women with RPL showed binding against phospholipids other than CL or LAC. In a larger earlier study, Yetman and Kutteh[5] determined the prevalence of aPL among 866 women with RPL. In this population, 150 of 866 (17.3%) women with RPL were positive for IgG and/or IgM aCL, whereas only 12 of 288 (4%) of control women without a history of poor obstetric outcome were positive for the same antibodies ($P<.001$). The same study identified 87 of 866 women with RPL who were negative for aCL but positive for 1 of the other aPL. Although this study was retrospective, it suggests that a significant number of women with RPL would not have been identified if they had been tested only for aCL. The same investigators recently reported on another group of 872 women with RPL.[76] Positive aCLs were detected in 132 of 872 women with RPL (15.1%), LAC was detected in 31 of 872 (3.6%), and aPS was identified in 49 of 872 (5.6%) women with RPL.[77] Anti-PS antibodies were found in women with 2 consecutive losses (18/391 or 4.6%), women with 3 consecutive losses (16/288 or 5.6%), and women with 4 or more consecutive losses (15/193 or 7.8%) and these antibodies were identified in several women who tested negative for aCL.[77]

The APLA 2010 aPL task force recognized that the lack of standardization among different laboratories has made it difficult for physicians to identify patients with APS and those at risk for a miscarriage. Yet, problems still exist when patients with pregnancy loss are referred to fertility clinics who may have had testing performed at different laboratories using different control values and cutoff values to determine positive results. Also, standard testing may exclude a population of patients with aPL who have had significant obstetric problems but test positive for other aPL and negative for the most commonly assayed aCL and LAC. Based on the evidence reviewed and further the aPL task force recognized that aPL antibodies directed to phospholipids other than PS may have clinical significance but the current level of evidence does not warrant any change in the existing classification criteria.

Antiprothrombin and antiprothrombin-PS antibodies There are some assays that, if found positive, could add diagnostic value to a single aPL positive result. This is the case for antiprothrombin antibodies (aPT), which could be a second-level aPL assay in isolated LAC positivity. The problem with aPT is the heterogeneity of the ELISAs and the lack of standardization, and uniform units of measurement, which include methods using prothrombin alone as an antigen or a phosphatidylserine-prothrombin (PS/PT) complex. According to a recent monocentric study, antibodies directed to the PS-PT complex seem related to increased thrombin generation, supporting a relevant biologic role of these antibodies.[78] Early attempts to compare the available methods gave poor results.[79–83] Considering the progress reached in the immunoassay technology, large collaborative studies comparing different available assays and standardizing the way to perform them could probably achieve a better consensus. If routinely available, anti-PT or anti-PS/PT could represent a logical extension of investigations in patients with isolated LAC positivity, allowing a more solid laboratory diagnosis.

IgA aCL and anti-β_2GPI antibodies IgA aCL and anti-β_2GPI measurements are not included in current criteria for diagnosis of APS, although IgA aCL has been known to affect thrombus formation in mice[84,85] and to be associated with certain clinical manifestations of APS.[76,86–91] Rather, IgA aCLs seem to identify subgroups of patients, such as African-American or pure obstetric APS. Previous studies raised the possibility that IgA anti-β_2GPI might be associated with clinical manifestations of APS; those observations showed that patients with SLE with APS are more prone to be positive for the IgA isotypes.[92–95] A concise report by Yamada and colleagues[96] also showed anti-β_2GPI positivity in the absence of IgG anti-β_2GPI in a subgroup of women with unexplained RPL (particularly in the first trimester). Similar findings were reported by Lee and colleagues,[97] indicating that IgA anti-β_2GPI positivity is more common in women who experience unexplained recurrent spontaneous abortion and unexplained fetal death whose initial test results for other isotypes and LAC were negative. In most cases, the IgA isotype is present together with IgG and/or IgM; however, there are several reports of APS clinical manifestations in patients with isolated IgA anti-β_2GPI positivity.[84,98,99] Recently, Kumar and colleagues[100] reported 5 isolated cases of women who were exclusively positive for IgA anti-β_2GPI and had concomitant clinical manifestations of APS, including fetal loss.

Altogether these data confirm that isolated IgA anti-β_2GPI antibody titers may identify additional patients who have clinical features of APS but who do not meet current diagnostic criteria. Hence, the APLA 2010 aPL task force concluded that because of the small prevalence of IgA aCL and anti-β_2GPI positivity alone in the absence of IgG and/or IgM aCL positivity, those tests should be recommended in patients in whom IgG and IgM isotypes are negative and there is strong suspicion of APS. The task force also recognized that well-designed studies that should include evaluation and comparison of multiple commercially available assays in larger and well-characterized populations of patients are needed to confirm the diagnostic value of isolated IgA anti-β_2GPI positivity, before this test can be included in the diagnostic criteria.

THE BOTTOM LINE FOR THE PRACTICING CLINICIAN ON NONCRITERIA APL TESTS

From a practical perspective, the topic of noncriteria aPL tests for the practicing clinician can be summarized easily: there are no definitive and compelling data. Thus, it is uncertain whether or not women with REM or second-trimester or third-trimester clinical features suggestive of APS have (1) an increased frequency of abnormal noncriteria aPL results or (2) a decreased incidence of adverse pregnancy outcomes (APOs) or thrombosis with antithrombotic therapy (namely heparin).

Some physicians and patients may be enticed by a few promising study results that support the use of noncriteria aPL tests to direct heparin therapy to improve live delivery rates in obstetric patients with REM with APS. These studies, which showed near-doubling of live delivery rates, were single-institution efforts of small sample size and suboptimal design.[74] These small studies have not been rigorously confirmed by others using proper study design or with the same testing methodology used in the original studies and these flaws are not recognized in published meta-analyses and practice guidelines. Internationally accepted, standard calibrating sera or monoclonals are not available for these assays, nor is it certain that the immunoassays used could be reliably repeated in other laboratories. The net result is a medical literature from which no sound conclusion can be drawn, and vehemence for or against use of noncriteria aPLs should be treated with skepticism. We are also keenly aware that practical advice is needed by the reader who may have patients whose care demands a rational approach to the management of the topic of noncriteria aPL testing. Thus, we currently recommend the following when dealing with the frustrated and emotional patient with a clinical problem such as REM and who has obtained positive results in a noncriteria aPL test:

1. Familiarize yourself with the important differences in definitions of trial design parameters (**Table 1**).

Table 1
Inconsistencies in definitions in REM obstetric APS diagnosis study design

Parameter	Possibilities	Definitions
Pregnancy	3+	Biochemical, <10 wk, 20–24 wk, and so forth
Number of losses	3	2, 3, or both
Exclusion	3+	Karyotyping of losses previously, other autoimmune conditions, other REM causes
Test choice	6+	aCL, LAC, anti-β_2GPI, antiphosphatidylserine, antiphosphatidylethanolamine, and so forth
Ig class	3	IgG, IgM, IgA
Methodology	3+	Calibrated to international standards, not calibrated, agreement with CAP, multiple diagnostic platforms, and so forth
Positive/abnormal	3	High, medium/high, intermediate
Retesting	3+	None, 6 wk, 12 wk, and so forth

2. Identify a clinical laboratory that (1) provides evidence that the testing provided is calibrated to an original clinical study supporting clinical utility (2) distinguishes meaningfully positive results from those of low positive or equivocal nature.
3. Ensure that your approach to identifying patients for testing, the choices of testing, and related therapy at least attempts to match as much as possible a clinical study that showed clinical utility, even if not an ideal study design. For those clinicians who are not comfortable in this area, consultation with an experienced specialist is important.
4. Be able to cite data for the risks of therapy (namely heparin) that would be considered should an abnormal noncriteria aPL test result be obtained.

In the spirit of the modern paradigm of the clinician-patient partnership, the decision to order noncriteria aPL testing should rest with an informed patient, one that has been adequately and frankly counseled regarding the various uncertainties that attend such testing. The litmus test for such a patient should be the ability of the patient to correctly describe in her own words why noncriteria aPL testing cannot be definitively recommended or refuted, as well as the type and frequency of side effects of heparin treatment. For those patients who arrive with abnormal test results, the recommendation is testing be repeated 12 weeks after the original result, as per mainstream guidelines, at your chosen laboratory. Should a patient arrive with an abnormal result that has already been confirmed through appropriately timed repetition, retesting is not recommended unless the laboratory providing the testing does not provide the calibration and reporting approach described earlier.

YESTERDAY'S LESSONS

The stalemate in which noncriteria aPL testing finds itself is not a new story. It is the classic tale of the breakdown in the conversion of medical art into medical science. Almost all prospective, randomized, double-blind, high-powered, clinical studies have their roots in anecdote and case series. The observation and acumen of the clinical practitioner interacting with a single patient is often a powerful driving force behind innovation and progress. However, many a pitfall lies between the clinical gut sense or keen patient observation and completing clinical studies that provide rigorously established, definitive practice guidelines. The central problem preventing this situation with respect to noncriteria aPL testing and obstetric APS is one of language.

The literature is full of multiple definitions for almost every term used to establish the diagnosis of obstetric APS. The definitional variations are not minor subtleties but rather substantial, outcome-changing differences. For example take REM as a form of obstetric APS. Although it may seem like there is not much room for variation in establishing the diagnosis with statements such as "three or more pregnancy losses before ten weeks' gestation in the presence of abnormal titers of antiphospholipid antibodies," there are vast differences in which patients would be identified depending on the interpretation of at least seven different definitions. First, many physicians, patients, and professional organizations accept two consecutive pregnancy losses as an indication for clinical evaluation. The term pregnancy is often defined differently as biochemical, ultrasound confirmed, or both. Third, the definition of abnormal titers depends on the calibration system used and the chosen cut points (eg, 95th vs 99th percentiles, or 2, 3, 4, or 5 standard deviations from mean). Fourth and fifth are the type of aPL antibody (eg, antiphosphatidylserine, antiphosphatidylethanolamine) and the isotype (IgG, IgM, IgA). Six and seventh are the requirement for retesting and the interval between tests (6, 8, 10, or 12 weeks). Thus, within the simple statement "3 or more losses before the 10th week of gestation in the presence of abnormal titers of aPL antibodies" exist hundreds of permutations, and this is simply for the REM subset of obstetric APS.

Even if one were to have maintained consistency in diagnosis (eg, with REM obstetric APS), the treatment trials suffer from similar permutation problems. A typical statement such as "women with REM obstetric APS can benefit from antithrombotic therapy to reduce maternal complications of pregnancy" has at least 6 areas of definitional ambiguity (**Table 2**). It has long been recognized that the belief that heparin treatment can reduce pregnancy loss in women with REM obstetric APS hinges on 2 studies with an aggregate of less than 150 patients.[5] These studies had specific approaches to identifying treatment candidate patients, drug selection, timing of therapy initiation, and duration of therapy, which later contradictory studies did not match. Approaches in the trials supporting the use of heparin for REM obstetric APS that were considered important by the Obstetric Task Force for the last International Congress on Antiphospholipid Antibodies (Galveston, TX, April, 2010) included selection of patients as follows: systematic exclusion of patients with accepted causes of REM, confirmation of abnormal aPL antibody results in a central laboratory, use of assays calibrated with internationally accepted standards, and an untreated, aspirin-only control patient population who had a suboptimal live delivery rate less than 50% (otherwise adequately powering the study to detect benefit would be difficult).[9]

Table 2		
Inconsistencies in definitions of REM obstetric APS treatment trials		
Parameter	**Possibilities**	**Description**
Exclusion	3+	<2 pregnancy losses, <3 losses, other causes of REM
Drug	3	UFH/aspirin, LMWH/aspirin, placebo/aspirin
Timing of treatment initiation	3	First appropriately rising β human chorionic gonadotropin level, 6 weeks gestation, mixed
Duration of treatment	2+	highly variable
Placebo group live delivery	3	<40%, 40%–70%, 70%

The Obstetric Task Force also discussed the timing of initiation of treatment, concluding that the best design would likely initiate treatment before 5 or 6 weeks once an appropriately rising hCG is shown. Two recent meta-analyses concluded that UFH might be superior to LMWH as a treatment choice.[101,102]

The lesson to be reinforced from the wasting of resources represented by the thousands of publications on aPLs is that great care should be taken to establish agreement on clear definitions of all parameters in studies that seek to extend the promising findings of case studies or small prospective trials.

TOMORROW'S HOPE

It is often said that the first step in addressing a problem is recognizing there is a problem, a tenet to which we hold. Thus, the *Report of the Obstetric APS Task Force: 13th International Congress on Antiphospholipid Antibodies, 13th April 2010*[9] likely marks a historic milestone of hope in obstetric APS. Instead of choosing to spend energy reliving the same debates about the same conflicting but noncomparable studies, the task force recognized that for progress to be made so that researchers could design a study that would definitively address the open questions related to noncriteria aPLs, consensus had to be achieved with respect to many of the items listed in **Table 1**. These criteria would include a multicenter effort to determine which noncriteria aPL tests are repeatedly abnormal in a clinically significantly higher proportion of women with the study feature of APS (eg, REM), compared with an appropriately matched, normal population.

In addition to working toward standardizing definitions for diagnosis and therapy, improvements in standardization of laboratory testing are also occurring, which pave the way for definitive studies to be implemented. Attesting to this progress, and coinciding with the increasing standardization of the anti-B2 GPI assay, is the recent addition to the 2011 ACOG Practice bulletin on Antiphospholipid Syndrome of an abnormal anti-B2GPI test (IgG or IgM) as a sufficient laboratory criterion to establish the diagnosis of APS when accompanied by the appropriate clinical signs. Standardization and improvement in testing consistency of anti-β_2GPI assays, fostered by increasing stringency of CAP requirements for laboratory testing and US Food and Drug Administration requirements for diagnostic kit clearance, likely helped this assay to move from the noncriteria aPL test category to the criteria aPL test category.

With both improvement in laboratory standards and consensus from thought leaders that definitions need to be agreed on, the stage is set for high-quality studies to be performed should the necessary resources become available.

Example Patient Scenario

In certain respects one can view this era of modern medicine as embracing another age of enlightenment, because not only have evidence-based approaches become the desired standard but the ethos of medicine has evolved to prioritize the patient's right to apply medical information to their own value system. The practical implication of this observation is that the clinician's role is to ensure a patient understands the areas of certainty, uncertainty, risks, and benefits but not to usurp the patient's right to chose their own course. This is undoubtedly a delicate balance. As it relates to non-criteria aPL testing, conveying the uncertainty in this area to the patient is especially important because it empowers the patient to choose their own path, which more often provides greater satisfaction than being told what level of certainty is acceptable. This approach is liberating for the patient and also for the frustrated clinician, who often feels they must personally shoulder the burden for the confusing state of the field rather than facing the uncertainty in partnership with the patient.

The author's acknowledge that distilling the information provided in reviews of thrombophilia such as this one may be difficult to practically distill into day to day patient interactions. Therefore, a specific example patient-clinician interaction is provided below as a practical application of the information in this review.

Ms X is a 36-year-old woman with 2 losses before 10 weeks' gestation by ultrasound within the last 24 months. She has not yet been tested for any aPLs.

Clinician: Ms X, as we have discussed, we need to make a decision about the extent of testing we should perform. As you know, this is a very confusing area of medicine because studies in this field were done using different lab tests and with low patient numbers due to the understandable difficulty enrolling women in trials when they are pregnant. That being said, I have done everything possible to maximize our chances getting useful information by selecting a laboratory which provides the same testing that was used in the studies which demonstrated improvement in delivery rates. We also will use the same treatment approaches as performed in these studies. My job here is to ensure that you have all the facts and understand the risks and benefits of having testing performed which is not recommended by practice guidelines as you are ultimately the one who must decide here. Would you mind sharing with me your understanding? Let me ask you some questions:

Clinician: Why are these additional tests currently not recommended by the professional medical societies?

Ms X: Medical studies not being repeated or saying different things.

Clinician: Why is there debate about which heparin (blood thinner) to use?

Ms X: Most studies showing better delivery rates used one type of heparin (UFH), whereas the studies that used the other type (LMWH) did not seem to work at all or as well as UFH, which may be due to the fact that UFH was given immediately at the start of pregnancy instead of at 6 weeks.

Clinician: Why do people use LMWH then?

Ms X: Slightly lower side effects such as bone loss and it is easier to use although the cost is much higher for LMWH.

Clinician: How many women have a bleeding event that may require a transfusion if heparin is used during pregnancy?

Ms X: About 1 in 50 women.

Clinician: Why do we ask that you have any abnormal tests repeated?

Ms X: Because the main studies that showed benefit with treatment, treated patients who had abnormal test results confirmed with repeat testing.

INHERITED THROMBOPHILIAS IN PREGNANCY

Recent attention has focused on certain inherited thrombophilic factors that may predispose to arterial and/or venous thromboses and their possible association with pregnancy complications, including early pregnancy loss. These factors include a group of mostly autosomal-dominant, inherited gene mutations which lead to a hypercoagulable state, such as factor V Leiden G1691A (FVL), factor II or prothrombin G20210A (PGM), and hyperhomocysteinemia associated with methyle-netetrahydrofolate reductase C677T mutation. In addition, deficiencies in protein S, protein C, and antithrombin can lead to a hypercoagulable state. Managing inherited thrombophilia in pregnancy merits special consideration because thrombosis is the leading cause of maternal death in the Western world and inherited thrombophilia is identified in 50% of pregnancy-associated venous thromboembolism (VTE). It is known that changes during normal pregnancy promote coagulation, decrease antico-agulation, and inhibit fibrinolysis[103] and there is a marked increase in most of the coag-ulation factors: II, VII, VIII, IX, X, and XII as well as fibrinogen and von Willebrand factor (**Table 3**). There is also a decrease of physiologic anticoagulants, with protein S levels decreasing to 40% to 60% starting in the first trimester and remaining decreased for 3 months postpartum. This situation is caused by an estrogen-induced decrease in total protein S and an increase in C4b, which binds protein S. The combined effect of decreased protein S and increased factor VIII leads to increased resistance to acti-vation of protein C.[103] VTE and pulmonary embolisms remain the leading cause of direct maternal deaths in developed countries, and accounts for about 20% of pregnancy-related deaths.[104] It has been reported that there is a 5-fold to 10-fold increase in the risk of VTE for pregnant women over nonpregnant women of compa-rable age, with an incidence of 0.6 to 1.3 events per 1000 deliveries. Two-thirds of DVTs occur at antepartum, with a relatively even distribution over all 3 trimesters. In contrast, 43% to 60% of pregnancy-related episodes of pulmonary embolism seem to occur in the 4-week to 6-week postpartum period.[104] Apart from a history of throm-bosis, thrombophilia is the most important individual risk factor for VTE in pregnancy.

Although some studies of patients with RPL with a positive test for an inherited thrombophilia are conflicting, a case-control study of untreated patients with recurrent miscarriage who were heterozygous for the FVL mutation revealed a lower pregnancy success rate than the controls, who had a history of idiopathic recurrent miscarriage.[105]

The risk of pregnancy-associated VTE conferred by the type of thrombophilia has been evaluated in a recent meta-analysis of 9 studies that showed a 34.4 odds ratio (OR) for FVL homozygosity, 24.4 OR for prothrombin G20210A homozygosity, 8.3 OR for FVL heterozygosity, 6.8 OR for prothrombin G20210A heterozygosity, 4.8 OR for protein C deficiency, 4.7 OR for antithrombin (AT) deficiency, 3.2 OR for protein S deficiency, and 0.7 OR for MTHFRC677T homozygosity. All inherited thrombophilias with the exception of homozygosity for MTHFRC677T variant were found to be

Table 3 Most important changes in hemostatic factors during pregnancy	
Parameter Change	Change
Platelet count	↓
Factors V, XIII	↑/↓
Antithrombin, protein C	=
Protein S	↓
Factor XI	=/↓
Fibrinogen, von Willebrand factor	↑
Factors VII, VIII, IX, X, XII	↑
Tissue plasminogen activator	↓
PAI-1, thrombin-activatable fibrinolysis inhibitor	↑
Factor II, AT III, D-dimer	↑

associated with a statistically significant increase in the risk of pregnancy-related VTE.[106] However, given that the incidence of VTE during pregnancy is 1 in 1000 deliveries, it seems that the absolute risk of VTE in women without a history of thrombosis is low in the presence of the most common thrombophilias such as FVL or PGM. In addition, the OR for thrombophilias that have traditionally been considered to be of high risk, such as protein C deficiency or antithrombin deficiencies, are lower than might be expected. The positive predictive value for the risk of pregnancy-related VTE corrected for prevalence of some inherited thrombophilias are indicated in **Table 4**.

When considering all these data together, women with homozygosity for FVL or PGM, double heterozygosity, or AT deficiency are those at the highest risk for VTE. It is then advised that when present these deficiencies should be handled more aggressively than other inherited thrombophilias.

In a recent review and meta-analysis by Robertson and colleagues[106] about the risks, for individual inherited and acquired thrombophilia, for VTE and various APOs (early pregnancy loss, late pregnancy loss, preeclampsia, placental abruption, intrauterine growth restriction), a total of 79 studies were analyzed (including case-control, cohort, and randomized clinical trials) and ORs stratified by thrombophilia type were calculated for each outcome. Except MTHFR homozygosity, all heritable thrombophilias were found to be significantly associated with an increased risk of VTE, in particular FVL homozygosity (OR = 34) reducing to 8.32 in heterozygous FVL carriers. Concerning APO almost all inherited thrombophilias were found to increase the risk of the various outcomes (in particular protein S deficiency for late pregnancy loss, with an OR of 20). However, despite the increase in relative risk, the absolute risk of VTE and APO remains modest because of the low overall incidence of VTE and adverse outcomes in pregnancy. Hence universal screening for thrombophilia in pregnancy cannot be justified clinically. Thrombophilia screening and VTE prevention with LMWH are suggested only for women with previous VTE events and/or with higher-risk thrombophilias. Widespread screening for inherited thrombophilia in patients with previous APO but no VTE is considered not cost-effective.

Managing inherited thrombophilias during pregnancy depends on first accurately assessing the risk. This is not always an easy task, because published data are often obtained from retrospective studies, meta-analysis, or case-control studies with variable VTE risk in the comparative populations. A careful consideration of other exogenous risk factors and personal and family history of VTE should be performed. Women with inherited thrombophilia who develop VTE during pregnancy should receive the same treatment as pregnant women with VTE and no thrombophilia. Treatment is full-intensity anticoagulation, usually with LMWH, adjusted for weight changes throughout pregnancy. Warfarin can be considered after the first trimester, but

Table 4
Positive predictive value (PPV) of inherited thrombophilia factors

Thrombophilia	PPV
FVL heterozygous	1:500
Prothrombin G20210A heterozygous	1:200
FVL and prothrombin G20210A heterozygous	4.6:100
Protein C deficiency	1:113
Type 2 antithrombin deficiency	1:42
Type 1 antithrombin deficiency	1:2.8

alternative management for delivery is required. Fondaparinux, a pentasaccharide anticoagulant, has also been used in pregnancy, particularly in women who are unable to tolerate LMWH. Fogerty and Connors[103] recommended classifying inherited thrombophilia into 3 risk categories: high (FVL homozygous, PGM homozygous, compound heterozygous, AT deficiency, any thrombophilia with personal VTE history), intermediate (low-risk thrombophilia with family VTE history), and low (FVL heterozygous, PGM heterozygous, protein C deficiency, protein S deficiency, no personal/family history of VTE). Personal and family history strongly influenced that risk assignment. The investigators recommended anticoagulation for 4 to 6 weeks post partum for all women with inherited thrombophilia. For antenatal management, an individual risk should be considered. For high-risk patients, the investigators recommended intermediate or therapeutic intensity dosing of LMWH; for intermediate-risk patients, a prophylactic dose of LMWH should be used and for low-risk patients surveillance and monitoring are advised. The effectiveness of prophylactic interventions (with UFH or LMWH plus aspirin, or aspirin alone) in pregnant women with thrombophilia was also evaluated. Aside from APS there is insufficient evidence on the benefit of antithrombotic intervention to prevent VTE and APO.

In a prospective study by Dizon-Townson and colleagues,[107] 134 patients heterozygous for FVL mutation were identified among 4885 gravidas without a personal history of thromboembolism. The incidence of thromboembolism and other APOs was compared between FVL mutation carriers and noncarriers. No thromboembolic events occurred among the FVL mutation carriers, and no differences in APOs were observed between mothers who were carriers of FVL mutation and controls. Only a weak association was found between the presence of fetal FVL mutation and preeclampsia.[107] Hence, among pregnant women with no history of thromboembolism, maternal heterozygous carriage of the FVL mutation is associated with no increased risk of VTE and APO. Therefore neither universal screening for FVL mutation nor prophylactic anticoagulation treatment of carriers during pregnancy is indicated. In 2010 in a meta-analysis of 10 prospective cohort studies, Rodger and colleagues[108] found only a small absolute increased risk of late pregnancy loss for FVL carriers (OR = 1.52). Women with FVL and PGM seem not to be at increased risk of preeclampsia or giving birth to small-for-gestational-age infants. Moreover, based on 2 recent randomized, controlled trials, prophylaxis with LMWH in unselected women with previous RPL not associated with APS is not warranted.[109,110] Investigators from the Thrombosis: Risk and Economic Assessment of Thrombophilia Screening (TREATS) study,[106] after reviewing all prospective and retrospective studies concerning the association between VTE, APO, and thrombophilia, concluded that universal thrombophilia screening in women during pregnancy is not supported by the evidence. The findings from this study show that selective screening based on previous VTE history is more cost-effective than universal screening.

SUMMARY

This review of current literature indicates that women with inherited thrombophilia are at increased risk of developing complications during pregnancy. However, despite the increase in relative risk, the absolute risk for VTE and adverse outcomes in pregnancy remains low. Current understanding indicates that a combination of risk factors, including multiple inherited thrombophilic defects associated with secondary hypercoagulable states, have a particularly strong association with APO. Therefore, universal screening for thrombophilia in pregnancy cannot be clinically justified.

Despite RPL in APS and prevention of VTE, there is insufficient evidence on the benefit of antithrombotic interventions. Controlled clinical trials are urgently needed to address these questions.

REFERENCES

1. Harris EN. Syndrome of the black swan. Br J Rheumatol 1987;26:324–6.
2. Miyakis S, Lockshin MD, Atsumi T, et al. International consensus statement on an update of the classification criteria for definite antiphospholipid syndrome (APS). J Thromb Haemost 2006;4:295–306.
3. Branch DW, Gibson M, Silver RM. Clinical practice. Recurrent miscarriage. N Engl J Med 2010;363:1740–7.
4. Rai RS, Regan L, Clifford K, et al. Antiphospholipid antibodies and beta 2-glyco-protein-I in 500 women with recurrent miscarriage: results of a comprehensive screening approach. Hum Reprod 1995;10:2001–5.
5. Yetman DL, Kutteh WH. Antiphospholipid antibody panels and recurrent pregnancy loss: prevalence of anticardiolipin antibodies compared with other antiphospholipid antibodies. Fertil Steril 1996;66:540–6.
6. Branch DW, Silver RM, Porter TF. Obstetric antiphospholipid syndrome: current uncertainties should guide our way. Lupus 2010;19:446–52.
7. Farquharson RG, Quenby S, Greaves M. Antiphospholipid syndrome in pregnancy: a randomized, controlled trial of treatment. Obstet Gynecol 2002;100: 408–13.
8. Laskin CA, Spitzer KA, Clark CA, et al. Low molecular weight heparin and aspirin for recurrent pregnancy loss: results from the randomized, controlled HepASA Trial. J Rheumatol 2009;36:279–87.
9. Branch D, The Obstetric Task Force. Report of the Obstetric APS Task Force: 13th International Congress on Antiphospholipid Antibodies. Lupus 2011;20:158–64.
10. Silver RM. Fetal death. Obstet Gynecol 2007;109:153–67.
11. Smith GCS, Crossley JA, Aitken DA, et al. First-trimester placentation and the risk of antepartum stillbirth. JAMA 2004;292:2249–54.
12. Oshiro BT, Silver RM, Scott JR, et al. Antiphospholipid antibodies and fetal death. Obstet Gynecol 1996;87:489–93.
13. Meis PJ, Goldenberg RL, Mercer BM, et al. The preterm prediction study: risk factors for indicated preterm births. Maternal-Fetal Medicine Units Network of the National Institute of Child Health and Human Development. Am J Obstet Gynecol 1998;178:562–7.
14. Clark EA, Silver RM, Branch DW. Do antiphospholipid antibodies cause preeclampsia and HELLP syndrome? Curr Rheumatol Rep 2007;9:219–25.
15. do Prado AD, Piovesan DM, Staub HL, et al. Association of anticardiolipin antibodies with preeclampsia. A systematic review and meta-analysis. Obstet Gynecol 2010;116:1433–43.
16. De Wolf F, Carreras LO, Moerman P, et al. Decidual vasculopathy and extensive placental infarction in a patient with repeated thromboembolic accidents, recurrent fetal loss, and a lupus anticoagulant. Am J Obstet Gynecol 1982;142:829–34.
17. Hanly JG, Gladman DD, Rose TH, et al. Lupus pregnancy. A prospective study of placental changes. Arthritis Rheum 1988;31:358–66.
18. Nayar R, Lage JM. Placental changes in a first trimester missed abortion in maternal systemic lupus erythematosus with antiphospholipid syndrome: a case report and review of the literature. Hum Pathol 1996;27:201–6.

19. Peaceman AM, Rehnberg KA. The effect of immunoglobulin G fractions from patients with lupus anticoagulant on placental prostacyclin and thromboxane production. Am J Obstet Gynecol 1993;169:1403–6.
20. Van Horn JT, Craven C, Ward K, et al. Histologic features of placentas and abortion specimens from women with antiphospholipid and antiphospholipid-like syndromes. Placenta 2004;25:642–8.
21. Rand JH. Molecular pathogenesis of the antiphospholipid syndrome. Circ Res 2002;11:29–37.
22. Rand JH, Wu XX, Guller S, et al. Reduction of annexin-V (placental anticoagulant protein-I) on placental villi of women with antiphospholipid antibodies and recurrent spontaneous abortion. Am J Obstet Gynecol 1994;171:1566–72.
23. Rand JH, Wu XX, Quinn AS, et al. The annexin A5-mediated pathogenic mechanism in the antiphospholipid syndrome: role in pregnancy losses and thrombosis. Lupus 2010;19:460–9.
24. Out HJ, Kooijman CD, Bruinse HW, et al. Histopathological findings in placentae from patients with intra-uterine fetal death and anti-phospholipid antibodies. Eur J Obstet Gynecol Reprod Biol 1991;41:179–86.
25. Di Simone N, Luigi MP, Marco D, et al. Pregnancies complicated with antiphospholipid syndrome: the pathogenic mechanism of antiphospholipid antibodies: a review of the literature. Ann N Y Acad Sci 2007;1108:505–14.
26. Sebire NJ, Fox H, Backos M, et al. Defective endovascular trophoblast invasion in primary antiphospholipid antibody syndrome-associated early pregnancy failure. Hum Reprod 2002;17:1067–71.
27. Di Simone N, Meroni PL, de Papa N, et al. Antiphospholipid antibodies affect trophoblast gonadotropin secretion and invasiveness by binding directly and through adhered beta2-glycoprotein I. Arthritis Rheum 2000; 43:140–50.
28. Katsuragawa H, Kanzaki H, Inoue T, et al. Monoclonal antibody against phosphatidylserine inhibits in vitro human trophoblastic hormone production and invasion. Biol Reprod 1997;56:50–8.
29. Adler RR, Ng AK, Rote NS. Monoclonal antiphosphatidylserine antibody inhibits intercellular fusion of the choriocarcinoma line, JAR. Biol Reprod 1995;53: 905–10.
30. Rote NS, Vogt E, DeVere G, et al. The role of placental trophoblast in the pathophysiology of the antiphospholipid antibody syndrome. Am J Reprod Immunol 1998;39:125–36.
31. Di Simone N, Marana R, Castellani R, et al. Decreased expression of heparin-binding epidermal growth factor-like growth factor as a newly identified pathogenic mechanism of antiphospholipid-mediated defective placentation. Arthritis Rheum 2010;62:1504–12.
32. Ornoy A, Yacobi S, Matalon ST, et al. The effects of antiphospholipid antibodies obtained from women with SLE/APS and associated pregnancy loss on rat embryos and placental explants in culture. Lupus 2003;12:573–8.
33. Matalon ST, Shoenfeld Y, Blank M, et al. Antiphosphatidylserine antibodies affect rat yolk sacs in culture: a mechanism for fetal loss in antiphospholipid syndrome. Am J Reprod Immunol 2004;51:144–51.
34. Borghi MO, Raschi E, Scurati S, et al. Effects of a toll-like receptor antagonist and anti-annexin A2 antibodies on binding and activation of decidual cells by anti-β2glycoprotein I antibodies. Clin Exp Rheumatol 2007;2:35.
35. Francis J, Rai R, Sebire NJ, et al. Impaired expression of endometrial differentiation markers and complement regulatory proteins in patients with recurrent

pregnancy loss associated with antiphospholipid syndrome. Mol Hum Reprod 2006;12:435–42.

36. Di Simone N, Di Nicuolo F, D'Ippolito S, et al. Antiphospholipid antibodies affect human endometrial angiogenesis. Biol Reprod 2010;83:212–9.

37. Holers VM, Girardi G, Mo L, et al. Complement C3 activation is required for antiphospholipid antibody-induced fetal loss. J Exp Med 2002;195:211–20.

38. Martinez de la Torre Y, Buracchi C, Borroni EM, et al. Protection against inflammation- and autoantibody-caused fetal loss by the chemokine decoy receptor D6. Proc Natl Acad Sci U S A 2007;104:2319–24.

39. Quigg RJ, Kozono Y, Berthiaume D, et al. Blockade of antibody-induced glomerulonephritis with Crry-Ig, a soluble murine complement inhibitor. J Immunol 1998;160:4553–60.

40. Girardi G, Berman J, Redecha P, et al. Complement C5a receptors and neutrophils mediate fetal injury in the antiphospholipid syndrome. J Clin Invest 2003; 112:1644–54.

41. Redecha P, Tilley R, Tencati M, et al. Tissue factor: a link between C5a and neutrophil activation in antiphospholipid antibody induced fetal injury. Blood 2007;110:2423–31.

42. Girardi G, Yarilin D, Thurman JM, et al. Complement activation induces dysregulation of angiogenic factors and causes fetal rejection and growth restriction. J Exp Med 2006;203:2165–75.

43. Girardi G, Redecha P, Salmon JE. Heparin prevents antiphospholipid antibody-induced fetal loss by inhibiting complement activation. Nat Med 2004;10:1222–6.

44. Galli M, Luciani D, Bertolini G, et al. Lupus anticoagulants are stronger risk factors for thrombosis than anticardiolipin antibodies in the antiphospholipid syndrome: a systematic review of the literature. Blood 2003;101:1827–32.

45. Shamonki JM, Salmon JE, Hyjek E, et al. Excessive complement activation is associated with placental injury in patients with antiphospholipid antibodies. Am J Obstet Gynecol 2007;196:167.e1–5.

46. Cavazzana I, Manuela N, Irene C, et al. Complement activation in antiphospholipid syndrome: a clue for an inflammatory process? J Autoimmun 2007;28:160–4.

47. Salmon JE, Girardi G. Theodore E. Woodward Award: antiphospholipid syndrome revisited: a disorder initiated by inflammation. Trans Am Clin Climatol Assoc 2007;118:99–114.

48. Brandt JT, Triplett DA, Alving B, et al. Criteria for the diagnosis of lupus anticoagulants: an update. On behalf of the Subcommittee on Lupus Anticoagulant/Antiphospholipid Antibody of the Scientific and Standardisation Committee of the ISTH. Thromb Haemost 1995;74:1185–90.

49. Pengo V, Tripodi A, Reber G, et al. Update of the guidelines for lupus anticoagulant detection. J Thromb Haemost 2009;10:1737–40.

50. Pierangeli SS, Harris EN. A protocol for determination of anticardiolipin antibodies by ELISA. Nat Protoc 2008;3:840–8.

51. Wilson WA, Gharavi AE, Koike T, et al. International consensus statement on preliminary classification criteria for definite antiphospholipid syndrome: report of an international workshop. Arthritis Rheum 1999;42:1309–11.

52. Pengo V, Ruffatti A, Legnani C, et al. Clinical course of high-risk patients diagnosed with antiphospholipid syndrome. J Thromb Haemost 2010;8:237–42.

53. Harris EN, Gharavi AE, Patel S, et al. Evaluation of the anticardiolipin antibody test: report of an international workshop held April 4 1986. Clin Exp Immunol 1987;68:215–22.

54. Harris EN. The Second International Anticardiolipin Standardization Workshop: the Kingston Anticardiolipin Antibody Study (KAPS) group. Am J Clin Pathol 1990;101:616–24.

55. Harris EN, Pierangeli S, Birch D. Anticardiolipin wet workshop report: Vth international symposium on antiphospholipid antibodies. Am J Clin Pathol 1994;101:616–24.

56. Pierangeli SS, Stewart M, Silva LK, et al. Report of an anticardiolipin workshop during the VIIth International Symposium on antiphospholipid antibodies. J Rheumatol 1998;25:156–62.

57. Reber G, Arvieux J, Comby D, et al. Multicenter evaluation of nine commercial kits for the quantitation of anticardiolipin antibodies. Thromb Haemost 1995;73:444–52.

58. Wong RCW, Wilson RJ, Pollock W, et al. Anticardiolipin antibody testing and reporting practices among laboratories participating in a large external quality assurance program. Pathology 2004;36:174–81.

59. Tincani A, Allegri F, Sanmarco M, et al. Anticardiolipin antibody assay: a methodological analysis for a better consensus in routine determinations–a cooperative project of the European Antiphospholipid Forum. Thromb Haemost 2001;86:575–83.

60. Bertolaccini ML, Amengual O, Atsumi O, et al. "Non-criteria" aPL tests: report of a task force and preconference workshop at the 13th International Congress on Antiphospholipid Antibodies, Galveston, TX, USA, April 2010. Lupus 2011;20:191–205.

61. Laroche P, Berard M, Rouquette AM, et al. Advantage of using both anionic and zwitterionic phospholipid antigens for the detection of antiphospholipid antibodies. Am J Clin Pathol 1996;106:549–54.

62. Bertolaccini ML, Roch B, Amengual O, et al. Multiple antiphospholipid tests do not increase the diagnostic yield in antiphospholipid syndrome. Br J Rheumatol 1998;37:1229–32.

63. Fialova L, Mikulikova L, Matous-Malbohan I, et al. Prevalence of various antiphospholipid antibodies in pregnant women. Physiol Res 2000;49:299–305.

64. Amoroso A, Mitterhofer AP, Del Porto F, et al. Antibodies to anionic phospholipids and anti-β_2GPI: association with thrombosis and thrombocytopenia in systemic lupus erythematosus. Hum Immunol 2003;64:265–73.

65. Tebo AE, Jaskowski TD, Phansalkar AR, et al. Diagnostic performance of phospholipid-specific assays for the evaluation of antiphospholipid syndrome. Am J Clin Pathol 2008;129:870–5.

66. Tebo AE, Jaskowski TD, Hill HR, et al. Clinical relevance of multiple antibody specificity testing in anti-phospholipid syndrome and recurrent pregnancy loss. Clin Exp Immunol 2008;154:332–8.

67. Matzner W, Chong P, Xu G, et al. Characterization of antiphospholipid antibodies in women with recurrent spontaneous abortions. J Reprod Med 1994;39:27–30.

68. Gilman-Sachs A, Lubinski J, Beer AE, et al. Patterns of anti-phospholipid antibody specificities. J Clin Lab Immunol 1991;35:83–8.

69. Campbell AL, Pierangeli SS, Wellhausen S, et al. Comparison of the effects of anticardiolipin antibodies from patients with the antiphospholipid syndrome and with syphilis on platelet activation and aggregation. Thromb Haemost 1995;73:529–34.

70. Merkel PA, Chang YC, Pierangeli SS, et al. Comparison between the standard anticardiolipin antibody test and a new phospholipid test in patients with a variety of connective tissue diseases. J Rheumatol 1999;26:591–6.

71. Harris EN, Pierangeli SS. A more specific ELISA assay for the detection of anti-phospholipid antibodies. Clin Immunol Newslett 1995;15:26–8.
72. Day HM, Thiagarajan P, Ahn C, et al. Autoantibodies to beta2-glycoprotein I in systemic lupus erythematosus and primary antiphospholipid antibody syndrome: clinical correlations in comparison with other antiphospholipid antibody tests. J Rheumatol 1998;25:667–74.
73. Franklin RD, Kutteh WH. Effects of unfractionated and low molecular weight heparin on antiphospholipid antibody binding in vitro. Obstet Gynecol 2003; 101:455–62.
74. Franklin RD, Kutteh WH. Antiphospholipid antibodies (APA) and recurrent pregnancy loss: treating a unique APA positive population. Hum Reprod 2002;17: 2981–5.
75. Branch DW, Silver R, Pierangeli S, et al. Antiphospholipid antibodies other than lupus anticoagulant and anticardiolipin antibodies in women with recurrent pregnancy loss, fertile controls, and antiphospholipid syndrome. Obstet Gynecol 1997;89:549–55.
76. Cucurull E, Gharavi AE, Diri E, et al. IgA anticardiolipin and anti-beta2-glycoprotein I are the most prevalent isotypes in African American patients with systemic lupus erythematosus. Am J Med Sci 1999;318:55–60.
77. Kutteh WH, Corey A, Jaslow CR. Antiphospholipid antibodies and recurrent pregnancy loss: prevalence of anticardiolipin antibodies, the lupus anticoagulant, and antiphosphatidyl serine antibodies [abstract]. Lupus 2010;19:C156.
78. Bertolaccini ML, Atsumi T, Khamashta MA, et al. Autoantibodies to human prothrombin and clinical manifestations in 207 patients with systemic lupus erythematosus. J Rheumatol 1998;25:1104–8.
79. Donohoe S, Mackie IJ, Isenberg D, et al. Anti-prothrombin antibodies: assay conditions and clinical associations in the anti-phospholipid syndrome. Br J Haematol 2001;113:544–9.
80. Vaarala O, Puurunen M, Manttari M, et al. Antibodies to prothrombin imply a risk of myocardial infarction in middle-aged men. Thromb Haemost 1996;75:456–9.
81. Horbach DA, van Oort E, Donders RC, et al. Lupus anticoagulant is the strongest risk factor for both venous and arterial thrombosis in patients with systemic lupus erythematosus. Comparison between different assays for the detection of antiphospholipid antibodies. Thromb Haemost 1996;76:916–24.
82. Galli M, Beretta G, Daldossi M, et al. Different anticoagulant and immunological properties of anti-prothrombin antibodies in patients with antiphospholipid antibodies. Thromb Haemost 1997;77:486–91.
83. Forastiero RR, Martinuzzo ME, Cerrato GS, et al. Relationship of anti beta2-glycoprotein I and anti prothrombin antibodies to thrombosis and pregnancy loss in patients with antiphospholipid antibodies. Thromb Haemost 1997;78: 1008–14.
84. Pierangeli SS, Liu XW, Barker JH, et al. Induction of thrombosis in a mouse model by IgG, IgM and IgA immunoglobulins from patients with the antiphospholipid syndrome. Thromb Haemost 1995;74(5):1361–7.
85. Lopez LR, Santos ME, Espinoza LR, et al. Clinical significance of immunoglobulin A versus immunoglobulins G and M anti-cardiolipin antibodies in patients with systemic lupus erythematosus. Correlation with thrombosis, thrombocytopenia, and recurrent abortion. Am J Clin Pathol 1992;98:449–54.
86. Molina JF, Gutierrez-Urena S, Molina J, et al. Variability of anticardiolipin antibody isotype distribution in 3 geographic populations of patients with systemic lupus erythematosus. J Rheumatol 1997;24:291–6.

87. Wong KL, Liu HW, Ho K, et al. Anticardiolipin antibodies and lupus anticoagulant in Chinese patients with systemic lupus erythematosus. J Rheumatol 1991;18: 1187–92.
88. Kalunian KC, Peter JB, Middlekauff HR, et al. Clinical significance of a single test for anti-cardiolipin antibodies in patients with systemic lupus erythematosus. Am J Med 1988;85:602–8.
89. Selva-O'Callaghan A, Ordi-Ros J, Monegal-Ferran F, et al. IgA anticardiolipin antibodies–relation with other antiphospholipid antibodies and clinical significance. Thromb Haemost 1998;79:282–5.
90. Alarcon-Segovia D, Delezé M, Oria CV, et al. Antiphospholipid antibodies and the antiphospholipid syndrome in systemic lupus erythematosus: a prospective analysis of 500 consecutive patients. Medicine (Baltimore) 1989;68:353–65.
91. Spadaro A, Riccieri V, Terracina S, et al. Class specific rheumatoid factors and antiphospholipid syndrome in systemic lupus erythematosus. Lupus 2000;9: 56–60.
92. Diri E, Cucurull E, Gharavi AE, et al. Antiphospholipid (Hughes') syndrome in African-Americans: IgA aCL and abeta2 glycoprotein-I is the most frequent isotype. Lupus 1999;8:263–8.
93. Bertolaccini ML, Atsumi T, Escudero-Contreras A, et al. The value of IgA antiphospholipid testing for the diagnosis of antiphospholipid (Hughes) syndrome in systemic lupus erythematosus. J Rheumatol 2001;28:2637–43.
94. Danowski A, Kickler TS, Petri M. Anti-beta2-glycoprotein I: prevalence, clinical correlations, and importance of persistent positivity in patients with antiphospholipid syndrome and systemic lupus erythematosus. J Rheumatol 2006;33: 1775–9.
95. Petri M. Update on anti-phospholipid antibodies in SLE: the Hopkins' Lupus Cohort. Lupus 2010;19:419–23.
96. Yamada H, Tsutsumi A, Ichikawa K, et al. IgA-class anti-beta2-glycoprotein I in women with unexplained recurrent spontaneous abortion. Arthritis Rheum 1999; 42:2727–8.
97. Lee RM, Branch DW, Silver RM. Immunoglobulin A anti-beta2-glycoprotein antibodies in women who experience unexplained recurrent spontaneous abortion and unexplained fetal death. Am J Obstet Gynecol 2001;185:748–53.
98. Lakos G, Kiss E, Regeczy N, et al. Isotype distribution and clinical relevance of anti-beta2-glycoprotein I (β_2GPI) antibodies: importance of IgA isotype. Clin Exp Immunol 1999;117:574–9.
99. Lee RM, Brown MA, Branch DW, et al. Anticardiolipin and anti-beta2-glycoprotein-I antibodies in preeclampsia. Obstet Gynecol 2003;102:294–300.
100. Kumar S, Papalardo E, Sunkureddi P, et al. Isolated elevation of IgA anti-beta2glycoprotein I antibodies with manifestations of antiphospholipid syndrome: a case series of five patients. Lupus 2009;18:1011–4.
101. Mak A, Cheung M, Cheak A, et al. Combination of heparin and aspirin is superior to aspirin alone in enhancing live birth in patients with recurrent pregnancy loss and positive anti-phospholipid antibodies: a meta-analysis of randomized controlled trials and meta-regression. Rheumatology 2010;49:281–8.
102. Ziakas P, Pavlov M, Voulgarelis M. Heparin treatment in antiphospholipid syndrome with recurrent pregnancy loss: a systematic review and metaanalysis. Obstet Gynecol 2010;115:1256–62.
103. Fogerty AE, Connors JM. Management of inherited thrombophilia in pregnancy. Curr Opin Endocrinol Diabetes Obes 2009;16:464–9.

104. Benedetto C, Marozio L, Tavella AM, et al. Coagulation disorders in pregnancy: acquired and inherited thrombophilias. Ann N Y Acad Sci 2010;1205:106–17.
105. Werner EF, Lockwood CJ. Thrombophilias and stillbirth. Clin Obstet Gynecol 2010;53:617–27.
106. Robertson L, Wu O, Langhorne P, et al. Thrombosis: Risk and Economic Assessment of Thrombophilia Screening (TREATS) Study. Thrombophilia in pregnancy: a systematic review. Br J Haematol 2005;132:171–96.
107. Dizon-Townson D, Miller C, Sibai B, et al. The relationship of the Factor V Leiden mutation in pregnancy outcomes for mother and fetus. Obstet Gynecol 2005; 106:517–24.
108. Rodger MA, Betancourt MT, Clark P, et al. The association of factor V Leiden and prothrombin gene mutation and placenta-mediated pregnancy complications: a systematic review and meta-analysis of prospective cohort studies. PLoS Med 2010;7(6):e1000292.
109. Clark P, Walker ID, Langhorne P, et al. SPIN (Scottish Pregnancy Intervention) study: a multicenter, randomized controlled trial of low-molecular-weight heparin and low-dose aspirin in women with recurrent miscarriage. Blood 2010;115: 4162.
110. Kaandorp SP, Goddijn M, van der Post JA, et al. Aspirin plus heparin or aspirin alone in women with recurrent miscarriage. N Engl J Med 2010;362:1586–96.

Pharmacotherapeutic Management of Nicotine Dependence in Pregnancy

Shannon M. Clark, MD*, Ramzy Nakad, MD

KEYWORDS

• Pregnancy • Smoking • Nicotine dependence • Management

Smoking among reproductive-aged women is associated with significant adverse pregnancy outcomes when it persists into the gestational period. As one of the few preventable causes of adverse pregnancy outcomes, smoking in pregnancy has become a significant public health concern. About 5% to 10% of perinatal deaths, 20% to 35% of birth of low-birth-weight (LBW) infants, and 8% to 15% of preterm deliveries (PTD) have been attributed to smoking.[1,2] Smoking is also associated with infertility, pregnancy loss, placental abruption, birth defects (heart defects, orofacial clefts), preterm premature rupture of membranes, and placenta previa. Preterm birth associated with LBW results in prolonged hospital admission and treatment in the neonatal intensive care unit for the neonate with an increase of approximately 66% in the health care costs.[3–5] Although the antenatal adverse effects can be immediately observed, there are postnatal effects that present themselves much later.

Postnatal morbidities, including neonatal death, neonatal respiratory distress syndrome, patent ductus arteriosus, intraventricular hemorrhage, necrotizing enterocolitis, retinopathy of prematurity, sudden infant death syndrome, respiratory infections, reactive airway disease, otitis media, and multiple others, are also associated with maternal smoking during pregnancy.[6,7] Furthermore, adverse effects can proceed into childhood and adulthood, whereby maternal smoking is associated with childhood cancers and cognitive deficits, as well as ischemic heart disease, hypertension, diabetes, lung disease, and cerebrovascular accidents in adults.[8,9] Despite these adverse effects, approximately 25% of reproductive-aged American women continue to smoke cigarettes.[3] According to the Centers for Disease Control and Prevention in 2009, 12.2% to 14.1% of pregnant women in the United States smoke, with an understanding that underreporting has a significant effect on data collection.[3,10,11]

The authors have nothing to disclose.

Division of Maternal-Fetal Medicine, Department of Obstetrics and Gynecology, University of Texas Medical Branch, 301 University Boulevard, Galveston, TX 77555, USA

* Corresponding author.

E-mail address: shclark@utmb.edu

The adverse effects of maternal smoking can be attributed to predominantly 3 events: impaired placental gas exchange, direct fetal toxicity, and activation of the fetal sympathetic nervous system. Impaired fetal oxygen delivery because of abnormal placental gas exchange as a result of nicotine exposure is caused by decreased capillary volume, increased villous membrane thickness, decreased inter-villous perfusion, and nicotine-induced vasospasm.[12,13] Nicotine causes vasocon-striction through the release of catecholamines and nitric oxide, which causes constriction of the uteroplacental blood vessels and impairs delivery of oxygen and nutrients to the developing fetus.[14] This is the main pathophysiologic process leading to uteroplacental insufficiency and thus potential intrauterine growth restriction and placental abruption. In addition, the development of carboxyhemoglobin from inhala-tion of carbon monoxide (CO) affects both maternal and fetal systemic oxygen delivery. In the fetus, carboxyhemoglobin competes with oxyhemoglobin during tissue oxygenation, further contributing to impaired fetal oxygenation.

Second, toxicity from more than 2500 substances found in cigarettes, including nicotine, cyanide, CO, and lead, contributes to the pathophysiologic alterations that lead to adverse fetal effects from smoking that can result in damage to the developing fetal central nervous system, heart, and lungs. After maternal inhalation, nicotine enters the fetus through the placenta and returns back to the maternal circulation for elimination.[15] Nicotine can be found in the fetal circulation at levels that exceed maternal plasma levels by 15%, and amniotic fluid levels are 88% higher than maternal plasma levels.[16] Nicotine reaches the amniotic fluid through fetal urine production or through the blood vessels of the amniochorionic membrane.[17] As a result, the fetus is continually exposed to nicotine through the swallowing of amniotic fluid, and exposure can continue even after maternal nicotine levels decline.[17] Primate animal models have also shown that nicotine impairs lung development in the fetus, leading to decreased lung weight and volume and increased airway resistance through interaction with the nicotinic acetylcholine receptors (nAChRs), which are abundant in the fetal lung tissue.[18,19] Regarding fetal brain development, studies in rodents have shown that nicotine stimulates the nicotinic cholinergic receptors at inappropriate times, interfering with the normal numbers of neurons in selected areas of the fetal brain.[20] Finally, nicotine activates the fetal sympathetic nervous system, leading to increased fetal heart rate and decreased breathing movements, both of which are used to assess fetal well-being during pregnancy.

Nicotine is the major pharmacologically active substance in tobacco and the most studied regarding adverse pregnancy outcomes. Nicotine binds to nicotinic cholin-ergic receptors located in the brain, autonomic ganglia, adrenal medulla, and neuro-muscular junctions.[21] Once nicotine binds to these receptors, a variety of neurotransmitters are released, including dopamine, noradrenaline, adrenaline, acetylcholine, and serotonin. The release of these neurotransmitters mediates the psychoactive actions of nicotine.[21] In particular, the increased dopamine release stim-ulates the brain-reward system and is the impetus for most pleasurable activities and drug addiction behaviors, making it responsible for the addictive properties of nicotine.[15,22] The rapid peak in plasma nicotine levels is quickly followed by a steady decline to the withdrawal stage, which triggers the next cigarette.[23] This repetitive cycle of stimulation and withdrawal relief is the basis of nicotine addiction in pregnant and nonpregnant smokers alike.

Higher maternal peak arterial blood concentrations are reached when nicotine is administered more quickly, such as through inhalation, resulting in more intense cardiovascular and subjective effects of nicotine exposure.[17] Avoidance of these peak plasma levels of nicotine is a goal when considering pharmacotherapy of smoking cessation in pregnancy. Tempering the withdrawal symptoms because of the lack of immediate gratification that occurs when maternal nicotine levels are at their highest can be accomplished through behavioral counseling and psychosocial intervention strategies. Nicotine addiction is no different in the pregnant patient when compared with the nonpregnant patient when considering its mechanism of action, addictive properties, and propensity for withdrawal. However, the potential for adverse effects on the fetus make smoking cessation during pregnancy a priority.

A higher proportion of women stop smoking during pregnancy than at any other time in their lives.[4] It is estimated that 20% to 30% of women stop smoking at some point during pregnancy and 80% to 85% of these women will remain abstinent throughout the pregnancy.[9,24] A majority of those who do quit have done so by their first prenatal visit (18%–40%), and those who do not stop by this time are likely to continue throughout pregnancy.[4,25] Concerns over the effects of smoking on the fetus and nausea and vomiting of pregnancy experienced in the first and, sometimes, the early second trimesters of pregnancy often contribute to a woman's increased motivation to stop smoking.[7] Despite these concerns, however, approximately 20% to 25% of women continue smoking during their pregnancies.[2,15] Furthermore, of the women who manage to stop during pregnancy, about 70% resume smoking within 6 months into the postpartum period.[9,26]

Smoking cessation at any point in pregnancy, including the third trimester, can be beneficial and result in the birth of higher birth weight infants and decrease the risk of adverse antenatal events attributed to smoking. Because pregnancy is a time when most women seek medical attention for prenatal care, medical intervention is quite feasible in all trimesters of pregnancy. In addition, pregnancy is the only time when some women seek routine medical care and are seen on a regular basis for an extended period. Thus, an obstetric provider can play a significant role in interventions that may lead to maternal smoking cessation. However, it is estimated that only 49% of obstetricians routinely counsel their patients about smoking cessation and offer follow-up and only 28% discuss actual strategies for cessation.[1] As a result, a significant opportunity for medical intervention is lost.

In 2008, the US Department of Health and Human Services (USDHHS) released the updated Clinical Practice Guidelines with recommendations concerning smoking cessation in pregnancy.[3,27] The first recommendation is that pregnant smokers be offered extended or augmented psychosocial interventions that exceed minimal advice to quit whenever possible. The USDHHS found that abstinence rates were higher in patients who received augmented intervention through advice from their physician, pregnancy-specific self-help materials, and counseling sessions with a health educator and who continued follow-up. The second recommendation is for physicians to offer effective smoking cessation interventions not only at the first prenatal visit but also throughout the entire pregnancy, even though abstinence early in pregnancy may have the greatest benefits to both the mother and fetus. It is estimated that more than 20% of low-birth-weight births could be prevented by eliminating smoking during pregnancy, therefore counseling and encouragement to quit smoking should be addressed throughout the pregnancy.[27] In addition, perinatal outcomes do not improve by merely decreasing the number of cigarettes smoked throughout pregnancy.[28,29] As a result, complete cessation of smoking is the recommended goal.[1]

The final recommendation that was included in the 2001 USDHHS recommendations is that pharmacotherapy should be considered when a pregnant smoker is unable to quit and the benefits of quitting outweigh the risks of pharmacotherapy.[3] Counseling alone is not effective in 80% of pregnant smokers and seems to be more successful in light to moderate smokers.[7,30,31] However, underutilization of pharmacotherapy in pregnant women occurs because of concerns of adverse fetal effects and consequences for breastfeeding. The risk/benefit ratio for the use of pharmacotherapy for smoking cessation in pregnancy is favorable especially in moderate to heavy smokers (>10 cigarettes/d) because with smoking, the fetus is exposed to higher doses of nicotine, CO, and multiple other toxins.[32] In addition, the moderate to heavy smoker is less likely to quit during pregnancy. This article discusses the current recommendations for the pharmacotherapeutic management of nicotine dependence in pregnancy for the moderate to heavy smoker.

NICOTINE REPLACEMENT THERAPY

At present, nicotine replacement therapy (NRT) is the pharmacologic treatment of choice in pregnancy, and the risk-benefit ratio for its use is favorable. The current US Food and Drug Administration (FDA)-approved NRT products are nicotine gum, transdermal nicotine patches, nicotine nasal spray, nicotine lozenge, and nicotine inhaler. Data from animal studies suggest that nicotine is harmful to the developing fetus, but the benefits may be acceptable despite the risks.[33] As a result, all NRT products, except for nicotine gum, are FDA pregnancy category D indicating that there is evidence of human fetal risk; nicotine gum is FDA pregnancy category C.[34] Because the total amount of nicotine exposure to the fetus is less with NRT than with continued moderate to heavy smoking, it is recommended that NRT be considered in pregnancy if efforts to quit without medication are unsuccessful.[35] In addition, with NRT, the developing fetus is not exposed to the other toxic substances found in cigarettes.

In 2005, the American College of Obstetricians and Gynecologists Technical Bulletin proposed the use of nicotine gum or transdermal patches in heavy smokers only when nonpharmacologic treatments have failed.[36] When compared with the other forms of NRT, transdermal patches produce lower, longer-lasting, steadier concentrations of nicotine rather than high concentrations for shorter periods. Limited pharmacokinetic studies have reported that NRT results in plasma cotinine and nicotine levels that are no higher than that observed with smoking more than 10 cigarettes per day, which is considered moderate to heavy smoking.[37,38] In contrast, nicotine gum and nasal spray can provide nicotine exposure similar to that of smoking when used regularly throughout the day.[39] As a result, the transdermal patches have less potential for addiction and lower levels of nicotine, making them the preferred NRT in pregnancy. At present, 26% to 44% of American and British obstetric providers recommend NRT to pregnant smokers.[40–42]

The goal of NRT is to provide a level of nicotine just above that associated with withdrawal symptoms by delivering nicotine at a more constant rate. NRT acts through stimulation of nicotinic receptors in the ventral tegmental area of the brain with subsequent release of dopamine in the nucleus accumbens.[43] This process, in addition to the peripheral actions of nicotine, causes a decrease in withdrawal symptoms during abstinence. Through preventing and/or minimizing the symptoms of withdrawal, patients can focus their efforts on behavioral and psychological changes necessary for long-term cessation.[34] NRT does not completely eliminate the withdrawal symptoms due to the rapid release and high levels of nicotine in the arterial system observed with inhalation of cigarette smoke when compared with the slow release of nicotine observed with NRTs.[43] Nicotine administered through NRT penetrates the central nervous system less rapidly and in lower concentrations than that through cigarette smoking, which does not provide the patient with the immediate reinforcing effects of nicotine administration associated with smoking.[34] The absence of the stimulation-withdrawal relief cycle described earlier because of the slow release of nicotine with the transdermal patch is what makes its potential for addiction minimal.[23]

The reported quit rates with NRT in nonpregnant patients are approximately 20% to 30% at 6 months and 20% to 40% at 1 year for all-comers, and compliance is higher and side effects lower with the transdermal patch than with the other NRTs.[44–46] Recent Cochrane reviews show that NRT doubles cessation rates when compared with nonpharmacologic intervention programs and placebo.[43,47,48] Finally, the odds of abstinence increase by 71% with NRT compared with placebo.[49] However, NRT is more successful when combined with behavioral modification support and most studies implement some form of such therapy when examining the efficacy of NRT, as seen in a study by Miller and colleagues.[50] This study showed greater quit rates after 6 months in individuals who received and used free nicotine patches in addition to brief telephone counseling (33%) compared with those who received telephone counseling alone (6%). Overall, implementation of any form of NRT should be done in conjunction with counseling in some form on smoking cessation strategies.

The more commonly studied NRTs in pregnancy are the transdermal nicotine patch and nicotine gum. However, for the reasons previously stated, the transdermal patch is the more commonly prescribed NRT in pregnancy. Because nicotine and cotinine (the main metabolites of nicotine) are metabolized more quickly during pregnancy, the efficacy of NRT at conventional doses may be insufficient.[51] Consequently, it has been hypothesized that NRT therapy in pregnancy may require higher doses to prevent withdrawal symptoms and relapse, thereby potentially increasing the risk to the fetus. However, the effect that pregnancy has on nicotine metabolism in each individual varies greatly, and therapeutic monitoring may be necessary to reach the optimal dosage of NRT. The amount of nicotine delivered to the fetus with NRT, and the potential adverse effects on the pregnancy and fetus are hard to quantify because of the lack of experimental studies on humans.

The transdermal patches come in 21-mg and 16-mg formulations for both the pregnant and nonpregnant smoker. The typical dosing regimen with the 21-mg patches is 21 mg/d for 4 to 6 weeks, then 14 mg/d for 2 weeks, and then 7 mg/d for 2 weeks, and this regimen is typically used with moderate to heavy smokers. The 16-mg patch is a single-dose patch applied for 16 h/d for 6 weeks without tapering.[21] It is recommended that the lowest effective dose of the NRT transdermal patch be prescribed in pregnancy, and the treatment usually lasts for 6 to 14 weeks. Furthermore, the 16-mg patch is recommended to avoid exposing the fetus during the nighttime.

A study by Dempsey and colleagues[51] on the metabolism of nicotine and cotinine in 10 pregnant smokers after the intravenous administration of nicotine and cotinine during pregnancy and postpartum showed that both are metabolized more rapidly and that the half-life of cotinine was significantly decreased. Even though renal blood flow is increased in pregnancy, the study did not show an increase in renal clearance of nicotine during pregnancy, indicating that the accelerated metabolism may be because of increased metabolism by the liver.[51] Despite the increased metabolism of nicotine, the daily intake of nicotine was unchanged during pregnancy, and the intake of nicotine from smoking seemed not to be influenced by its increased metabolism in pregnancy.[51] As a result, plasma levels of nicotine with NRT will not accumulate to a greater degree in pregnancy when compared with the nonpregnant subject, and altered dosing of the transdermal patch and other forms of NRT is not necessary because standard dosing during pregnancy seems to be in the same therapeutic range for nonpregnant individuals. Furthermore, maternal venous nicotine levels are generally lower than with active smoking, and the high arterial peak levels seen in smokers are not found in NRT users. For reasons stated earlier, the 21-mg patch has been shown to result in no greater exposure to nicotine and no exposure to tobacco-related toxins and CO.[52] It is still recommended, however, that pregnant women use the 16-hour rather than the 24-hour transdermal patch, or the lowest effective transdermal patch dose. NRT should be reserved for women who are moderately or highly dependent (>10 cigarettes per day) secondary to unanswered questions regarding safety in pregnancy.

Because of the paucity of data on NRT in pregnancy, its efficacy is still unknown. In a randomized controlled trial by Wisborg and colleagues[52] on NRT transdermal patches in 250 healthy women smoking more than 10 cigarettes per day, there was no difference in successful quit attempts at all stages and at 1 year postpartum when compared with placebo, but the study was small and underpowered. However, infants born to mothers in the NRT group had significantly higher birth weights (186 g) than the placebo group, indicating that intrauterine growth restriction secondary to smoking could be a result of the multiple other compounds found in cigarettes and not a result of nicotine exposure alone.[52] Although these findings could be an indication that the nicotine in NRT does not have a significant effect of infant birth weight, the results of this study warrant further investigation because rodent data have consistently shown that nicotine can cause growth restriction. To date, there is no clear and consistent evidence that NRT is efficacious for smoking cessation in pregnancy.

The common side effects of the transdermal patch include skin irritation (50% of users) and sleep disturbance. If patients experience sleep disturbances, the 16-hour rather than the 24-hour patch should be used. Contraindications to their usage include systemic eczema, unstable angina, arrhythmias, pregnancy, and myocardial infarction of less than 1-month duration. The safety of NRT over cigarette smoking is predominantly the result of nonexposure to the harmful and toxic substances found in tobacco.[43] Finally, although the NRT transdermal patch is contraindicated in pregnancy, its use is recommended in moderate to heavy smokers for the reasons previously discussed.

BUPROPION SUSTAINED RELEASE

Bupropion (amfebutamone), an aminoketone antidepressant related to the phenylethylamines, was initially developed for the treatment of depression. It has since been developed as a nonnicotine aid for smoking cessation in the formulation bupropion sustained release (SR), or Zyban, and is the first nonnicotine medication approved for smoking cessation. Its effect on nicotine dependence seems to be separate from its antidepressant effect because it is effective in subjects without depression.[53] It is considered an alternative for persons who cannot tolerate NRT or who prefer nonnicotine treatment. Bupropion SR can also be prescribed to pregnant women who smoke more half a pack per day or who fail NRT.[54] As with NRT, the risk-benefit ratio for the use of bupropion in pregnancy is favorable. However, its use in pregnancy is still limited because of the lack of safety data on the fetus and uncertainty regarding the optimal dosage and duration of treatment.

The clinical effects of bupropion are mediated by the blockage of the reuptake of dopamine, norepinephrine, and serotonin in the mesolimbic dopaminergic system and the locus ceruleus of the brain.[55,56] It is also thought that bupropion acts as a brain nicotinic receptor antagonist in the nucleus accumbens, thus blocking the effects of nicotine.[57] These actions may reduce the cravings for nicotine and alleviate the symptoms of withdrawal.[58] Bupropion has an advantage over NRT in that there is the absence of nicotine exposure to the fetus while decreasing withdrawal symptoms.[7] The recommended dose of bupropion in both pregnant and nonpregnant subjects is 300 mg/d in 2 divided doses. It is recommended that bupropion be started 2 weeks before the anticipated quit date for smoking with 150 mg/d for 3 days and then 150 mg twice daily. At present, there is no evidence that bupropion is metabolized more quickly in pregnancy, and pharmacokinetic data are limited.

As with NRT, bupropion treatment results in quit rates that are almost double that of placebo.[47,48] In a randomized controlled trial by Jorenby and colleagues,[59] bupropion SR was found to have higher abstinence rates when compared with placebo and nicotine transdermal patch. In this study of 893 nondepressed, nonpregnant smokers randomized into 4 groups (placebo, NRT alone, bupropion SR alone or bupropion SR plus NRT), the 1-year quit rate was 16% in the placebo group, 16% in the NRT group, 30% in bupropion group, and 36% in bupropion plus NRT group. These results are similar to those of another study by Hurt and colleagues[60] that showed abstinence of 27% at 6 months when compared with 16% abstinence with placebo. In 4 randomized controlled trials, the absolute risk of quitting smoking with bupropion was 21% when compared with placebo.[61] However, many of these studies have also shown that cessation rates decline as the duration of follow-up is extended. In addition, smoking cessation rates seem to increase with increased duration of treatment, usually more than 7 weeks. Because bupropion is an antidepressant and smoking rates are increased in persons with depression, these studies have excluded persons with a history of major depression. This exclusion ensured that any effects observed during the studies were independent of the antidepressant effects of bupropion.

Bupropion is an FDA pregnancy category C drug, indicating that animal studies have demonstrated adverse effects on the fetus, but there are no controlled studies in women, or no studies are available in either animals or humans.[33,34] All information on bupropion in pregnancy is based on animal studies at 10 to 45 times human exposure and a small number of human studies, and it seems to have a better safety profile than nicotine.[33] Furthermore, studies in rats and rabbits at doses up to 14 times and 10 times the human dose, respectively, have shown no increased risk of teratogenicity.[62] GlaxoSmithKline, the manufacturer, has kept a registry on its use in pregnancy. In March 2008, when the final report was released, 1597 pregnancies were exposed to bupropion, with 994 pregnancies analyzed for 1005 outcomes.[63] Birth defects, largely including defects of the heart and great vessels, were found in 3.6% of fetuses exposed in the first trimester. This result was no different than that seen in first trimester exposures to other antidepressants.

In a 2005 prospective comparative study by Chun-Fai-Chan and colleagues[64] on 136 pregnant women in the first trimester already taking bupropion for depression or smoking cessation, no increase in the rates of malformation was observed in the 105 live births included in the study at 4 months and 1 year after delivery. There was also no difference in birth weight or neonatal death. However, the spontaneous abortion rate was higher in the bupropion-treated group, but was similar to that in 4 other studies on the safety of antidepressants in pregnancy in which the results were not statistically significant because of small sample size.[62] Because of concern over bupropion's association with cardiac malformations, Cole and colleagues[65] performed a retrospective epidemiologic study of the United States health care database. They found that in the 1213 women exposed to bupropion during the first trimester and in the 1049 women exposed after the first trimester, the incidence of cardiac malformations was similar to the rate found in users of other antidepressants. However, Alwan and colleagues[66] conducted a retrospective case-control study of birth defects risk factors on 6853 infants with major heart defects and 5869 controls who were exposed to bupropion in the first trimester of pregnancy for the treatment of depression. They found a positive association between early pregnancy exposure to bupropion and left outflow tract heart defects, although the results were not conclusive and recommendation for further studies was made. Despite these findings, the concern over whether bupropion is associated with birth defects and spontaneous abortion remains, and further studies are warranted.

The common side effects of bupropion are insomnia and dry mouth, both of which are dose related, and to a lesser extent headache, nausea, and anxiety. The most serious side effect with bupropion as well as many other antidepressants is the dose-related incidence of seizures. The incidence of seizures with bupropion is reported to be 0.1% to 0.4%, similar to the incidence with other antidepressants, and is more common with the immediate release form rather than the SR form.[67] No seizures have been reported in clinical trials of bupropion SR. However, bupropion is contraindicated in patients with seizure disorder, concurrent use of other forms of bupropion, anorexia/bulimia, medications that may lower the seizure threshold, severe hepatic cirrhosis, and in patients undergoing abrupt discontinuation of alcohol or sedatives.[34]

Bupropion has also been associated with treatment-emergent hypertension in earlier studies in patients with and without preexisting hypertension.[68] It seems that this finding occurs exclusively in patients receiving NRT plus bupropion; no reports exist with NRT or bupropion alone.[68] Bupropion also inhibits metabolism of drugs by liver cytochrome P458 2D6 (antipsychotics, β-blockers, type 1C antiarrhythmics), therefore physicians should use caution if a patient is taking one of these drugs.[69] A majority of the serious side effects did not occur in clinical trials but rather in various case reports. Finally, hypersensitivity reactions with bupropion SR can occur and are usually manifested as a skin rash, which occurs in 0.1% patients.[68] Other hypersensitivity reactions include a serum sicknesslike reaction and erythema multiforme.[70,71]

VARENICLINE

Varenicline, a cytisine analogue, is an α4β2 neuronal nicotinic acetylcholine partial agonist and α7 neuronal nicotinic acetylcholine full agonist that binds with high affinity and selectivity at these receptors, which are upregulated by long-term nicotine exposure and are implicated in nicotine addiction.[15,24,72] The efficacy of varenicline is thought to be the result of low-level agonist activity at the α4β2 receptor site, which is found predominantly in the human brain, in addition to the competitive inhibition of nicotine binding.[34] Varenicline binds to nicotine receptors more readily than nicotine, and these receptors ultimately become blocked by the drug.[73] Furthermore, the partial agonist activity induces modest receptor stimulation that decreases the symptoms of nicotine withdrawal by inducing 30% to 60% of the dopamine flow produced by nicotine, minimizing craving and withdrawal symptoms in abstinent subjects.[34,74,75]

By blocking the ability of nicotine to activate α4β2 nAChRs, varenicline inhibits the surge of dopamine release that is thought to be responsible for the reinforcement and reward associated with exposure to nicotine, which is a full agonist at the receptor sites.[73,76,77] As a result, if abstinent smokers resume smoking after varenicline therapy, the expected response seen with smoking is not experienced by the smoker because inhaled nicotine cannot attach to the nAChRs to cause the sudden release of dopamine.[77] Finally, smokers gain less pleasure from the nicotine contained in a cigarette, experience less craving and withdrawal, and are better able to achieve abstinence.[72] The ability of varenicline to decrease the craving and withdrawal symptoms experienced by smokers makes it an ideal drug for smoking cessation in pregnancy. However, because of the lack of data on varenicline in pregnancy, it is not recommended.

Varenicline seems to have greater abstinence rates than NRT and shows greater reduction in the cravings and feelings of withdrawal seen with smoking than with NRT.[15] It has been hypothesized that the α4β2 partial agonists are more effective as a smoking cessation aid than other therapies.[15] It seems this receptor could stimulate the release of enough dopamine to reduce craving and withdrawal symptoms while acting as a partial antagonist for nicotine.[15] The duration of treatment with varenicline at 1 mg twice daily is typically 12 weeks, and providers commonly extend treatment by 12 weeks in those who achieve abstinence. During the first week of treatment, the dose is titrated to 0.5 mg daily on days 1 to 3, 0.5 mg twice daily on days 4 to 7, and then 1 mg twice daily on day 8, which is the target quit date.[78] Subjects may remain on a lower dose if they cannot tolerate 1 mg twice daily. It has been shown that treatment with varenicline at 2 mg/d for 12 weeks results in 2 to 3 times higher abstinence rates than placebo 12 months after treatment.[72]

In randomized trials, varenicline at 1 mg twice daily increased the chances of stopping smoking by 2- to 3-fold when compared with placebo, even beyond the treatment phase.[74] Two phase 3 randomized trials on the efficacy, tolerability, and safety of varenicline, each containing more than 1000 subjects, showed that at 1 mg twice daily for 12 weeks, varenicline is significantly more effective than bupropion SR (150 mg twice daily) and placebo for smoking cessation.[79,80] The CO-confirmed continuous abstinence rates (CARs) in a pooled analysis of these 2 trials were higher with varenicline than with bupropion SR or placebo during the last 4 weeks of treatment (weeks 9–12).[79,80] In addition, the CO-confirmed CARs for weeks 9 to 52 were higher with varenicline than with placebo in both trials.[79,80] Furthermore, smoking satisfaction was reduced in subjects who continued to smoke while taking varenicline.[80] In a phase 3 randomized trial comparing 12 weeks of varenicline with 10 weeks of the NRT transdermal patch, the CO-confirmed CARs were higher with varenicline than with NRT (55.9% vs 43.2%) during the last 4 weeks of treatment, cravings and withdrawal symptoms were reduced, smoking satisfaction was reduced, and more subjects remained abstinent at 1 year.[81] Overall, at 1 mg twice daily, varenicline improves the chances of quitting by almost 50% when compared with bupropion SR and NRT.[74]

Varenicline is an FDA pregnancy category C drug and should be used in pregnancy only if the potential benefit justifies the potential risk to the fetus.[34] There are currently no data on the effect of varenicline use on fetal development when consumed during pregnancy and lactation.[15] Animal studies in rats and rabbits at doses 36 to 50 times that of human exposure have failed to show evidence of teratogenicity.[33] There are no data on the safety profile of varenicline or information on whether the drug is more rapidly metabolized in pregnancy.[77] There is no current opinion on the safety or effectiveness of varenicline in pregnancy.[77] It is contraindicated for use during pregnancy and lactation until evidence of its safety in pregnant and nursing women is available.[82]

Side effects of varenicline include gastrointestinal and sleep disorders and headache. Insomnia, abnormal dreams, constipation, dry mouth, and flatulence are also reported side effects.[83] Nausea is the most commonly reported side effect and seems to diminish with continued use of varenicline. There is currently a warning because of the potential risks of serious neuropsychiatric events in patients taking varenicline, including agitation, depressed mood, suicidal ideation, and worsening of preexisting psychiatric illness.[84] These adverse effects were seen in subjects experiencing nicotine withdrawal and subjects who were still smoking.[82] As a result, any history of psychiatric illness, such as, major depressive disorder, panic disorder, psychosis, bipolar disorder, and suicidal attempt/ideation, should be discussed before initiating therapy with varenicline. Clinicians should monitor for changes in mood and behavior during treatment if a patient reports a history of any of these disorders. It is unclear whether these side effects are associated with varenicline or nicotine withdrawal. For subjects who have significant side effects, a lower dose of varenicline may be prescribed.

SUMMARY

Smoking in pregnancy is a common serious comorbid condition that should be treated as an addiction. That smoking in pregnancy is truly an addiction is supported by the fact that pregnant women often continue to smoke despite having been counseled by their heath care provider regarding the adverse effects of smoking on the pregnancy and fetus. Furthermore, women who continue to smoke despite these risks are likely to be more highly addicted (>10 cigarettes per day). Because pregnancy is a time when some women seek routine medical care for an extended period, medical intervention is possible. However, there are a significant number of women who do not receive adequate counseling regarding smoking cessation and may not even be offered pharmacotherapy if it is warranted. Improvement in physician awareness of adequate counseling and treatment options for smoking cessation in pregnancy is necessary. Overall, both physician and patient knowledge of the medications available to aid in smoking cessation is lacking.

Any medication given to the pregnant woman is assumed to have some risk because there are unknowns with every medication when considering the effects on the developing fetus. As a result, psychosocial interventions and involvement in smoking cessation programs should be the first step toward achieving smoking cessation in the pregnant patient. When these interventions fail, pharmacotherapy can and should be considered, especially in the moderate to heavy smoker. It has also been suggested that the more highly addicted smokers may require larger doses of smoking cessation therapies. In addition, the physiologic changes in pregnancy may further affect the pharmacokinetic profile of these medications, which could alter both the timing and the dosing of medications. However, data are still lacking in this area, and the optimal timing and dosage of these medications in pregnancy is unknown.

Because there is data on the safety of these medications in pregnancy are lacking; physicians are still hesitant to prescribe pharmacotherapy for smoking cessation because of the potential adverse fetal effects. For the most part, we can assess and quantify adverse effects on the mother. However, unless adverse effects on the fetus present antenatally or immediately postpartum, adverse fetal outcomes may not be observed until much later in life. More trials on the safety and effectiveness of the current pharmacotherapies available for smoking cessation are needed, and data on the long-term outcomes of the infants exposed to these medications during all trimesters of pregnancy are necessary. Until more data are available, the risks versus benefits of prescribing these medications must be considered and the patient must be counseled appropriately.

Despite the uncertainties regarding the medications available to aid in smoking cessation in pregnancy, the fact remains that smoking exposes the pregnant woman to multiple chemicals and toxins besides nicotine that can adversely affect the pregnancy and fetal development. As a result, reducing or avoiding exposure to the harmful substances in cigarettes would result in improved outcomes for the mother and fetus both antenatally and postnatally. Although NRT exposes the pregnancy to nicotine, a potential teratogen, avoidance of exposure to other harmful substances in cigarettes is still beneficial for the pregnancy. Because of the findings of animal studies, there are concerns that nicotine may affect human fetal brain development. As a result, the lowest dose of nicotine that is adequate to achieve smoking cessation is recommended. Although whether NRT is effective for smoking cessation in pregnancy is still uncertain, NRT is the preferred pharmacotherapy in pregnancy when nonpharmacotherapeutic interventions have failed.

Women may be hesitant to take bupropion not only because of concerns of birth defects and spontaneous abortion but also because an oral medication during the first and early second trimesters of pregnancy when nausea and vomiting may occur poses an additional problem. Bupropion is prescribed in pregnancy when NRT has failed and sometimes as first-line therapy for smoking cessation in pregnancy, and it has even been proposed that bupropion plus NRT may be an alternative for the problem smoker. As with NRT, the safety and effectiveness of bupropion for smoking cessation in pregnancy warrants further study. Varenicline is a promising new therapy for smoking cessation and has been shown to be more effective than NRT, bupropion, and placebo. However, because of the lack of studies in pregnancy, it is not currently prescribed in the pregnant patient. Although studies of NRT, bupropion, and varenicline have shown that they are effective for smoking cessation in the nonpregnant patient, there is no clear evidence that any are effective in pregnancy. Further studies, especially with bupropion and varenicline, are necessary to provide valid alternatives as nonnicotine pharmacotherapies for smoking cessation in pregnancy.

- As one of the few preventable causes of adverse pregnancy outcomes, smoking in pregnancy has become a significant public health concern. About 5% to 10% of perinatal deaths, 20% to 35% of LBW, and 8% to 15% of PTD have been attributed to smoking.[1,2]
- The adverse effects of maternal smoking can be attributed to predominantly 3 events: impaired placental gas exchange, direct fetal toxicity, and activation of the fetal sympathetic nervous system.
- Nicotine addiction is no different in the pregnant subject when compared with the nonpregnant patient, when considering its mechanism of action, addictive properties, and propensity for withdrawal. However, the potential for adverse effects on the fetus make smoking cessation during pregnancy a priority.
- Because the total amount of nicotine exposure to the fetus is less with NRT than with continued moderate to heavy smoking, it is recommended that NRT be considered in pregnancy if efforts to quit without medication are unsuccessful.[35] In addition, with NRT, the developing fetus is not exposed to the other toxic substances found in cigarettes.
- It has been hypothesized that NRT therapy in pregnancy may require higher doses to prevent withdrawal symptoms and relapse, thereby potentially increasing the risk to the fetus. However, the effect that pregnancy has on nicotine metabolism in each individual varies greatly, and therapeutic monitoring may be necessary to reach the optimal dosage of NRT.
- Concern over whether bupropion is associated with birth defects and spontaneous abortion remains, and further studies are warranted.
- The partial agonist activity of varenicline induces modest receptor stimulation that decreases the symptoms of nicotine withdrawal by inducing 30% to 60% of the dopamine flow produced by nicotine, minimizing craving and withdrawal symptoms in abstinent subjects, making it a promising alternative as a nonnicotine pharmacotherapy for smoking cessation in pregnancy.[34,74,75] There is no current opinion on the safety or effectiveness of varenicline in pregnancy.[77] It is contraindicated for use during pregnancy and lactation until evidence of its safety in pregnant and nursing women is available.[82]

REFERENCES

1. The Surgeon General's 1990 Report on The Health Benefits of Smoking Cessation. Executive Summary. Anonymous Morbidity & Mortality Weekly Report Recommendations & Reports 1990;39(RR-12):i–xv, 1–12. Available at: http://ovidsp.tx.ovid.com/sp-3.3.1a/ovidweb.cgi?&S=JNPAFPBNPLDDJGFANCCLNEMCHPECAA00&Complete+Reference=S.sh.14%7c4%7c1. Accessed February 28, 2011.
2. Fang WL, Goldstein AO, Butzen AY, et al. Smoking cessation in pregnancy: a review of postpartum relapse prevention strategies. J Am Board Fam Pract 2004;17(4):264–75.
3. U.S. Department of Health and Human Services. Women and smoking: a report of the Surgeon General, vol. 17. Rockville (MD): U.S. Department of Health and Human Services, Public Health Service, Office of the Surgeon General; 2001. 2002. p. 264–75.
4. Lumley J, Oliver SS, Chamberlain C, et al. Interventions for promoting smoking cessation during pregnancy. Cochrane Database Syst Rev 2004;4:CD001055.
5. Centers for Disease Control and Prevention (CDC). Medical care expenditures attributable to cigarette smoking during pregnancy-United States. MMWR Morb Mortal Wkly Rep 1997;46(44):1048–50.
6. Brown HL, Hopf SK. Clinical perspectives on smoking during pregnancy. Female Patient 1998;23:59.
7. Crawford JT, Tolosa JE, Goldenberg RL. Smoking cessation in pregnancy: why, how, and what next. Clin Obstet Gynecol 2008;51:419–35.
8. Raymond EG, Cnattingius S, Kiely JL. Effects of maternal age, parity, and smoking on the risk of stillbirth. Br J Obstet Gynaecol 1994;101(4):301–6.
9. Higgins S. Smoking in pregnancy. Curr Opin Obstet Gynecol 2002;14:145–51.
10. Lumley J, Oliver S, Waters E. Interventions for promoting smoking cessation during pregnancy. (Cochrane Review) (1999). Cochrane Database Syst Rev 2000;2:CD001055. Update Software, Oxford (UK).
11. CDC. Trends in smoking before, during, and after pregnancy-Pregnancy Risk Assessment Monitoring System (PRAMS) 2009, United States, 31 sites, 2000–2005. Surveillance summaries. MMWR Morb Mortal Wkly Rep 2009;58:1–36.
12. Larsen LG, Clausen HV, Jonsson L. Stereologic examination of placentas from mothers who smoke during pregnancy. Am J Obstet Gynecol 2002;186:531–7.
13. Lehtovirta P, Forss M. The acute effect of smoking on intervillous blood flow of the placenta. Br J Obstet Gynaecol 1978;85:729.
14. Benowitz NL, Gourlay SG. Cardiovascular toxicity of nicotine: implications for nicotine replacement therapy. J Am Coll Cardiol 1997;29:1422–31.
15. Maritz GS. Are nicotine replacement therapy, varenicline or bupropion options for pregnant mothers to quit smoking? Effects on the respiratory system of the offspring. Ther Adv Respir Dis 2009;3:193–210.
16. Andres RL, Day MC. Perinatal complications associated with maternal tobacco use. Semin Neonatol 2000;5:231–41.
17. Benowitz NL, Dempsey DA. Pharmacotherapy for smoking cessation during pregnancy. Nicotine Tob Res 2004;6(Suppl 2):S189–202.
18. Sekhon HS, Jia Y, Raab R, et al. Prenatal nicotine increases pulmonary alpha7 nicotinic receptor expression and alters fetal lung development in monkeys. J Clin Invest 1999;103:637–47.
19. Sekhon HS, Keller JA, Benowitz NL, et al. Prenatal nicotine exposure alters pulmonary function in newborn rhesus monkeys. Am J Respir Crit Care Med 2001;164(6):989–94.

20. Slotkin TA, Cho H, Whitmore WL. Effects of prenatal nicotine exposure on neuronal development: selective actions on central and peripheral catecholaminergic pathways. Brain Res Bull 1987;18:601–11.
21. Dempsey DA, Benowitz NL. Risks and benefits of nicotine to aid smoking cessation in pregnancy. Drug Saf 2001;24:277–322.
22. Tomkins DM, Sellers EM. Addiction and the brain: the role of neurotransmitters in the cause and treatment of drug dependence. CMAJ 2001;4:817–21.
23. Pontieri FE, Tanda G, Orzi G, et al. Effects of nicotine on the nucleus accumbens and similarity to those of addictive drugs. Nature 1996;382(6588):255–7.
24. Mas R, Escriba V, Colomer C. Who quits smoking during pregnancy? Scand J Soc Med 1996;24:102–6.
25. Lumely J. Stopping smoking. Br J Obstet Gynaecol 1987;94:289–92.
26. Coleman T. Special groups of smokers. BMJ 2005;328:575–7.
27. U.S. Department of Health and Human Services. Clinical Practice Guideline. Treating tobacco use and dependence: 2008 update. Rockville (MD): U.S. Department of Health and Human Services, Public Health Service, Office of the Surgeon General; 2008.
28. Li CQ, Windsor RA, Perkins L, et al. The impact on infant birth weight and gestational age of cotinine-validated smoking reduction during pregnancy. JAMA 1993;269:1519–24.
29. Dolan-Mullen P, Ramirez G, Groff JY. A meta-analysis of randomized trials of prenatal smoking cessation interventions. Am J Obstet Gynecol 1994;171: 1328–34.
30. Lancaster T, Stead LF. Physician advice for smoking cessation. Cochrane Database of Systematic Reviews 2004;4:CD000165.
31. Benowitz NL, Dempsey DA, Goldenberg RL, et al. The use of pharmacotherapies for smoking cessation during pregnancy. Tob Control 2000;9:iii91–4.
32. Rigotti NA, Park ER, Chang Y, et al. Smoking cessation medication use among pregnant and postpartum smokers. Obstet Gynecol 2008;111:348–55.
33. Oncken CA, Kranzler HR. What do we know about the role of pharmacotherapy for smoking cessation before or during pregnancy? Nicotine Tob Res 2009; 11(11):1265–73.
34. Hudmon KS, Corelli RL, Prokhorov AV. Current approaches to pharmacotherapy for smoking cessation. Ther Adv Respir Dis 2010;4:35–47.
35. Benowitz NL. Nicotine replacement therapy during pregnancy. JAMA 1991; 266(22):3174–7.
36. ACOG committee opinion. Smoking cessation during pregnancy. ACOG Committee on Health Care for Underdeserved Women. ACOG Committee on Obstetric Practice. Obstetrics & Gynecology 2005;106(4):883–8. Available at: http://ovidsp.tx.ovid.com/sp-3.3.1a/ovidweb.cgi?&S=JNPAFPBNPLDDJGFANCCLNEMCHPECAA00&Link+Set=S.sh.57%7c1%7csl_10. Accessed February 28, 2011.
37. Oncken CA, Hatsukami DK, Lupo VR, et al. Effects of short-term use of nicotine gum in pregnant smokers. Clin Pharmacol Ther 1996;59:654–61.
38. Ogburn PL Jr, Hurt RD, Croghan IT, et al. Nicotine patch use in pregnant smokers: nicotine and cotinine levels and fetal effects. Am J Obstet Gynecol 1999;181:736–43.
39. Coleman T, Britton J, Thornton J. Nicotine replacement therapy in pregnancy. BMJ 2004;328:965–6.
40. Herbert R, Coleman T, Britton J. UK general practitioners' beliefs, attitudes, and reported prescribing of nicotine replacement therapy in pregnancy. Nicotine Tob Res 2005;7:541–6.

41. Price JH, Jordan TR, Drake JA. Obstetricians and gynecologists' perceptions and use of nicotine replacement therapy. J Community Health 2006;31: 160–75.

42. Oncken CA, Pbert L, Ockene JL, et al. Nicotine replacement prescription practices of obstetric and pediatric clinicians. Obstet Gynecol 2000;96:261–5.

43. Molyneaux A. Nicotine replacement therapy. BMJ 2004;328:454–6.

44. Fiore MC, Smith SS, Jorenby DE, et al. The effectiveness of the nicotine patch for smoking cessation. JAMA 1994;271:1940–7.

45. Hajek P, West R, Foulds J, et al. Randomized comparative trial of nicotine polacrilex, a transdermal patch, nasal spray, and an inhaler. Arch Intern Med 1999; 159:2033–8.

46. Fiore MC, Novotny TE, Pierce JP, et al. Methods used to quit smoking in the United States. JAMA 1990;263:3244–54.

47. Hughes JR, Stead LF, Lancaster T. Antidepressants for smoking cessation. Cochrane Database Syst Rev 2007;1:CD000031.

48. Stead LF, Perera R, Bullen C, et al. Nicotine replacement therapy for smoking cessation. Cochrane Database Syst Rev 2008;1:CD000146.

49. Silagy C, Mant D, Fowler F, et al. Nicotine replacement therapy for smoking cessation. Cochrane Database Syst Rev 2000;3:CD000146.

50. Miller N, Frieden TR, Liu SY, et al. Effectiveness of a large-scale distribution programme of free nicotine patches: a prospective evaluation. Lancet 2005;365: 1843–54.

51. Dempsey D, Jacob P III, Benowitz NL. Accelerated metabolism of nicotine and cotinine in pregnant smokers. J Pharmacol Exp Ther 2002;301:594–8.

52. Wisborg K, Henrikson TB, Jespersen LB, et al. Nicotine patches for pregnant smokers: a randomized controlled study. Obstet Gynecol 2000;96:967–71.

53. Galanti LM. Tobacco smoking cessation management: integrating varenicline in current practice. Vasc Health Risk Manag 2008;4:837–45.

54. Rayburn WF, Bogenschutz MP. Pharmacotherapy for pregnant women with addictions. Am J Obstet Gynecol 2004;191:1885–97.

55. Ferris RM, Cooper BR, Maxwell RA. Studies of bupropion's mechanism of antidepressant activity. J Clin Psychiatry 1983;44:74–8.

56. Ascher JA, Cole JO, Colin JN, et al. Bupropion: a review of its mechanism of antidepressant activity. J Clin Psychiatry 1995;56:395–401.

57. Slemmer JE, Martin BR, Damaj MI. Bupropion is a nicotinic antagonist. J Pharmacol Exp Ther 2000;295:321–7.

58. Fiore MC, Jaen CR, Baker TB, et al. Treating tobacco use and dependence: 2008 update US public health service practice guideline executive summary. Respir Care 2008;55:1217–22.

59. Jorenby DE, Leishow SJ, Nides MA, et al. A controlled trial of sustained-release bupropion, a nicotine patch, or both for smoking cessation. N Engl J Med 1999; 340:685–91.

60. Hurt RD, Sachs DPL, Glover ED, et al. A comparison of sustained-release bupropion and placebo for smoking cessation. N Engl J Med 1997;337:1195–202.

61. Hughes J, Stead L, Lancaster T. Antidepressants for smoking cessation. Cochrane Database Syst Rev 2000;4:CD000031.

62. Goldstein MG. Bupropion sustained release and smoking cessation. J Clin Psychiatry 1998;56:68–72.

63. GlaxoSmithKline. The bupropion pregnancy registry: final report, 1 September 1997 through 31 March 2008. Available at: http://pregnancyregistry.gsk.com/documents/bup_report_final_2008.pdf. Accessed February 28, 2011.

64. Chun-Fai-Chan B, Koren G, Fayez I, et al. Pregnancy outcome of women exposed to bupropion during pregnancy: a prospective comparative study. Am J Obstet Gynecol 2005;192:932–6.
65. Cole JA, Modell JG, Haight BR, et al. Bupropion in pregnancy and the prevalence of congenital malformations. Pharmacoepidemiol Drug Saf 2007;16:474–84.
66. Alwan S, Reefhuis J, Botto LD, et al. Maternal use of bupropion and risk for congenital heart defects. Am J Obstet Gynecol 2010;203:52, e1–6.
67. Hays JT, Ebbert JO. Bupropion sustained release for treatment of tobacco dependence. Mayo Clin Proc 2003;78:1020–4.
68. Hays JT, Hurt RD, Rigotti NA, et al. Sustained-release bupropion for pharmacologic relapse prevention after smoking cessation: a randomized, controlled trial. Ann Intern Med 2001;135:423–33.
69. Holm K, Spencer C. Bupropion: a review of its use in the management of smoking cessation. Drugs 2003;59:1007–24.
70. Peloso PM, Baillie C. Serum sickness-like reaction with bupropion [letter]. JAMA 1999;282:1817.
71. Lineberry TW, Peters GE Jr, Bostwick JM. Bupropion-induced erythema multiforme. Mayo Clin Proc 2001;76:664–6.
72. Crunelle CL, Miller ML, Booij J, et al. The nicotinic acetylcholine receptor partial agonist varenicline and the treatment of drug dependence: a review. Eur Neuropsychopharmacol 2010;20:69–79.
73. Coe JW, Brooks PR, Vetelino MG, et al. Varenicline: an alpha4beta2 nicotinic receptor partial agonist for smoking cessation. J Med Chem 2005;48:3474–7.
74. Cahill K, Stead L, Lancaster T. A preliminary benefit-risk assessment of varenicline in smoking cessation. Drug Saf 2009;32:119–35.
75. Rao J, Shankar PK. Varenicline: for smoking cessation. Kathmandu Univ Med J (KUMJ) 2009;7:162–4.
76. Foulds J. The neurobiological basis for partial agonist treatment of nicotinic dependence: varenicline. Int J Clin Pract 2006;60:571–6.
77. Coleman T. Recommendations for the use of pharmacological smoking cessation strategies in pregnant women. CNS Drugs 2007;21:983–93.
78. Tonstad S, Rollema H. Varenicline in smoking cessation. Expert Rev Respir Med 2010;4(3):291–9 Health Reference Center Academic. Wed. 18 Oct 2010.
79. Jorenby DE, Taylor H, Rigotti NA, et al. Efficacy of varenicline, an α4β2 nicotinic acetylcholine receptor partial agonist, vs placebo or sustained-release bupropion for smoking cessation. JAMA 2006;296:56–63.
80. Gonzales D, Rennard SI, Nides M, et al. Varenicline, an α4β2 nicotinic acetylcholine receptor partial agonist, vs placebo or sustained release bupropion for smoking cessation. JAMA 2006;296(1):47–55.
81. Aubin H-J, Bobak A, Britton JR, et al. Varenicline versus transdermal nicotine patch for smoking cessation: results from a randomized open-label trial. Thorax 2008;63:717–24.
82. Hays JT, Ebbert JO. Varenicline for tobacco dependence. N Engl J Med 2008; 359:20182024.
83. Keating FM, Leyseng-Williamson KA. Varenicline: a pharmacoeconomic review of its use as an aid to smoking cessation. Pharmacoeconomics 2010;28:231–54.
84. Center for Drug Evaluation and Research. Varenicline (marketed as Chantix) information: FDA alert. Rockville (MD): food and Drug Administration; 2008.

Controversies in the Management of Placenta Accreta

Luis D. Pacheco, MD[a,b,*], Alfredo F. Gei, MD[c]

KEYWORDS

• Pregnancy • Hemorrhage • Placenta accreta • Transfusion

Hemorrhagic shock is the most common form of shock encountered in common obstetric practice. In 2005, in the United States, hemorrhage was the third leading cause of maternal death due to obstetric factors.[1]

Historically, the most frequent indication for a peripartum hysterectomy has been uterine atony. Recent literature suggests that this is not the case anymore, with abnormal placentation becoming the most common condition requiring such operation.[2,3] The incidence of placenta accreta is estimated at 1 in 533 pregnancies.[4] With the currently increasing cesarean section rate, as well as a decrease in vaginal birth after cesarean section, this number is likely to increase in the near future.

In this article, the authors address some of the controversies surrounding the diagnosis and treatment of placental accreta. The term placenta accreta will be used to include all variants of the disease (accreta, increta, percreta).

WHICH IMAGING MODALITIES ARE NECESSARY FOR THE DIAGNOSIS OF PLACENTA ACCRETA?

In the vast majority of cases, placenta accreta may be diagnosed on the basis of ultrasound alone. Sonographic findings suggestive of accretism include the presence of placental lacunae giving a Swiss cheese appearance, loss of the normal retroplacental

The authors have nothing to disclose.

[a] Division of Maternal Fetal Medicine, Department of Obstetrics & Gynecology, The University of Texas Medical Branch at Galveston, 3400 John Sealy Annexure, 301 University Boulevard, Galveston, TX 77555-0587, USA

[b] Division of Surgical Critical Care, Department of Anesthesiology, The University of Texas Medical Branch at Galveston, 3400 John Sealy Annexure, 301 University Boulevard, Galveston, TX 77555-0587, USA

[c] Division of Maternal Fetal Medicine, Department of Obstetrics and Gynecology, The Methodist Hospital, 6550 Fannin, Suite 901, Smith Tower, Houston, TX 77025, USA

* Corresponding author. Division of Surgical Critical Care, Department of Anesthesiology, The University of Texas Medical Branch at Galveston, 301 University Boulevard, Galveston, TX 77555-0587.

E-mail address: ldpachec@utmb.edu

hypoechoic space, and increased vascularity with uterine wall vessel invasion as noted by the use of color Doppler.

In recent years, there has been increased interest in magnetic resonance imaging (MRI) for the evaluation of patients with suspected placenta accreta since it can provide information on depth of invasion and may be particularly useful in the diagnosis of posteriorly located placentas.[5] MRI findings suggestive of placenta accreta include lower uterine bulging, heterogeneous placenta, and dark intraplacental linear bands on T2-weighted images.[6]

In a multicenter historical cohort study, Dwyer and colleagues[7] compared the accuracy of both ultrasound and MRI in the diagnosis of placental accretism. The sensitivities for the diagnosis of placenta accreta for ultrasound and MRI were 93% and 80%, respectively. Specificities (negative study in the absence of the condition) were 71% and 65%, respectively. Neither difference achieved statistical significance. The accuracy for the diagnosis may be increased by complementing the abdominal ultrasound with transvaginal sonography.[7]

The use of paramagnetic contrast media in MRI (gadolinium) likely would improve the diagnostic performance of MRI; however, the agent crosses the placenta, and the effects on the fetus are unknown.

At present, it appears that the diagnostic abilities of both ultrasound and MRI are similar. In cases where the diagnosis is unclear, MRI and ultrasound may be used as complementary tests.

In patients with suspected placenta percreta, the authors recommend a complementary MRI to better define the extent to adjacent organs (eg, bladder, bowel) so that appropriate preoperative planning may be undertaken (eg, placement of ureteral stents).

HOW IS PRENATAL CARE DIFFERENT IN THE PATIENT WITH PLACENTA ACCRETA?

Once the diagnosis is established, patients should receive iron or folic acid as needed to maintain normal hemoglobin values. Occasionally, patients may require recombinant erythropoietin as adjuvant therapy. Patients should ideally be referred to a center with capacities to care for them. Such centers should have a multidisciplinary team available including maternal fetal medicine, general surgery, urology, vascular surgery, interventional radiology, blood bank, and neonatology.

Recent evidence questions the need for serial fetal growth ultrasounds in the setting of placenta previa without accretism, as this does not increase the risk of intrauterine growth restriction.[8] In the setting of suspected accretism, however, the authors recommend sonographic follow up every 3 to 4 weeks to evaluate placental location, depth of invasion, and fetal growth.

Occasionally, patients may benefit from preoperative autologous blood donation. Patients will donate units of their own blood during pregnancy, and such products will be stored in the blood bank and used on the day of the surgery. Theoretically, the hemoglobin will recover (patients will be on iron supplements) between donations.[9] In practice, however, anemia is a limiting factor, and patients usually may only donate a limited number of units throughout pregnancy. This technique will not prevent the risks associated with blood collection, storage, and administration, and is not acceptable for Jehovah's Witnesses.[9] Overall, the technique is not cost-effective and is recommended only for patients with rare blood types or alloimmunization to rare antibodies, for whom immediate availability of allogeneic blood products is foreseen to be difficult.[9]

Timing of delivery is a controversial subject. A recent decision analytical model suggested that delivery at 34 weeks of gestation may be optimal and that amniocentesis for determination of fetal lung maturity does not improve outcomes and is not recommended.[10] Advanced planning and interdisciplinary collaboration are fundamental, and as gestational age increases, so does the risk of emergent bleeding. The authors concur with the latter recommendation; patients with suspected accretism should be delivered between 34 and 37 weeks. Recent evidence suggests that patients with placenta previa and a cervical length less than 30 mm have a higher risk of acute hemorrhage.[11] If debate exists on whether to deliver at 34 weeks or a couple of weeks later (no later than 37 weeks), clinicians may consider obtaining a cervical length by transvaginal ultrasound. If the cervix is less than 30 mm and the gestational age more than 34 weeks, the authors favor delivery as opposed to waiting a few more weeks to prevent emergent bleeding and emergent deliveries.

WHICH PREOPERATIVE INTERVENTIONS ARE BENEFICIAL FOR PATIENTS WITH SUSPECTED ACCRETISM TO DECREASE TRANSFUSION NEEDS?

Acute normovolemic hemodilution (ANH) may be undertaken in the operative room before starting the case. A central line is placed, and blood is collected from the patient into citrated blood bags from the blood bank. Patients should have both a hemoglobin level above10 gr/dL and no history of cardiovascular disease. On average, 500 to 1000 mL of whole blood may be collected, and the patient will receive either colloid (1:1 ratio) or crystalloid (3:1 ratio) to maintain hemodynamics. Once surgical bleeding is controlled, the patient will receive the blood previously collected so that a smaller amount of red cells are lost during the acute bleeding episode. The collected blood may be stored at room temperature for up to 6 hours.[9] This technique is acceptable for some Jehovah's Witnesses as long as the collection bag is connected to the central venous line at all times (avoid circuit disconnections). Overall, there is minimal evidence to suggest that ANH alone spares significant amounts of allogeneic blood.[9]

Preoperative bilateral common iliac artery balloon catheter placement with inflation after delivery of the fetus has been reported in the literature. Theoretically, balloon inflation leads to bilateral vessel occlusion, limiting total blood loss. The efficacy of the latter approach has been questioned.[12,13] Another option described involves preoperative placement of femoral access by interventional radiology with selective embolization of uterine vessels at the time of delivery using polyvinyl alcohol, gel, foam, or coils.[14]

In the authors' institution, the use of balloon occlusion catheters in the pelvic circulation did not reduce transfusion requirements compared with historic controls.[15] The authors do not use this technique.

WHAT IS THE OPTIMAL ANESTHETIC TECHNIQUE FOR PATIENTS WITH PLACENTAL ACCRETISM?

When massive blood loss is expected, a complete sympathectomy (eg, spinal anesthesia) could impair the patient's ability to cope with sudden hypovolemia, as the capacity to vasoconstrict and increase systemic vascular resistances will be limited. However, regional anesthesia with a continuous epidural technique is safe and may be appropriate for patients with placental accretism. Emergent situations with active bleeding may be better served with general anesthesia.

CAN THE CELL SAVER BE USED IN THESE CASES?

Intraoperative cell salvage has been used successfully in obstetric hemorrhage. Blood is aspirated from the surgical field and filtered into a collecting reservoir. Filters in the device will remove molecules like tissue factor, alpha fetoprotein, platelets, and circulating procoagulants.[16] After filtration, packed red cells with a hematocrit of 55% to 80% will be obtained and may be readministered to the patient.

Patients who are Rh negative should receive anti-D immunoglobulin as soon as possible with a dose given according to results of a Kleihauer Betke stain to prevent alloimmunization.[9] This step is necessary, since the filters will not remove fetal red blood cells that are aspirated from the surgical field. A theoretical concern with the use of the cell saver in obstetrics is the occurrence of iatrogenic amniotic fluid embolism (AFE), since small amounts of amniotic fluid will bypass the filters of the device and be present in the packed red cells. However, more than 400 cases of cell saver use in obstetrics have been published, and no evidence of iatrogenic AFE exists. This technique is safe and effective in obstetric cases where massive blood loss is expected.[17]

IS THERE A ROLE FOR CONSERVATIVE TREATMENT IN PLACENTAL ACCRETISM?

The definite treatment for placental accretism is cesarean hysterectomy, ideally without attempts to remove the placenta.[14] In cases in which the placenta has been distorted and massive hemorrhage ensues, the authors do not recommend attempts for conservative measures, as delays in definite treatment (hysterectomy) may seriously compromise maternal hemodynamics. Patients with no interest in future childbearing likely will also benefit from hysterectomy without delay. In selected cases, including women who desire to have more children or cases with placenta percreta invading adjacent organs (eg, bladder, ureter, bowel), a conservative approach may be attempted.[18] Different techniques have been described. In cases involving only focal accretism found incidentally at the time of surgery, attempts to place local haemostatic sutures may control bleeding after placental removal. Alternatively, the placenta may be partially left in situ. When a conservative approach is attempted, a vertical incision in the skin is recommended to facilitate a high uterine incision (sometimes even fundal or posterior) that avoids the placenta.[19] Once the baby is delivered, if no active hemorrhage is noted, the uterine incision may be closed and the placenta left in situ. The main complications associated with conservative management are delayed bleeding requiring either hysterectomy or curettage and sepsis. In a recent series of 167 patients with placenta accreta, conservative management was successful in 78.4% of the cases. Severe maternal morbidity occurred in 6% of cases.[18] No convincing evidence exists to use adjuvant methotrexate, and the authors do not recommend it. The conservative approach may be combined with administration of uterotonics, intraoperative uterine devascularization, or pelvic arterial embolization by interventional radiology. The use of prophylactic antibiotics may be considered, despite lack of clinical data. These patients should be followed closely, as postpartum hemorrhage may happen up to 105 days after the initial procedure.[18] No guidelines exist regarding the optimal postdelivery follow-up of patients treated with this approach. The authors recommend serial ultrasounds to assess placental involution and frequent visits to screen for delayed hemorrhage and early signs of sepsis.

IS THERE A ROLE FOR THE USE OF RECOMBINANT FACTOR VII A?

Recombinant factor VII a (rFVIIa) is licensed for use in patients with hemophilia and inhibitory alloantibodies.[20] It is increasingly being used for off-license indications, including trauma, heart surgery after cardiopulmonary bypass, vascular surgery, warfarin reversal, and obstetric hemorrhage. More than 75% of level 1 trauma centers in the United States recommend the use of rFVIIa in their massive transfusion protocols.

Once endothelial injury has occurred, subendothelial collagen and tissue factor are exposed to the circulation. Factor VII (endogenous and exogenously administered) will bind to tissue factor and activate the clotting cascade, leading to local fibrin deposition. Systemically, rFVIIa will also bind activated platelets, leading to fibrin formation away from the site of injury. Despite having a very short half-life (2–6 hours), concerns about thromboembolism as a complication are real. rFVIIa is not a first-line treatment for bleeding, and it will only be effective once major sources of bleeding have been controlled. The use of this product should be combined with best practice use of blood products.[21] Prior to administration, the patient should ideally have a platelet count greater than 50,000/mm^3, fibrinogen greater than 50 to 100 mg/dL, temperature greater than 32°C, pH greater than 7.2, and normal ionized calcium.[21] The latter will facilitate adequate functioning of the clotting cascade.

Seventeen randomized controlled trials have been reported in different subgroups of patients in which rFVIIa was used to control hemorrhage. Four of them found a reduction in transfusion requirements or blood loss, and none reported a survival benefit.[22] Overall, it looks like rFVIIa is effective in limiting the amount of blood products transfused, but data on survival benefit are lacking.

The obstetric literature has numerous case reports and case series involving the use of this product. Publication bias is a major concern, and the authors are not aware of any published randomized trials involving rFVIIa in obstetric practice. The optimal dose is still unknown. Many reports in obstetric hemorrhage have used a dose of 90 μg/kg. If used in cases of placenta accreta, the authors recommend aggressive postpartum deep venous thrombosis prophylaxis once the bleeding risk is considered to be low.

WHICH MECHANISMS LEAD TO ACUTE COAGULOPATHY?

Classically, hemorrhage resuscitation has been centered on administration of crystalloids and packed red blood cells (PRBC). Use of other blood products, like fresh frozen plasma, cryoprecipitates, and platelets, is indicated if laboratory values are abnormal (eg, platelet count <50,000/mm^3, fibrinogen <100 mg/dL, prothrombin time [PT] or activated partial thromboplastin time [aPTT >1.5 × normal). These current transfusion guidelines fail to prevent coagulopathy in massive bleedings.[23] Patients with crystalloid/PRBC-based resuscitation will frequently develop dilution of clotting factors and platelets, leading to the so called dilutional coagulopathy. The latter may be complicated by hypothermia and acidosis, both of which lead to coagulation dysfunction.

Massive crystalloid resuscitation may actually worsen bleeding before achieving surgical control of hemorrhage due to increases in intravascular hydrostatic pressures and dislodgement of fresh clots in sites of endothelial injury.[24]

Recent evidence has shown that early coagulopathy may occur before hemodilution and before consumption of clotting factors takes place. This mechanism of early coagulopathy has mainly been studied in trauma; however, obstetric hemorrhage may share some of the mechanisms involved.[24] Early tissue hypoperfusion leads to endothelial upregulation of the receptor thrombomodulin. This receptor interacts with thrombin, leading to activation of the protein C pathway. Protein C is a natural anticoagulant that will irreversibly inhibit factors Va and VIIIa and also enhance fibrinolysis through inhibition of plasminogen activator inhibitor 1.[25] Increased fibrinolytic activity has been described in obstetric hemorrhage secondary to uterine atony, placental abruption, and accretism.[24] These new mechanisms of coagulopathy have challenged the current resuscitation guidelines, suggesting that early clotting factor replacement and early identification of excessive fibrinolysis could be associated with improved outcomes.

WHAT IS HEMOSTATIC RESUSCITATION, AND DOES IT IMPROVE OUTCOMES?

Hemostatic resuscitation is a new concept that mainly involves 3 aspects:

1. Limited early aggressive use of crystalloids and consideration of permissive hypotension
2. Early administration of fresh frozen plasma and platelets (with concomitant packed red blood cells) achieving a ratio of 1:1:1
3. Early use of rFVIIa.

Aggressive crystalloid resuscitation is avoided to prevent hemodilution and early clot dislodgement secondary to increases in blood pressure as a result of volume expansion. Prior to surgical control of hemorrhage, permissive hypotension with systolic blood pressures between 80 and 100 mmHg may be optimal to limit ongoing blood loss.[24] Permissive hypotension may be considered in patients with postpartum hemorrhage; however, no data are available during the antenatal period, as uterine perfusion pressure may be compromised.

As previously discussed, resuscitation based on crystalloid and PRBC often only leads to dilutional coagulopathy. Haemostatic resuscitation involves the early administration of fresh frozen plasma and platelets with PRBC in a ratio of 1:1:1. The latter approach prevents the early development of coagulopathy. Retrospective military and civilian papers have demonstrated overall absolute mortality reductions of 15% to 62% with the use of higher ratios of FFP:PRBC.[26] A significant limitation of the available literature on this topic is the presence of survival bias. On average, the median time to obtaining the first unit of PRBC is 18 minutes, as opposed to more than 1 hour for fresh frozen plasma (needs to be thawed).[27] Sicker patients will likely die before availability of fresh frozen plasma, while less sick patients will survive to the moment when fresh frozen plasma is available. The latter may explain why patients with high FFP:PRBC ratios had better survival. A few studies have specifically addressed the survivorship bias in high FFP:RBC studies. When early deaths were excluded, no survival benefit for higher ratios was noted.[28] Prospective trials are required to validate the benefit of early fresh frozen plasma administration. Despite the lack of prospective data, many centers in the United States have adopted massive transfusion protocols involving the use of high FFP:PRBC ratios and early use of rFVIIa. These massive transfusion protocols are frequently used in massive obstetric hemorrhage.

Administration of large amounts of blood products could lead to a higher incidence of transfusion-related acute lung injury (TRALI) and transfusion-related immunomodulation (TRIM).[29] Others suggest the opposite, with the rationale that early administration of fresh frozen plasma and platelets achieves hemostasis earlier, thus decreasing the total number of blood products given.[23]

HOW CAN HEMOSTASIS BE MONITORED?

Conventional plasma-based coagulation analyses like the PT, aPTT, and international normalized ratio (INR) are poor predictors for transfusion requirements and are unable to identify specific coagulation anomalies.[30] The thromboelastograph (TEG) is an easy test that provides information regarding the specific component of the coagulation process that may be affected. It can easily be performed at the bedside. A small amount of blood is placed into a cuvette, and the blood is stirred with an agitator connected to a strain gauge. As the movement of the agitator is inhibited, the strain gauge depicts a graphic representation of the strength of the clot. **Fig. 1.** depicts the main components of the TEG. Both the reaction time/clotting time and the alpha angle reflect the activity of clotting factors. Once the clot is formed, the maximum amplitude correlates with platelet function. Lastly, the velocity at which the amplitude decreases correlates with fibrinolytic activity. Obstetric hemorrhage often has a significant component of enhanced fibrinolysis. Conventional clotting tests will fail to identify such anomaly, while the TEG may easily detect it, leading to a change in management where antifibrinolytic agents like tranhexamic acid or epsilon aminocaproic acid should be administered. Where available, the authors recommend the use of the TEG to guide transfusion therapy.

WHAT IS ABDOMINAL COMPARTMENT SYNDROME?

In cases where massive resuscitation takes place, several factors may contribute to increase the pressure in the abdominal compartment. Any space-occupying mass, like a hematoma, will increase intra-abdominal pressure. Both crystalloid and colloid administration lead to third spacing of fluid (crystalloid will third space earlier than colloid). Consequently, bowel edema and ascitis may ensue. Extensive surgical procedures are commonly associated with ileus, which may also favor intra-abdominal hypertension. Put together, all these factors may increase the intra-abdominal pressure to a point where compression of the abdominal and retroperitoneal vessels will compromise preload to the heart, leading to a drop in cardiac output and, consequently, in blood pressure. Another important component of this syndrome is oliguria, as the kidney is poorly perfused not only due to compromised cardiac output, but also due to compression by the increased extravascular pressure, leading to a decrease in the gradient of perfusion. Cephalad displacement of the diaphragm leads to bibasal atelectacies, with more right-to-left shunt and consequent hypoxemia. Patients on mechanical ventilators will display sudden increases in airway pressures. Central vascular pressure (central venous pressures or pulmonary pressures recorded by

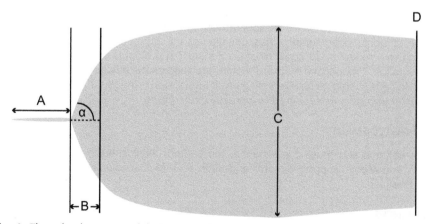

Fig. 1. Thromboelastogram. (A) Corresponds to the reaction time. (B) Indicates clotting time. A, B, and the α angle reflect the function of clotting factors. In cases of clotting factor deficiency, both times will be prolonged. (C) The maximum amplitude of the clot, and it correlates with platelet function. The amplitude is proportional to platelet function. (D) Indicates fibrinolysis. Cases of hyperfibrinolysis will show rapid resolution of the clot, giving a teardrop appearance.

means of a pulmonary artery catheter) will also be elevated, as the intrathoracic pressure rises secondarily to the upward displacement of the diaphragm.

Obstetricians need to be familiar with this complication, as the administration of more fluid in an attempt to increase blood pressure and urine output will only worsen intra-abdominal pressures and hemodynamics. If the condition is suspected, a bladder pressure should be obtained at the bedside as a surrogate of abdominal pressure.[31] Bladder pressure should be measured with the patient in the supine position and the bladder distended with 25 mL of saline after the urinary catheter has been clamped.[31] Normal abdominal pressures are 0 to 10 mm Hg. Abdominal hypertension is defined as an intra-cavitary pressure greater than 12 mm Hg. Finally, abdominal compartment syndrome includes a pressure greater than 20 mm Hg and at least 1 organ compromised.[31]

Normal values of intra-abdominal pressure in the postpartum period are not known. A recent publication involving women after a cesarean section found mean intra-abdominal pressures of 6.4 plus or minus 5.2 mm Hg. Interestingly, and likely due to higher risk of third spacing, patients with a cesarean section and preeclampsia had mean values of 11 plus or minus 9 mm Hg.[32]

Once the diagnosis is established, most patients will require surgical decompression, and the open abdomen may be managed with a vacuum-assisted closure or a Bogota bag or silo.[31] Enteral feeding and limitation of fluid therapy are beneficial. If fluids are required, the use of colloids (eg, albumin) is recommended over crystalloids. Limited evidence suggests that temporal use of paralytic agents while the abdomen is open may help achieve primary fascial closure.[33]

SUMMARY

Obstetric hemorrhage is one of the most common causes of maternal morbidity and mortality worldwide. Abnormal placentation, including placenta accreta, is currently the most common indication for peripartum hysterectomy. Prenatal identification of these cases and early referral to centers with the capability to manage them will likely result in improved outcomes. Interventions that may limit transfusion requirements include normovolemic hemodilution, selective embolization of pelvic vessels by interventional radiology, conservative management of accretism in a few selected cases, and the use of the cell saver intraoperatively. Current understanding of the mechanisms of acute coagulopathy has questioned the current transfusion guidelines, leading to a tendency to apply massive transfusion protocols based on hemostatic resuscitation. Prospective trials are required to validate the efficacy of this approach. Obstetricians should be familiar with current transfusion protocols, as the incidence of placental accretism is expected to increase in the future.

ACKNOWLEDGMENTS

For editorial and graphic assistance, the authors thank the Ob/Gyn Publication, Grant, and Media Support director and staff: R.G. McConnell, LeAnne Garcia, and Alan Sheffield.

REFERENCES

1. Kung HC, Hoy DL, Murphy SL. Deaths: final data for 2005. Hyattsville (MD): National Center for Health Statistics; 2008.
2. Kwee A, Bots ML, Visser GH, et al. Emergency peripartum hysterectomy: a prospective study in The Netherlands. Eur J Obstet Gynecol Reprod Biol 2006;124:187–92.

3. Smith J, Mousa HA. Peripartum hysterectomy for primary postpartum haemorrhage: incidence and maternal morbidity. J Obstet Gynaecol 2007;27:44–7.

4. Wu S, Kocherginsky M, Hibbard JU. Abnormal placentation: twenty-year analysis. Am J Obstet Gynecol 2005;192:1458–61.

5. Baughman WC, Corteville JE, Shah RR. Placenta accreta: spectrum of US and MR imaging findings. Radiographics 2008;28(7):1905–16.

6. Teo TH, Law YM, Tay KH, et al. Use of magnetic resonance imaging in evaluation of placental invasion. Clin Radiol 2009;64(5):511–6.

7. Dwyer BK, Belogolovkin V, Tran L, et al. Prenatal diagnosis of placenta accreta: sonography or magnetic resonance imaging? J Ultrasound Med 2008;27(9):1275–81.

8. Harper LM, Odibo MO, Macones GA, et al. Effect of placenta previa on fetal growth. Am J Obstet Gynecol 2010;203(4):330.e1–5.

9. Catling S. Blood conservation techniques in obstetrics: a UK perspective. Int J Obstet Anesth 2007;16:241–9.

10. Robinson BK, Grobman WA. Effectiveness of timing strategies for delivery of individuals with placenta previa and accreta. Obstet Gynecol 2010;116(4):835–42.

11. Stafford IA, Dashe JS, Shivvers SA, et al. Ultrasonographic cervical length and risk of hemorrhage in pregnancies with placenta previa. Obstet Gynecol 2010;116(3):595–600.

12. Levine AB, Kuhlman K, Bonn J. Placenta accreta: a comparison of cases managed with and without pelvic artery balloon catheters. J Matern Fetal Med 1999;8:173–6.

13. Mok M, Heidemann B, Dundas K, et al. Interventional radiology in women with suspected placenta accreta undergoing cesarean section. Int J Obstet Anesth 2008;17:255–61.

14. Angstmann T, Gard G, Harrington T, et al. Surgical management of placenta accreta: a cohort series and suggested approach. Am J Obstet Gynecol 2010;202:38.e1–9.

15. Zacharias N, Gei AF, Suarez V, et al. Balloon tip catheter occlusion of the hypogastric arteries for the management of placenta accreta. Am J Obstet Gynecol 2003;189(6):S128.

16. Tawes RL Jr. Clinical applications of autotransfusion. Semin Vasc Surg 1994;7:89–90.

17. Rainaldi MP, Tazzari PL, Seagliarini G, et al. Blood salvage during cesarean section. Br J Anaesth 1998;80:196–8.

18. Sentilhes L, Ambroselli C, Kayem G, et al. Maternal outcome after conservative treatment of placenta accreta. Obstet Gynecol 2010;115(3):526–34.

19. Wright JD, Bonanno C, Shah M, et al. Peripartum hysterectomy. Obstet Gynecol 2010;116(2):429–34.

20. Stanworth SJ, Birchall J, Doree CJ, et al. Recombinant factor VIIa for the prevention and treatment of bleeding in patients without haemophilia. Cochrane Database Syst Rev 2007;2:CD005011.

21. Spahn DR, Cerny V, Coats TJ, et al. Management of bleeding following major trauma: a European guideline. Crit Care 2007;11(1):R17.

22. Johansson PI, Ostrowski SR, Secher NH. Management of major blood loss: an update. Acta Anaesthesiol Scand 2010;54:1039–49.

23. Nascimento B, Callum J, Rubenfeld G, et al. Clinical review: fresh frozen plasma in massive bleedings-more questions than answers. Crit Care 2010;14:2002.

24. Brigitte E. Fluid and blood transfusion management in obstetrics. Eur J Anaesthesiol 2010;27(12):1031–5.

25. Brohi K, Cohen MJ, Davenport RA. Acute coagulopathy of trauma: mechanism, identification, and effect. Curr Opin Crit Care 2007;13:680–5.

26. Cotton BA, Gunter OL, Isbell J, et al. Damage control hematology: the impact of a trauma exsanguination protocol on survival and blood product utilization. J Trauma 2008;64:1177–82.

27. Snyder CW, Weinberg JA, McGwin G, et al. The relationship of blood product ratio to mortality: survival benefit or survival bias? J Trauma 2009;66:358–62.

28. Scalea TM, Bochicchio KM, Lumpkins K, et al. Early aggressive use of fresh frozen plasma does not improve outcome in critically injured trauma patients. Ann Surg 2008;248:578–84.

29. Gonzalez EA, Moore FA, Halcomb JB, et al. Fresh frozen plasma should be given earlier to patients requiring massive transfusion. J Trauma 2007;62:112–9.

30. Reikvam H, Steien E, Hauge B, et al. Thromboelastography. Transfus Apher Sci 2009;40:119–23.

31. Cheatham ML. Abdominal compartment syndrome. Curr Opin Crit Care 2009; 15(2):154–62.

32. Abdel-Razeq SS, Campbell K, Funai EF, et al. Normative postpartum intra-abdominal pressure: potential implications in the diagnosis of abdominal compartment syndrome. Am J Obstet Gynecol 2010;203(2):149, e1–4.

33. Abouassaly CT, Dutton WD, Zaydfudim V, et al. Postoperative neuromuscular blocker use is associated with higher primary fascial closure rates after damage control laparotomy. J Trauma 2010;69(3):557–61.

Operative Vaginal Deliveries: Practical Aspects

Alfredo F. Gei, MD[a],*, Luis D. Pacheco, MD[b,c]

KEYWORDS

• Operative vaginal delivery • Instrumental deliveries
• Forceps • Vacuum

Human delivery is not an easy process.[1] Women have delivered for thousands of years with various degrees of assistance from fellow human beings. From an anthropological point of view, the essence of our specialty (the assistance of the delivering mother) seems to be one of the social behaviors that differentiate humans from other animal species.[1]

Forceps, vacuum, and cesarean section (CS) are relatively recent additions to the obstetrician's armamentarium.[2] As new tools and advances in the field become available and as we refine our knowledge of which interventions are beneficial and which are harmful and to whom, the role of our tools has evolved. The art of modern obstetrics is one that mandates from obstetricians the attentive vigilance of the development of natural processes and an active intervention when such processes fall outside normally accepted standards. What constitutes the "normal process" and the "accepted standard" is subject to discussion, and international variations in obstetric practice are in part the reflection of such controversies.[2]

The declining trend of instrumented deliveries in the second stage of labor contrasted with an increasing number of CSs continues to fuel the perception that instruments are potentially harmful for fetuses and mothers, and that a cesarean delivery is preferable in most circumstances.[3] The decrease in the number of physicians with the training and required skill to perform these procedures as well as fear of litigation compounds the problem of declining instrumental use even further.[3–6]

In this article we present a practical approach to the contemporary issue of instrumental deliveries, outlining, when available, the supporting evidence for their

[a] Division of Maternal-Fetal Medicine, Department of Obstetrics and Gynecology, The Methodist Hospital of Houston, Smith tower 6550 Fannin, Suite 901, Houston, TX 77025, USA
[b] Division of Maternal Fetal Medicine, Department of Obstetrics & Gynecology, University of Texas Medical Branch at Galveston, 3400 John Sealy Annexure, 301 University Boulevard, Galveston, TX 77555-0587, USA
[c] Division of Surgical Critical Care, Department of Anesthesiology, University of Texas Medical Branch at Galveston, 3400 John Sealy Annexure, 301 University Boulevard, Galveston, TX 77555-0587, USA
* Corresponding author.
E-mail address: agei@tmhs.org

Obstet Gynecol Clin N Am 38 (2011) 323–349
doi:10.1016/j.ogc.2011.03.002
0889-8545/11/$ – see front matter © 2011 Elsevier Inc. All rights reserved.

obgyn.theclinics.com

recommendations, and the most current position of professional colleges in obstetrics and gynecology.

DO WE STILL NEED INSTRUMENTS FOR DELIVERY? CAN OBSTETRICS DO WITHOUT THEM?

Most women wish to have a spontaneous vaginal delivery.[7] Yet in the countries included in **Table 1**, 1 in 3 women will face an operative delivery and 1 in 9 an assisted vaginal delivery.[8–13] Given the current lack of patient popularity of prophylactically assisted vaginal deliveries and of elective shortenings of the second stage, most of these procedures have presumably a medical (maternal, obstetric, or fetal) indication.[2]

The various rates of operative vaginal deliveries (OVDs) and CSs suggest that the approach to similar clinical situations is radically different among specialists of different latitudes, resulting in different behaviors and obstetric interventions.[14] These national differences have also been observed within different regions of several countries.[15,16]

With the rationale that an unplanned operative delivery may have major physical and psychological sequelae and affect the mother and her child, even if physical trauma does not occur, if it was possible to predict emergency operative deliveries one might consider offering women a CS instead.[17] Identification of antenatal risk factors for such intervention would hold promise in terms of reducing somatic and psychological trauma as well as the cost of service delivery, especially in primigravid women.[18]

Unfortunately, although multiple clinical factors have been associated with an increased risk of a CS or even an OVD, our means of predicting different outcomes of labor (spontaneous vaginal delivery [SVD], CS, or OVD) are not sufficiently powerful to allow modification of current obstetric practice,[17,19] adding to the uncertainty of which patients will undergo which delivery.

WHAT ARE THEIR USES?

Forceps and obstetric vacuums are employed to assist a vaginal delivery for their potential to do 3 things:

1. Increase the expelling force (adding or replacing the maternal expelling forces)
2. Decrease the resistance force of the maternal birthing canal by modifying the perimeter of the fetal head (correction of malpositions, asynclitism, and deflection)
3. Decrease the resistance of the birthing canal by increasing the perimeter of the soft pelvis (in the case of forceps).[20,21]

Table 1
Prevalence of assisted delivery in selected countries by total number of deliveries (shown as percentages)

	Vacuum-Assisted Deliveries (%)	Forceps-Assisted Deliveries (%)	Cesarean Deliveries (%)	Total Assisted Deliveries (%)	Births (year)	Ref.
Scotland	3.3	9.7	26.1	39.1	57,945 (2009)	8
Ireland	12	4	25.0	39	71,963 (2007)	9
Canada	10.3	4.6	25.6	40.5	333,974 (2004)	10
Australia	7.5	3.6	30.9	42	289,496 (2007)	11
England	7.0	3.3	22.7	33.0	575,900 (2004)	12
USA	3.5	0.8	31.8	36.1	4,316,233 (2007)	13

Different professional societies propose different indications for the use of OVDs to its members (**Table 2**). It is imperative for the practitioner to have a clear understanding of the purpose of the OVD in each particular case. As a result of the mechanical actions of instruments, the authors favor the division of the reasons for an instrumented delivery into prophylactic (**Tables 3** and **4**) and therapeutic indications (**Box 1**), and furthermore, into maternal or fetal.

This classification allows for the appropriate planning and preparation of the particular procedure (eg, prophylactic outlet vacuum or forceps delivery for maternal cardiac disease vs a 90° rotation and delivery for a transverse arrest of descent). It also provides physicians with a simple framework to improve communication with expectant families eager for information regarding the need for assistance in their deliveries.[2]

Practical Tips

- It is central to the success of all OVDs for the obstetrician to diagnose, understand, and document the indication.
- It is important for the patient (and family) to understand the rationale for the use of instrument on her delivery.
- The preparations of the OVD should be concordant with the indications for the procedure.

WHERE TO DO THE DELIVERY?

There are no randomized controlled trials comparing a trial of instrumental vaginal delivery (vacuum extraction or forceps) with immediate CS in an operating room environment for women with failure to progress in the second stage of labor.[25]

The Royal College of Obstetricians and Gynaecologists (RCOG) recommends that considering that fetal injuries have been attributed to delay between a failed OVD and a CS and that higher rates of failure are anticipated in cases of maternal obesity, presumed fetal macrosomia, occipitoposterior (OP) positions of the fetal head, and midpelvic procedures, such deliveries should be performed as a trial of instrumental delivery in the setting of an operating room.[26]

Operative deliveries that are anticipated to have a higher rate of failure, therefore, should be considered a trial of labor and conducted in a place where immediate recourse to CS can be undertaken. The report by Lowe[27] recorded a 7-minute longer second stage of labor for 61 women of unexpected failed instrumental delivery compared with 47 women of failed instrumental delivery conducted as a trial of delivery in the operating theater, with full preparations in place to proceed to an immediate CS. In the study by Lowe involving only cases of dystocia without fetal distress, the rate of failed trial was 39%.[27,28]

There is little evidence of increased maternal or neonatal morbidity following failed OVD compared with immediate CS where immediate recourse to CS is available.[26,29]

According to Loudon and colleagues,[14] the chances of requiring a cesarean delivery in these circumstances is approximately 6%.

Recommendation

Operative vaginal births that have a higher rate of failure should be considered a trial and conducted in a place where an immediate recourse to CS can be undertaken.

Practical Tips

- The authors recommend the attempt at OVD to be performed in the operating room with a double setup for a possible CS if a rotation greater than 45° is

Table 2
Indications of operative vaginal deliveries

Indication	ACOG	RCOG	SOGC	RANZCOG
Fetal	Suspicion of imminent or potential fetal compromise	Presumed fetal compromise	Nonreassuring fetal status	Fetal compromise suspected or anticipated
Maternal/Medical	Shortening of the second stage for maternal benefit	Indications to avoid Valsalva Examples: • cardiac disease Class III or IV, • hypertensive crises, • cerebral vascular disease, • myasthenia gravis, • spinal cord injury	Medical indications to avoid Valsalva Examples: • cerebral vascular disease, • cardiac conditions	Maternal effort contraindicated Examples: • aneurysm, • risk of aortic dissection, • proliferative retinopathy, • severe hypertension, or • cardiac failure
Obstetric	Prolonged second stage: • Nulliparous women: lack of continuing progress for 3 h with regional anesthesia, or 2 h without regional anesthesia • Multiparous women: lack of continuing progress for 2 h with regional anesthesia, or 1 h without regional anesthesia	Inadequate progress: • Nulliparous women: lack of continuing progress for 3 h (total of active and passive second stage of labor) with regional anesthesia, or 2 h without regional anesthesia • Multiparous women: lack of continuing progress for 2 h (total of active and passive second-stage labor) with regional anesthesia, or 1 h without regional anesthesia • Maternal fatigue/exhaustion	Inadequate progress: • Adequate uterine activity documented • No evidence of cephalopelvic disproportion • Lack of effective maternal effort	Delay in the second stage of labor: There is no clear demarcation as to an appropriate length of time to wait before embarking on instrumental delivery for failure to progress It is a matter for the clinician and patient given the particular circumstance

Abbreviations: ACOG, American Congress of Obstetricians and Gynecologists; RANZCOG, Royal Australian and New Zealand College of Obstetricians and Gynaecologists; RCOG, Royal College of Obstetricians and Gynaecologists; SOGC, Society of Obstetricians and Gynaecologists of Canada.
Data from Refs.[21,26,45,47]

Table 3
Prophylactic indications of operative vaginal deliveries

Type of Indication	Purpose	Condition Treated	Examples
Maternal	Prevention of Valsalva maneuver and maternal decompensation	Cardiovascular diseases	• Class III–IV valvulopathies • Symptomatic cardiomyopathies • Active rheumatic or lupic pericarditis
	Prevention of Valsalva maneuver and potential rupture of aneurysms	Cerebrovascular abnormalities	• H/O subarachnoid bleeding • H/O berry aneurysms
	Prevention of Valsalva and worsening of hypoxemia	Respiratory diseases	• Severe asthma • Pulmonary fibrosis • COPD
Fetal	Prevention of IC hemorrhage in prematures[a]	Avoid sudden decompression of the fetal head	• Prematurity
	Prevention of head deflection and spinal trauma	Avoid head entrapment and cervical spine trauma	• Breech vaginal delivery

Abbreviations: COPD, chronic obstructive pulmonary disease; H/O, history of; IC, intracerebral.
[a] Controversial study results; an effect seems to be present for the prevention of late IC hemorrhages in a subset of infants less than 1500 g.

Table 4
Therapeutic indications of forceps-assisted deliveries

Purpose	Condition Treated	Examples
Correction of fetal head attitude	Abnormalities of fetal head: 1. Position 2. Flexion 3. Synclitism 4. Combinations of the above	• Transverse arrest of descent • Persistent occipitoposterior position • Face presentation (mentoanterior)
Addition to the extracting vector	Lack of pushing effort	• Maternal exhaustion • Psychomotor agitation (psychosis/drugs) • Spinal cord injuries
Addition to the extracting vector	Nonreassuring fetal status	• Fetal bradycardia • Intrapartum bleeding • Intrapartum cord prolapse
Addition to the extracting vector	Arrested delivery (with normal mechanism)	• Prolonged second stage • Arrest of descent
Replacement of extracting vector	Acute maternal compromise with or without fetal compromise	• Eclampsia intrapartum • Amniotic fluid embolism intrapartum • Abruptio placentae • Psychotic states (and general anesthesia)

Box 1
Vacuum versus forceps: some generalities

- Vacuum
  - Easier to apply
  - Slower delivery
  - More likely to result in scalp trauma
  - Associated with increased rates of intracranial trauma
  - Higher likelihood of failure
  - Not recommended under 34 weeks
- Forceps
  - More difficult to apply
  - Faster delivery
  - Increased maternal soft tissue trauma
  - More prone to potential injury
  - Requires better analgesia
  - May be used at any gestational age

Data from Refs.[22–24]

---

planned, a mid-pelvic procedure will be attempted, the fetus is large, or the electronic fetal monitoring is nonreassuring.
- An experienced operator or supervisor should be present for all attempts at rotational, mid-cavity, and trial of OVD.[26]
- Inform the patient, the family, and the delivering team (including anesthesia, nursing, and surgical technician) of the possibility of a safe and successful attempt at a vaginal delivery and of the possibility of a CS if the trial is deemed potentially traumatic or difficult, or does not succeed.

FORCEPS OR VACUUM?

Though frequently used interchangeably, forceps and vacuum denote both a rather large group of mechanically dissimilar instruments and the procedure of delivering fetuses with them. From the mechanical standpoint, forceps are modified clamps that grasp the fetal head and vacuums are pulling devices that attach to the fetus through the generation of a vacuum between a closed attaching system (cup) and the fetal head. Both types of instruments are applied to the fetus within the birth canal to assist in the extraction of the fetal head by replicating the natural mechanism of delivery.[2,20,30,31]

Experts often provide conflicting evidence for and against the use of these procedures.[21,30,31] The literature discussing the use of vacuum and forceps includes prospective randomized trials comparing the outcomes after forceps-assisted and vacuum-assisted births.[32–35] These trials do not use the same inclusion criteria or the same instruments, or look at the same outcomes, making comparison of the techniques difficult. Neonatal mortality and serious morbidity related to spontaneous vaginal birth, vacuum or forceps, or CS have also been reviewed in large retrospective studies.[36–41] None of these prospective or retrospective studies discuss specifics of the technique used for vacuum or forceps procedures, the time required, or the criteria for abandonment of the procedure.[21] In addition, the analysis of morbidities (particularly long-term) associated with the use of instruments is fraught with bias (selection/ascertainment/response/recall), lack of power to find true differences by route of delivery, lack of prepregnancy baseline data, lack of long-term follow-up, inconsistencies, unaddressed covariables, and an incomplete understanding of physiologic processes being evaluated.[42]

A meta-analysis of studies comparing the use of vacuum and forceps has suggested that a vacuum delivery is the method of choice for an instrumented delivery.[32]

Although vacuum deliveries are more likely to fail, the overall CS rate in the meta-analysis by Johnson and Menon is still lower when the vacuum device is used rather than forceps.[32,43] The reason for this is not entirely clear.[43] It may have to do with patient selection or with the fact that a failed vacuum-assisted delivery (VAD) was typically followed by an attempted forceps-assisted delivery (FAD) ("as a rescue"), whereas a failed FAD was more likely to be followed by a CS.[14,43] The latter hypothesis is favored by the recent study by Baskett and colleagues[44] on 1000 vacuum procedures. In Baskett's report the overall success of the vacuum assistance in achieving a vaginal delivery was 87.1%, with a significant difference between nulliparous (84.7%) and parous women (92.3%) ($P = .001$). In 9.8% of the cases where a vacuum was applied, the delivery was ultimately accomplished by forceps after an unsuccessful vacuum attempt. In this study an additional 2% of women had a CS after a failed vacuum procedure. As a result of the different failure rates in nulliparous versus parous women, the CS rate was significantly higher in nulliparous women who had a vacuum procedure ($P = .002$).[44]

In a 10-year analysis of operative deliveries during the second stage in two hospitals in the United Kingdom, Loudon and colleagues[14] noted a secular trend of increasing failure rates of OVDs, which was correlated with the increased failure rates of vacuums.

As far as morbidities, each type of instrument has a different profile of complications.[32,45,46] The generalities of the instruments and the patterns of morbidity tend to be consistent, and are outlined in **Box 1**.

The meta-analysis of FAD versus VAD is not able to resolve the issue according to the indication of the procedure: prophylactic versus therapeutic; nor according to the specific interventions required from its use: correction of malrotation, correction of asynclitism, correction of deflection, and/or replacement or addition to the expelling vectors. An additional confounding factor is related to the experience of the operators using the instruments. It becomes difficult to interpret a meta-analysis of forceps versus vacuum when it is not known whether the practitioners participating in the trials included are equally trained, equally inclined, and equally proficient in the use of one instrument versus another. Differences in training and proficiency with one instrument or the other can result in operator bias even in the most carefully conducted randomized trial.

Comments on the Available Evidence

The information available is of insufficient quality to recommend one instrument over the other in each specific case. Given an indication for OVD the choice of instruments depends of: the particular indication for the procedure, the anesthesia (in place or available), the availability of instruments, the training and experience of the obstetrician, and the preference of the patient.

Recommendations

The choice of intervention needs to be individualized, as one technique is not clearly safer or more effective than the other.[21] The clinician should select the instrument based on his or her clinical experience and the clinical circumstances.[45]

Practical Tips

Some clinical suggestions for the selection of instruments are included in **Box 2**.

HOW SHOULD WE USE INSTRUMENTS FOR DELIVERY?

Any medical intervention has the potential for additional morbidity and even mortality. The individual and social success of the assistance of the birthing process is the outcome of the healthiest mother and child. In cases of OVDs, a true failure is not when a vaginal delivery is not accomplished but when a preventable injury is inflicted.[27]

To substantiate the need of a medical procedure that may have maternal and neonatal implications, one needs to weigh the risks versus the benefits of the intervention with the patient or the couple. When an operative intervention is required in the second stage of labor, the options, risks, and benefits of vacuum, forceps, and CS must be considered and weighed up. Therefore an instrumented vaginal delivery deserves as much consideration, thought, and preparation as its alternative: the abdominal delivery. The safety and success of these procedures hinges on a systematic approach to the issue. The stepwise approach like the one proposed in **Box 3** and **Fig. 1** offers a rational use of the means of assisting a vaginal delivery. This guideline for clinical practice follows specific instructions to ensure not only that the procedure is performed under the right circumstances, but also sets its performance under conditions that would minimize the potential for maternal or fetal morbidity.[46]

Preliminary evidence shows that minimal changes in policy toward the preparation for an OVD may decrease not only its rates but also the incidence of traumatic births, with a relative increase in the number of trials of instrumental deliveries in the operating room and a relative decrease in the number of CSs performed for no progress of labor or during the second stage without a trial of forceps or vacuum.[48] Leung and colleagues[48] speculate that these changes were the result of operator improvement in performance, possibly resulting from the awareness of being evaluated, a phenomenon known as the "Hawthorne effect."

A careful adherence to clinical guidelines, conditions, and steps recommended could improve the outcome and decrease the potential for morbidity associated with the use of forceps.[49,50]

Recommendations

Operative vaginal delivery should not be attempted unless the criteria for safe delivery have been met (see **Boxes 4** and **5**).[26]

Practical Tips

- A clinical algorithm proposing a systematic approach to the potential need and performance of an OVD is included in **Fig. 1**.
- The indications, contraindications, prerequisites of use, appropriate steps in application (including abandonment of the procedure), and postpartum conduct are important steps in the clinical decision-making and execution of the procedure.

EPISIOTOMY OR NOT?

Routine episiotomy has not been demonstrated to be an effective way to shorten the second stage of labor.[21,51] The routine use of episiotomies has not been shown to decrease the duration of the second stage or the rates of shoulder dystocia associated

> **Box 2**
> **Clinical criteria for the selection of forceps instruments**
>
> - In principle, choose an instrument that will accomplish all the functions required for that case (avoidance of multiple instruments)
> - Other criteria:
>   - Primiparity: consider vacuum or a forceps with overlapping shanks to minimize vulvar distension
>   - Elliot forceps
>   - Tucker-McLane forceps
>   - Naegele forceps
>   - Indication
>   - Prophylactic:
>   - Rounded heads (ie, nonmolded) (vacuum or forceps with greater cephalic curvature):
>   - Tucker-McLane forceps
>   - Salas forceps
>   - Modeled heads (shallow vacuum cups or forceps with lesser cephalic curvature):
>   - Simpson forceps
>   - Elliot forceps
>   - Correction of asynclitism:
>   - Kielland forceps
>   - Luikart forceps
>   - Salinas forceps
>   - Salas forceps
>   - Correction of deflection:
>   - Any except for divergent forceps (Salinas, Salas, Laufe, Suzor)
>   - Correction of malrotation disorders of the fetal head:
>   - Kielland forceps
>   - Salinas forceps
>   - Salas forceps
>   - Leff forceps
>   - Luikart forceps (for smaller degrees of malrotation)
>   - Aftercoming head of breech presentation:
>   - Laufe forceps
>   - Piper forceps
>   - Kielland forceps

with OVD.[51,52] In a meta-analysis of the studies evaluating the routine use of episiotomy versus a restrictive policy for it, the restrictive policy was associated with more anterior vulvar trauma, but less posterior perineal trauma, less suturing, and fewer healing complications, and had no effect on severe perineal or vaginal trauma,

---

Box 3
Contraindications for the use of forceps

- Nonconsenting or uncooperative patient
- Patient and/or fetus with established hemorrhagic diathesis or at significant risk for it (including thrombocytopenias)
- Osteogenesis imperfecta
- Unengaged head
- Unknown position of the fetal head[a]
- Mid-transverse arrest with posterior asynclitism
- Dead fetus or known lethal anomaly in the fetus[b]

[a] Position of the head needs to be established if possible through the clinical palpation of both fontanelles. Although recently the use of ultrasound to diagnose position in cases of difficult ascertainment has been recommended, the presence of a large caput or bone overlap with obliteration of fontanelles is a clinical marker for difficulty of the procedure.
[b] In general there is no reason to expose the mother to potential injuries, if the fetus is not viable.
Note: Macrosomia is not a contraindication for OVD; caution should be used because of the increased risk of shoulder dystocia in this situation.[47]

---

dyspareunia, urinary incontinence, or severe pain measures. No difference was noted when median episiotomies were compared with mediolateral episiotomies.[53]

Despite the strong positions encountered in the literature, the most recent Cochrane review concluded that the studies comparing median and mediolateral episiotomies were of poor methodological quality as to draw definitive conclusions over which technique is better.[53] A 2005 systematic review did not report a difference in sphincter tears between midline and mediolateral episiotomies, as sphincter tear events were rare, and relevant studies were consistent in reporting no benefit in preventing fecal incontinence.[54] Of note is that neither supported the use of routine episiotomy. Recent literature has not provided any further conclusive evidence.[55] Midline episiotomies have been associated with an increased risk of external rectal sphincter lacerations, particularly when associated with an OVD (including VAD).[44,52,56] In a recent prospective study of 1000 vacuum deliveries, third-degree or fourth-degree tears were also seen more often in women who had an episiotomy than in those who did not, regardless of parity.[44]

A retrospective case-control study from Sweden of 5435 primiparous women found an association between OVD (VAD odds ratio [OR] 5.4, 95% confidence interval [CI] 2.8–10.3; FAD OR 10.2, 95% CI 2.2–6.8; and fetal head circumference OR 1.4, 95% CI 1.1–1.8) and sphincter tears. Most interestingly, they found mediolateral episiotomy (OR 0.3, 95% CI 0.1–0.6) and epidural anesthesia (OR 0.3, 95% CI 0.2–0.6) to be protective.[57] As a result of the low frequency of performance, no comment on median episiotomy was made.[55,57] Like the Swedish study, another retrospective report found mediolateral episiotomy to be protective (OR 0.4, 95% CI 0.2–0.7).[57,58] In a case-control study of 100 primigravidas, Eogan and colleagues[59] demonstrated a 50% relative decrease in risk of having a third-degree tear for every 6° of separation from the perineal midline that an episiotomy was cut.

Anal sphincter lacerations at the time of delivery may be complicated by future fecal incontinence in up to 57% of patients, despite immediate identification and repair, and are to be dutifully avoided.[2,26]

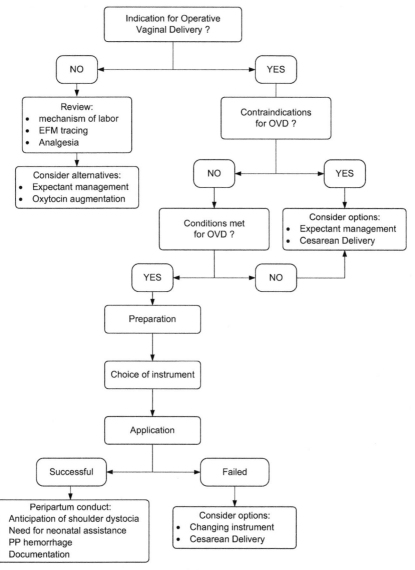

Fig. 1. Systematic approach to vaginal delivery. The contraindications, conditions (or prerequisites), and preparation of the patient for instrumental deliveries are outlined in Boxes 3, 4, and 5, respectively. EFM, electronic fetal monitoring; OVD, operative vaginal delivery; PP, postpartum.

Of interest, increased rates of both OVDs and perineal lacerations (even when controlled by the use of forceps) have been reported among women with a shortened perineal body, suggesting for the first time an association between biological characteristics of the women's pelvis and soft tissue and the need to use forceps, and not a causal effect between the forceps and the perineal lacerations.[60,61] This suggestion would be supported by a study by Poggi and colleagues[62] showing that birth size as evidenced by fetal weight, and not the force exerted by the clinician during delivery, is the main factor responsible for the perineal trauma.

Box 4
Conditions for operative vaginal deliveries

1. Full cervical dilatation

2. Membranes ruptured

3. Engagement of the fetal head

4. Head is vertex or mentoanterior

5. Variety of position must be known

6. No disproportion between head size and pelvic size (mid-pelvis)

7. Empty bladder

8. Adequate analgesia

9. Operator familiar with labor course and the clinical assessment of pelvis and fetal size

10. Experienced operator (or supervisor)

11. Knowledge of advantages and techniques of different instruments

12. Operator prepared to abandon procedure

13. Capability of performing a CS if difficulties encountered

Data from Gei AF, Belfort MA. Forceps-assisted vaginal delivery. Obstet Gynecol Clin North Am 1999;26:345–70; and Sentilhes L, Gillard P, Descamps P, et al. Indications et prérequis à la réalisation d'une extraction instrumentale: quand, comment et où? J Gynecol Obstet Biol Reprod 2008;37:S188–201 [in French].

Recommendations

Episiotomy has not been proved to be an essential part of an assisted vaginal birth, as it does not reduce and may increase the incidence of maternal trauma.[21,63] The available evidence suggests that the use of episiotomy is harmful and can increase the

---

Box 5
Preparation of the patient

- Position: dorsal lithotomy[a] Walcher position

- Prepping and draping

- Bladder catheterization[b]

- Revision of instruments[c]/Preparation for episiotomy

- Disposition about pediatrician

- Preliminary examination[d]

- Anesthesia

[a] The feet should be at the level of the buttocks or even lower to prevent excessive distention of the perineum, which will increase the potential for lacerations and/or extension of episiotomies.
[b] Occasionally supporting the urethra between index and middle finger will facilitate the catheter introduction (urethral splinting).
[c] Particularly important to check that the blades match and to review the lock (easy slide in Kielland and modified Kielland).
[d] Recheck station, position, flexion, and synclitism, in particular if the patient has been moved from a labor room to a delivery room.

---

rates of perineal lacerations in patients undergoing instrumented deliveries (both vacuum and forceps). In the uncommon case where the perineum is preventing delivery, an episiotomy may expedite a vaginal birth (although no prospective evidence is currently available). Median episiotomies are associated with an increased risk of severe perineal (third-degree or fourth-degree) lacerations.[21,51,63]

Practical Tips

- Do not cut an episiotomy before the presentation is at the level of the pelvic floor (if one is deemed necessary) and after the forceps blades have been removed from the pelvis.
- If an episiotomy is needed in association with an OVD, a mediolateral is preferable to a midline episiotomy.
- The authors favor the incision of the perineum beginning at the vulvar fourchette at the time of vulvar distension during a uterine contraction with an angle of at least 30° from the midline.

ANTIBIOTICS OR NOT?

A Cochrane review on the effect of prophylactic antibiotics on infectious morbidity after OVDs included only one randomized trial.[64] There were 7 women with endomyometritis in the group given no antibiotics and none in the prophylactic antibiotic group. This difference did not reach statistical significance, but the relative risk (RR) reduction was 93% (RR 0.07; 95% CI 0.00–1.21).[64,65] There is also not enough evidence at this time to recommend the use of prophylactic antibiotics in cases of fourth-degree perineal lacerations.[66]

Recommendation

There is not enough evidence to recommend practice.

Practical Tips

- In the setting of OVDs the use of prophylactic antibiotics is reasonable in cases of manual exploration of the uterus, manual removal of the placenta, and extensive repair of lacerations including fourth-degree perineal lacerations.
- Good standards of hygiene and aseptic techniques are recommended.[26]

ARE INSTRUMENTAL ROTATIONS OUT OF THE QUESTION?

At this time there are no randomized controlled trials comparing rotation with expectant management or instrumental rotations to CSs.[25]

The important points that have to be considered in this analysis are the relative difficulty of these procedures, and the potential morbidity associated with the natural history of fetal head malpositions or that associated with instrumental rotations.

One of the arguments in favor of rotations to occipitoanterior (OA) are the higher rates of perineal trauma encountered with deliveries in posterior varieties of presentation. In a retrospective study of 588 forceps procedures by Benavides and colleagues,[67] anal sphincter injury occurred significantly more often in the OP group (51.5%) than in the OA group (32.9%) (OR 2.2; 95% CI 1.3–3.6). In a logistic regression model that controlled for OP position, maternal body mass index, race, length of second stage, episiotomy, birth weight, and rotational forceps, an OP head position was 3.1 times more likely (95% CI 1.6–6.2) to be associated with an anal sphincter injury than an OA head position. The neonatal morbidity appears also to be increased in OVDs in the OP position when compared with OVDs in the OA position.[68]

The role of rotational forceps in fetal-neonatal morbidity is controversial.[21,69,70] Hankins and colleagues[69] did not find an increase in maternal or neonatal morbidity outcomes when forceps rotations of 90° or more were compared with lesser degrees of rotation. In a study evaluating more than 140 rotations, Schiff and colleagues[71] found similar maternal and neonatal outcomes in a comparison with a matched control group of VADs. Feldman and colleagues[70] reported higher rates of admission to the neonatal intensive care unit, which were unrelated to the mode of delivery. These investigators also noted lower rates of maternal morbidity associated with forceps rotations with the Leff forceps when compared with traditional low or outlet forceps, a difference likely reflecting the expertise of the operators with this particular instrument.[70] Similarly, Al-Suhel and colleagues[72] report that the use of Kielland forceps had maternal outcomes no different than nonrotational vacuums and lower rates of adverse neonatal outcomes than all other forms of instrumental delivery. In a report of VADs applied to 167 cases of OP presentation, Neri and colleagues[73] reported a 79.6% success rate of the instrument in effecting an "autorotation" to OA.[74]

Recommendations

The aforementioned findings suggest that perineal trauma could be diminished by rotating the fetus to occiput anterior instead of performing a direct occiput posterior delivery. Deciding on whether to proceed with a rotation greater than 90° depends not only on the experience of the obstetrician but, in addition, to the patient's parity, size of the fetus, size and conformation of the pelvis, station of the presentation, presence of plastic phenomena (molding, caput), fetal well-being assessment, and availability of instruments.[26,69,75,76] Such procedures should be performed as a trial of forceps and abandoned if the rotation is deemed difficult or potentially traumatic.[27,48,75]

Practical Tips

- A manual rotation might prevent an instrumental rotation.[21,77]
- Rotational forceps deliveries should not be attempted in hospitals not equipped to perform an immediate CS unless exceptional circumstances exist (RANZCOG [Royal Australian and New Zealand College of Obstetricians and Gynaecologists] rotation).
- Consider rotations of the presentation in all cases of OP position with the exception of the occipitosacral at the low to outlet stations.
- Malrotations of the fetal head are frequently associated of asynclitism and deflection, which need to be corrected before (asynclitism) and after (deflection) the rotation of the fetal head.
- Rotation of the fetal head should only be attempted between contractions (RANZCOG rotation).
- In most cases the proper alignment of fetal head into the maternal pelvis is the only intervention required to resolve a mechanical dystocia or even an abnormal fetal heart rate tracing (**Fig. 2**).
- In the authors' centers, after a successful rotation the patient is encouraged to push her fetus after disarticulation of the branches and removal of the forceps.[76]

WHEN TO ABANDON THE PROCEDURE?

There are no randomized trials looking at this issue. Different operational criteria have been proposed for the abandonment of an OVD.[64] The RCOG proposes to abandon a FAD when the forceps' blades cannot be applied easily, the handles do not easily approximate, a rotation is not easily effected with gentle torque, or there is no

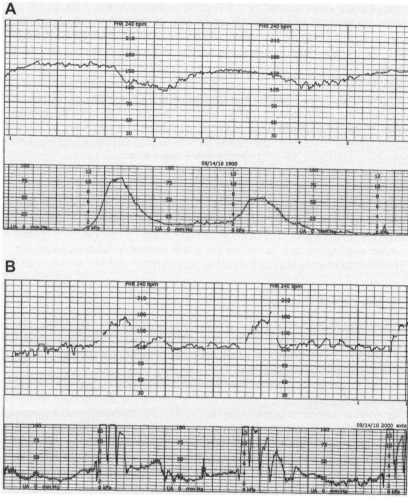

Fig. 2. Electronic fetal monitoring tracing of a primigravid at term. Right occipitoposterior position with anterior asynclitism. (*A*) Before trial of OVD. (*B*) After Kielland forceps rotation and correction of asynclitism.

evidence of progressive descent with each pull or when delivery is not imminent following 3 pulls of a correctly applied instrument by an experienced operator.[26] The Canadian guidelines propose to consider abandonment of the vacuum and/or forceps when it fails to achieve delivery of the fetus in a reasonable time, although no operational criteria are provided.[21]

The threshold for abandoning an instrumental delivery and resorting to an alternative mode of delivery is likely to differ between clinicians and the clinical circumstances.[45,78]

In a report by Murphy and colleagues,[79] 82% of OVDs were completed within 3 pulls. More than 3 pulls at attempted OVD was associated with increased neonatal trauma for both completed and failed deliveries; the majority of these deliveries were accomplished by "less experienced trainees" with 1 to 5 years of obstetric experience.

In comparing the need for 0 to 2 pulls with 3 or more pulls with a vacuum, nulliparous women required significantly more pulls than parous women ($P = .001$).[44] In this study more than 3 pulls were required by 4.9% of the nulliparous and 2.6% of the parous women. In the study of vacuum by Vacca,[80] 84% of the patients required 4 pulls or fewer. In his report 5 pulls or more were required in 40% of cases where the cup was deflexing, 29% of the mid-pelvic extractions, and 16% of the rotational procedures.

Recommendations

Most operative deliveries, including the application of a vacuum, should be considered a trial. Unless the practitioner is certain that an OVD is going to be successful, the possibility of failure needs to be anticipated. In these circumstances, an alternative plan that will result in a safe and expeditious birth must be in place and implemented promptly if the planned operative birth is unsuccessful.[21]

Practical Tips

- An experienced operator or supervisor needs to be in attendance for all OVDs.
- The obstetrician needs to be prepared to abandon a forceps or vacuum procedure if the instrument cannot be applied properly, if there is no progress after proper application, or if further attempts are deemed potentially traumatic.
- The number of pulls should not be the only criterion used to abandon an OVD.

WHAT IF ONE OF THEM FAILS?

There are no randomized trials available to answer this question. Two different considerations are pertinent in the clinical decision regarding the best course of action: (a) the factors associated with the failure of an instrument, and (b) the morbidity associated with the combination of instruments.

Factors that reduce the chances of a failed vaginal delivery include greater maternal age, greater body mass index, diabetes, greater gestational age, greater fetal weight, induction of labor, abnormal or prolonged labor, and OP presentations.[81] Factors associated with a failed trial of instrumental vaginal delivery include nulliparity, malposition of the fetal head, high level of the head, deflexed head, and reduced pelvic capacity.[82]

When analyzed by the instrument used, forceps are more likely to be successful than vacuum in both OA and OP applications.[83] When stratified by fetal station at the time of instrument application, forceps are significantly more successful at mid and low positions, whereas there is no difference with outlet stations.[83]

The literature available is consistent regarding the fact that the sequential use of forceps and vacuum carries a higher risk of morbidity for the neonate than either instrument alone.[37,41,82,84] The combined use of instruments increases the risk of intracranial hemorrhage, brachial plexus injury, facial nerve injury, need for mechanical ventilation, and depressed 5-minute Apgar scores, and has the potential for more maternal trauma as well.[36,37,41]

In a recent study of 1000 vacuum deliveries by Baskett and colleagues,[44] the majority (76.0%) of the 129 cases in which the vacuum failed to achieve delivery were subsequently delivered by forceps, according to the investigators, "without any untoward neonatal sequelae."

Fetal injuries have also been attributed to the delay between a failed OVD and a CS.[21]

Recommendations

The decision to proceed with another instrument or a CS after failure of one instrument should be weighed carefully and decided with respect to the unique circumstances of the individual case.[26,37,85,86] The American Congress of Obstetricians and

Gynecologists sanctions such use in specific conditions when a compelling and justifiable reason exists.[47]

Practical Tips

- If a second instrument is being considered after a failed instrumental application, reevaluate the indications, contraindications, and conditions for an OVD before the application of a second instrument. If a forceps delivery has failed it is unlikely that a vacuum will succeed.
- Adequate documentation of the rationale for the sequential use of instruments and the circumstances for its use are highly desirable.
- Peer review of the sequential use of instruments for the assistance of a vaginal delivery has been recommended (RCOG).

WHAT TO EXPECT FROM INSTRUMENTS? WHAT ARE THE COMPLICATIONS?

One of the most important factors in the decline of instrumental deliveries and of forceps in particular has been the perceived morbidity of these instruments.[87–89] For years instrumental deliveries have been the subject of intense medical scrutiny that has associated its use to outcomes ranging from maternal sexual dissatisfaction to pediatric dental malocclusion of the fetuses exposed to them.[90,91] The available information to evaluate the contribution of these procedures to maternal, fetal, or neonatal morbidity is of variable quality, has a wide range of reported outcomes, and for the most part does not take into account either the indications for its use or the comorbid conditions (prolonged second stage for example) associated with it. Yet when controlled by other clinical variables associated with difficult deliveries, some of the perceived associations with the use of instrument do not remain significant.[92]

The use of instruments in a delivery is in itself a good surrogate parameter of difficulty in the birthing process.[41,81] Large epidemiologic studies have shown that when compared with spontaneous vaginal deliveries, the women who required a FAD are older, nulliparous, have heavier fetuses, are more frequently postdates, more frequently are induced, have dystocia of their labors (including longer labors, abnormal uterine contractility patterns, and fetal malpositions), and have more diagnoses of fetal distress, pregnancy-induced hypertension, abruptio of the placenta, and chorioamnionitis.[38,41]

The risks attributed to the use of the instruments are therefore difficult to differentiate from the effects of the indication that prompted their use. In the case of OVD literature, association and causation are frequently confused.[93,94]

Because few studies have prospectively evaluated the elective use of forceps when seemingly no assistance was required, it is difficult to ascertain what proportion of the morbidity over the baseline the instruments are actually responsible for (their attributable risk).[95–97]

It is not surprising that the outcomes of OVDs in different parts of the world, by different operators with variable experience, associated with the use of different instruments for different indications and in different circumstances, are as widely variable as the ones summarized in **Boxes 1** and **2**. These considerations also explain why, in expert hands and in the absence of a medical indication, the morbidity associated with the use of forceps and vacuums is negligible.[44,95]

WHAT SHOULD WE TELL PATIENTS?

Despite its significant prevalence, the need for assistance with a vaginal delivery is rarely recognized by patients and the options to assist problems at the time of delivery are seldom discussed with them by their obstetricians.[96] Many patients who are presented with the option of an OVD during a prolonged second stage of labor, when the fetus is having deep variable decelerations, are already frustrated and overwhelmed with the situation; they are afraid about potential injury to the fetus or themselves by instruments they generally know very little about and about which they have only heard appalling (and frequently not substantiated) stories. With such a high prevalence of unpredictable obstetric events during labor, the role of obstetricians in prenatal patient education is paramount. Recently the RCOG has put forth both OVD Consent Advice and a pamphlet containing general information for patients contemplating the possibility of an assisted vaginal delivery (available at the RCOG Web site).[98,99] This

---

Box 6
Postpartum documentation

- *From the mother:*
  - Gravidity/Parity/Gestational age
  - Indication for use of forceps
  - Evaluation of the pelvis
  - Anesthesia used
- *From the fetus:*
  - Presentation/Station/Flexion/Synclitism
  - Presence and degree of plastic phenomena
- *From the delivery process:*
  - Type of forceps or vacuum
  - Application/Grip and symmetry achieved
  - Degree of traction and technique
  - Time of disarticulation
  - Time of delivery of fetus and placenta
  - Episiotomy if performed
  - Intrapartum findings
  - Mechanism of third stage
- *From the newborn:*
  - Weight
  - Apgar scores (if low, results of cord gases)
  - Presence of anomalies
  - Evaluation of gestational age and adequacy/Gestational age
  - Evaluation of the fetal application of the instrument (grip or forceps/placement of chignon)
- *From the parturient:*
  - Evaluation of birth canal
  - Episiorrhaphy or perineorrhaphy if performed
  - Estimated blood loss
  - Disposition of the mother and condition on transfer

Table 5
Maternal morbidity associated with spontaneous vaginal and assisted vaginal deliveries:
Demissie et al[41] (New Jersey, 1989–93)

Maternal Morbidity	Unassisted (n = 327, 373)	Forceps (n = 26, 491)	Vacuum (n = 19, 120)
Third-degree perineal tear	12359 (377.5)	3316 (1251.7)	1840·(962.3)
Adjusted odds ratio (95% CI)	0.39 (0.38–0.41)	1.00	0.78 (0.73–0.83)
Fourth-degree perineal tear	6626 (202.4)	2584 (975.4)	1199 (627.1)
Adjusted odds ratio (95% CI)	0.28 (0.27–0.30)	1.00	0.64 (0.60–0.69)
Postpartum hemorrhage	4734 (144.6)	517 (195.1)	458 (239.5)
Adjusted odds ratio (95% CI)	0.79 (0.72–0.87)	1.00	1.22 (1.07–1.39)

Abbreviation: CI, confidence interval.
Data from Demissie K, Rhads GG, Smulian JC, et al. Operative vaginal delivery and neonatal and infant adverse outcomes: population based retrospective analysis. BMJ 2004;329:1–6.

information was developed by the Patient Information Subgroup of the RCOG Guidelines and Audit Committee, with input from the Consumers' Forum, the authors of the clinical guideline, and women attending clinics.[99]

OVD can be associated with fear of subsequent childbirth, and in a severe form may manifest as a posttraumatic stress type syndrome that has been termed "tokophobia."[100–104] There is no evidence to support the use of formal debriefing in reducing the risk of subsequent postnatal depression for women who have experienced OVD. Nonetheless, women report the need for a review following delivery to

Table 6
Maternal morbidity associated with spontaneous vaginal and assisted vaginal deliveries:
Gardella et al[37] (Washington state, 1996)

	Incidence Among Spontaneous Vaginal Deliveries (N = 11,223)[a]	Assisted Vaginal Deliveries			
		Vacuum (N = 3741)		Forceps (N = 3741)	
		Incidence[a]	RR	Incidence[a]	RR
Vaginal laceration					
Nulliparas	17.1	22.9	1.3 (0.9–1.9)	47.0	2.7 (2.1–3.7)
Multiparas	6.2	10.9	1.8 (0.9–1.0)	19.1	3.1 (1.8–5.3)[c]
Third-degree laceration					
Nulliparas	72.8	140.0	1.9 (1.7–2.2)	157.7	2.2 (1.9–2.5)
Multiparas	12.8	57.4	4.5 (3.3–6.1)[d]	55.3	4.3(3.1–6.0)[d]
Fourth-degree laceration					
Nulliparas	23.7	36.9	1.6(1.2–2.1)	35.7	1.5(1.2–2.0)
Multiparas	3.5	9.3	2.7 (1.3–5.5)[e]	12.8	3.7 (1.9–7.4)
Cervical laceration[b]	2.3	4.8	1.7 (0.9–3.3)	5.9	2.2 (1.2–3.8)
Postpartum hemorrhage[b]	23.4	31.3	1.2 (1.0–1.5)	25.9	0.9 (0.7–1.2)

[a] The incidence is expressed as the number of cases per 1000 deliveries.
[b] Adjusted for parity.
[c] $P = .8$.
[d] $P = .001$.
[e] $P = .2$.

Table 7
Maternal morbidity associated with spontaneous vaginal and assisted vaginal deliveries: Wen et al[38] (Quebec, Canada, 1991/1992–1995/1996)

Adverse Outcomes	Vacuum vs Unassisted		Forceps vs Unassisted	
	OR	95% CI	OR	95% CI
Third-/fourth-degree perineal laceration	3.9	3.8, 4.1	8.4	8.0, 8.7

Abbreviations: OR, odds ratio; CI, confidence interval.
Data from Wen SW, Liu S, Kramer MS, et al. Comparison of maternal and infant outcomes between vacuum extraction and forceps deliveries. Am J Epidemiol 2001;153:103–7.

discuss the indication for delivery, the management of any complications, and the implications for future deliveries.[26,100] The optimal timing, setting, and health care professional for postdelivery review require further evaluation.[26] When compared with women who had CSs, women who underwent an OVD were more likely to prefer a vaginal delivery 1 year after the event and to actually have a vaginal delivery in subsequent pregnancies.[105] This fact may have an impact on the current epidemic of cesarean deliveries.

Recommendations

Ideally all women in labor should have had general information about instrumental delivery in the course of antenatal education, and should have had prior knowledge of the 1-in-10 chance (or whichever the local figure is) of having an instrumental delivery (**Box 6, Tables 5–10**).[46]

Practical Approach

- During prenatal care women need to be informed that complications can occur during her delivery and that a CS or an OVD might be required.

Table 8
Neonatal morbidity associated with spontaneous vaginal and assisted vaginal deliveries: Demissie et al[41]

Neonatal Morbidity	Unassisted (n = 327, 373)	Forceps (n = 26, 491)	Vacuum (n = 19, 120)
Cephalohematoma[a]	5457 (166.7)	1681 (634.6)	2135 (1116.6)
Facial nerve injury	78 (2.4)	98 (37.0)	10 (5.2)
Intracranial hemorrhage	122 (3.7)	45 (17.0)	31 (16.2)
Adjusted odds ratio (95% CI)[b]	0.29 (0.20–0.41)	1.00	0.96 (0.62–1.52)
Mechanical ventilation	768 (23.5)	83 (31.3)	77 (40.3)
Adjusted odds ratio (95% CI)	0.84 (0.66–1.06)	1.00	1.27 (0.92–1.74)
Retinal hemorrhage	597 (18.2)	51 (19.3)	30 (15.7)
Adjusted odds ratio (95% CI)	0.87 (0.65–1.18)	1.00	0.78 (0.50–1.24)

[a] Number of cases per 10,000 deliveries.
[b] Adjusted for birth weight, gestational age, deep transverse arrest, persistent occipitoposterior position, long labor, fetal distress, cord prolapse, placental abruption, and intrapartum bleeding.
Data from Demissie K, Rhads GG, Smulian JC, et al. Operative vaginal delivery and neonatal and infant adverse outcomes: population based retrospective analysis. BMJ 2004;329:1–6.

Table 9
Neonatal morbidity associated with spontaneous vaginal and assisted vaginal deliveries:
Gardella et al[37]

	Incidence Among Spontaneous Vaginal Deliveries (N = 11,223)[a]	Assisted Vaginal Deliveries			
		Vacuum (N = 3741)		Forceps (N = 3741)	
		Incidence[a]	RR	Incidence[a]	RR
Intracranial hemorrhage[b]	0.9	1.9	2.4 (0.9–6.2)	1.1	1.3 (0.4–4.1)
Facial nerve injury[c]	0.2	0.3	0.8 (0.1–9.0)	2.9	9.3 (3.1–27.4)
Brachial plexus injury[b]	1.5	3.7	2.3 (1.1–4.5)	5.3	2.8 (1.4–5.6)
Scalp injury					
Nulliparas	39.1	120.0	3.1 (2.6–3.7)	80.1	2.0 (1.7–2.5)
Multiparas	13.6	85.0	6.3 (4.8–8.3)§	43.6	3.2 (2.2–4.6)
Seizures[b]	0.2	0.8	4.4 (0.6–34.5)	0.5	2.9 (0.6–33.5)
Five-minute Apgar score ≤6[b]	8.3	17.0	1.8 (1.3–2.5)	11.0	1.1 (0.8–1.6)

[a] The incidence is expressed as the number of cases per 1000 infants.
[b] Adjusted for birth weight and parity.
[c] Adjusted for parity.
Data from Gardella C, Taylor M, Benedetti T, et al. The effect of sequential use of vacuum and forceps for assisted vaginal delivery on neonatal and maternal outcomes. Am J Obstet Gynecol 2001;85:896–902.

- If it has not occurred prior, it is suggested to begin the discussion of route and methods of delivery at 30 to 32 weeks. Specific questions and preferences of the patient and/or couple can be prospectively addressed and documented.
- After an OVD provide immediate debriefing of the couple regarding the need for the instrumental delivery, feedback of the application of the instrument on the fetus (after examination with the pediatrician or neonatologist), and expectations regarding neonatal outcome.
- A formal (Edinburgh Postpartum Depression score) and informal assessment of depressive symptoms is recommended for all deliveries.

Table 10
Neonatal morbidity associated with spontaneous vaginal and assisted vaginal deliveries:
Wen et al[38]

	Vacuum vs Unassisted		Forceps vs Unassisted	
Adverse Outcomes	OR	95% CI	OR	95% CI
Intracranial hemorrhage	4.5	3.0, 6.6	5.0	3.3, 7.7
Cephalhematoma	9.9	9.4, 10.5	5.9	5.5, 6.3
Facial-nerve injury	2.3	1.6, 3.4	9.8	7.3, 13.1
Convulsions	1.8	1.3, 2.4	2.0	1.4, 2.7
Neonatal in-hospital death	0.9	0.4, 2.1	1.0	0.4, 2.3

Data from Wen SW, Liu S, Kramer MS, et al. Comparison of maternal and infant outcomes between vacuum extraction and forceps deliveries. Am J Epidemiol 2001;153:103–7.

SUMMARY

OVDs are meant to facilitate and expedite delivery for mother and infant, not to complicate or injure either of them. A significant portion of the attributed morbidity to the instruments is the inherent morbidity of the process the instrument is called upon to assist. An appropriate use of instruments calls for a systematic approach to its potential need, a keen understanding of what processes are responsible for the problem, and how they are to be corrected with instruments. In developed countries at least a third of pregnant women require assistance during their birthing process in the form of obstetric forceps, obstetric vacuum, or cesarean delivery (see **Table 1**). Unfortunately, the lack of such obstetric interventions in nondeveloped countries explains in great measure the large disparities observed in maternal, fetal, and neonatal morbidity and mortality between developed and developing countries.[106,107]

As long as the vaginal route is an option for human delivery, forceps and vacuums will continue to assist women and children to carry out the delivery process unharmed.

REFERENCES

1. Rosenberg K, Trevathan W. Birth, obstetrics and human evolution. BJOG 2002; 109:1199–206.
2. Alfredo F, Gei AF, Pacheco LD. Forceps: still an option? Curr Womens Health Rev 2008;4:56–75.
3. Pierre F, Jousse M. Aspects medico-legaux de l'extraction instrumentale. J Gynecol Obstet Biol Reprod 2008;37:S276–87 [in French].
4. Dupuis O. Formation et apprentissage des extractions. J Gynecol Obstet Biol Reprod 2008;37:S288–96 [in French].
5. Chinnock M, Robson S. An anonymous survey of registrar training in the use of Kjelland's forceps in Australia. Aust N Z J Obstet Gynaecol 2009;49:515–6.
6. Ennen CS, Satin AJ. Training and assessment in obstetrics: the role of simulation. Best Pract Res Clin Obstet Gynaecol 2010;24:747–58.
7. Patel RR, Murphy DJ. Forceps delivery in modern obstetric practice. BMJ 2004; 328:1302–5.
8. Information and Statistics Division, Scotland. Births in Scottish hospitals, financial year 2008/2009. 2009. Available at: http://www.isdscotland.org. Accessed October 18, 2010.
9. Perinatal Statistics Report 2007. Health Research and Information Division. Dublin (Ireland): ESRI (The Economic and Social Research Institute); 2009. Available at: http://www.esri.ie. Accessed October 2, 2010.
10. Canadian perinatal health report, 2008 edition. Ottawa (Canada): Public Health Agency of Canada; 2008. Available at: http://www.phac-aspc.gc.ca/publicat/2008/cphr-rspc/pdf/cphr-rspc08-eng.pdf. Accessed October 2, 2010.
11. Australian Institute of Health and Welfare. Australia's health 2010. Australia's health series no. 12. Cat. no. AUS 122. Canberra (Australia): AIHW; 2010. Available at: www.aihw.gov.au/publications. Accessed October 2, 2010.
12. Department of Health. NHS Maternity Statistics, England: 2003–2004. Statistical Bulletin 2005/10. 2005. Crown copyright, reproduced with permission. [Cesarean rates are taken from the Maternity Tail data in Table 33. Where this is missing, the data is taken from the procedure coded HES record core data in Table 33]. Available at: www.dh.gov.uk. Accessed October 2, 2010.
13. Martin JA, Hamilton BE, Sutton PD, et al. Births: Final data for 2007. National vital statistics reports, vol. 58. Hyattsville (MD): National Center for Health Statistics; 2010.

14. Loudon JA, Groom KM, Hinkson L, et al. Changing trends in operative delivery performed at full dilatation over a 10-year period. J Obstet Gynaecol 2010;30: 370–5.
15. Clark SL, Belfort MA, Hankins GD, et al. Variation in the rates of operative delivery in the United States. Am J Obstet Gynecol 2007;196:526.e1–5.
16. Hanley GE, Janssen PA, Greyson D. Regional variation in the cesarean delivery and assisted vaginal delivery rates. Obstet Gynecol 2010;115:1201–8.
17. Nader R, Shek KL, Dietz HP. Predicting the outcome of induction of labour. Aust N Z J Obstet Gynaecol 2010;50:329–33.
18. Dietz HP, Lanzarone L, Simpson JM. Predicting operative delivery. Ultrasound Obstet Gynecol 2006;27:409–15.
19. Van De Pol G, De Leeuw JR, Van Brummen HJ, et al. Psychosocial factors and mode of delivery. J Psychosom Obstet Gynaecol 2006;27:231–6.
20. Gei AF, Belfort MA. Forceps-assisted vaginal delivery. Obstet Gynecol Clin North Am 1999;26:345–70.
21. Society of Obstetricians and Gynaecologists of Canada. SOGC clinical practice guidelines: guidelines for operative vaginal birth. Int J Gynaecol Obstet 2005; 88:229–36.
22. Williams MC. Vacuum-assisted delivery. Clin Perinatol 1995;22:933–52.
23. Schaal JP, Equy V, Hoffman P. Comparaison ventouse forceps. J Gynecol Obstet Biol Reprod 2008;37:S231–43 [in French].
24. Lurie S, Glezerman M, Baider C, et al. Decision-to-delivery interval for instrumental vaginal deliveries: vacuum extraction versus forceps. Arch Gynecol Obstet 2006; 274(1):34–6, p. 1–3.
25. Majoko F, Gardener G. Trial of instrumental delivery in theatre versus immediate caesarean section for anticipated difficult assisted births. Cochrane Database Syst Rev 2008;4:CD005545.
26. Operative vaginal delivery. Clinical Guideline 26. RCOG; 2005. Available at: http://www.rcog.org.uk/womens-health/clinical-guidance/operative-vaginal-delivery-green-top-26. Acccessed October 5, 2010.
27. Lowe B. Fear of failure: a place for the trial of instrumental delivery. Br J Obstet Gynaecol 1987;94:60–6.
28. Revah A, Ezra Y, Farine D, et al. Failed trial of vacuum or forceps—maternal and fetal outcome. Am J Obstet Gynecol 1997;176:200–4.
29. Olagundoye V, MacKenzie IZ. The impact of a trial of instrumental delivery in theatre on neonatal outcome. BJOG 2007;114:603–8.
30. American College of Obstetricians and Gynecologists. Delivery by vacuum extraction. ACOG Committee Opinion No. 208. Washington, DC: ACOG; 1998.
31. Chalmers JA, Chalmers I. The obstetric vacuum extractor is the instrument of first choice for operative vaginal delivery. Br J Obstet Gynaecol 1989;96(5): 505–6.
32. Johanson R, Menon V. Vacuum extraction versus forceps for assisted vaginal delivery. Cochrane Database of Systematic Reviews 1999;2:CD000224 [Editorial group: Cochrane Pregnancy and Childbirth Group 2009;1:1–28].
33. O'Mahony F, Hofmeyr GJ, Menon V. Choice of instruments for assisted vaginal delivery. Cochrane Database of Systematic Reviews 2010;11:CD005455 [Editorial group: Cochrane Pregnancy and Childbirth Group; 2010. p. 1–100].
34. Johanson RB, Heycock E, Carter J, et al. Maternal and child health after assisted vaginal delivery: five-year follow up of a randomized controlled study comparing forceps and ventouse. Br J Obstet Gynaecol 1999;106(6): 544–9.

35. Johanson RB, Rice C, Doyle M, et al. A randomised prospective study comparing the new vacuum extractor policy with forceps delivery. Br J Obstet Gynaecol 1993;100:524–30.
36. Towner D, Castro MA, Eby-Wilkens E, et al. Effect of mode of delivery in nulliparous women on neonatal intracranial injury. N Engl J Med 1999;341(2): 1709–14.
37. Gardella C, Taylor M, Benedetti T, et al. The effect of sequential use of vacuum and forceps for assisted vaginal delivery on neonatal and maternal outcomes. Am J Obstet Gynecol 2001;85:896–902.
38. Wen SW, Liu S, Kramer MS, et al. Comparison of maternal and infant outcomes between vacuum extraction and forceps deliveries. Am J Epidemiol 2001;153: 103–7.
39. De Leeuw JW, Struijk PC, Vierhout ME, et al. Risk factors for third degree perineal ruptures during delivery. BJOG 2001;108:383–7.
40. Handa VL, Danielsen BH, Gilbert WM. Obstetric anal sphincter lacerations. Obstet Gynecol 2001;98:225–30.
41. Demissie K, Rhoads GG, Smulian JC, et al. Operative vaginal delivery and neonatal and infant adverse outcomes: population based retrospective analysis. BMJ 2004;329:1–6.
42. Wax JR, Cartin A, Pinette MG, et al. Patient choice cesarean: an evidence-based review. Obstet Gynecol Surv 2004;59:601–16.
43. Ali UA, Norwitz ER. Vacuum-assisted vaginal delivery. Rev Obstet Gynecol 2009;2(1):5–17.
44. Baskett TF, Fanning CA, Young DC. A prospective observational study of 1000 vacuum assisted deliveries with the omnicup device. J Obstet Gynaecol Can 2008;30(7):573–80.
45. Royal Australian and New Zealand College of Obstetricians and Gynaecologists. Instrumental vaginal delivery. College Statement No. C-Obs 16. Melbourne (Australia): RANZCOG; 2004. Available at: www.ranzcog.edu.au/publications/statements/C-obs16.pdf. Accessed October 5, 2010.
46. Edozien LC. Towards safe practice in instrumental vaginal delivery. Best Pract Res Clin Obstet Gynaecol 2007;21:639–55.
47. Operative vaginal delivery. Reaffirmed 2009. Danvers (MA): ACOG Practice Bulletin 17; 2000.
48. Leung WC, Lam HS, Lam KW, et al. Unexpected reduction in the incidence of birth trauma and birth asphyxia related to instrumental deliveries during the study period: was this the Hawthorne effect? BJOG 2003;110:319–22.
49. O'Mahony F, Settatree R, Platt C, et al. Review of singleton fetal and neonatal deaths associated with cranial trauma and cephalic delivery during a national intrapartum-related confidential enquiry. BJOG 2005;112:619–26.
50. Sentilhes L, Gillard P, Descamps P, et al. Indications et prérequis à la réalisation d'une extraction instrumentale: quand, comment et où? J Gynecol Obstet Biol Reprod 2008;37:S188–201 [in French].
51. Myers-Helfgott MG, Helfgott AW. Routine episiotomy in modern obstetrics: should it be performed? Obstet Gynecol Clin North Am 1999;26(2):305–25.
52. Youssef R, Ramalingam U, Macleod M, et al. Cohort study of maternal and neonatal morbidity in relation to use of episiotomy at instrumental vaginal delivery. BJOG 2005;112:941–5.
53. Carroli G, Mignini L. Episiotomy for vaginal birth. Cochrane Database Syst Rev 2009;1:CD000081.

54. Hartmann K, Viswanathan M, Palmieri R, et al. Outcomes of routine episiotomy: a systematic review. JAMA 2005;293:2141–8.
55. Wheeler TL II, Richter HE. Delivery method, anal sphincter tears and fecal incontinence: new information on a persistent problem. Curr Opin Obstet Gynecol 2007;19:474–9.
56. Helwig JT, Thorp JM Jr, Bowes WA Jr. Does midline episiotomy increase the risk of third- and fourth-degree lacerations in operative vaginal deliveries? Am J Obstet Gynecol 1993;82:276–9.
57. Dahl C, Preben K. Obstetric anal sphincter rupture in older primiparous women: a case–control study. Acta Obstet Gynecol Scand 2006;85:1252–8.
58. Aukee P, Sundström H, Kairaluoma MV. The role of mediolateral episiotomy during labour. Analysis of risk factors for obstetric anal sphincter tears. Acta Obstet Gynecol Scand 2006;85:856–60.
59. Eogan M, Daly L, O'Connell P, et al. Does the angle of episiotomy affect the incidence of anal sphincter injury? BJOG 2006;113:190–4.
60. Deering SH, Carlson N, Stitely M, et al. Perineal body length and lacerations at delivery. J Reprod Med 2004;49:306–10.
61. Lurie S, Boaz M, Sadan O. Using anovaginal distance at the beginning of labor to predict the likelihood of instrumental delivery. J Reprod Med 2005;50:759–63.
62. Poggi SH, Allen RH, Patel C, et al. Effect of epidural anaesthesia on clinician-applied force during vaginal delivery. Am J Obstet Gynecol 2004;191:903–6.
63. Steed H, Corbett T, Mayes D. The value of routine episiotomy in forceps deliveries. J Soc Obstet Gynaecol Can 2000;22(8):583–6.
64. Liabsuetrakul T, Choobun T, Peeyananjarassri K, et al. Antibiotic prophylaxis for operative vaginal delivery. Cochrane Database Syst Rev 2004;3:CD004455.
65. Heitmann JA, Benrubi GI. Efficacy of prophylactic antibiotics for the prevention of endomyometritis after forceps delivery. South Med J 1989;82:960–2.
66. Buppasiri P, Lumbiganon P, Thinkhamrop J, et al. Antibiotic prophylaxis for fourth-degree perineal tear during vaginal birth. Cochrane Database Syst Rev 2005;4:CD005125.
67. Benavides L, Wu JM, Hundley AF, et al. The impact of occiput posterior fetal head position on the risk of anal sphincter injury in forceps-assisted vaginal deliveries. Am J Obstet Gynecol 2005;192:1702–6.
68. Pearl ML, Roberts JM, Laros RK, et al. Vaginal delivery from the persistent occiput posterior position. Influence on maternal and neonatal morbidity. J Reprod Med 1993;38:955–61.
69. Hankins GD, Leicht T, Van Hook J, et al. The role of forceps rotation in maternal and neonatal injury. Am J Obstet Gynecol 1999;180:213–4.
70. Feldman DM, Borgida AF, Sauer F, et al. Rotational versus nonrotational forceps: maternal and neonatal outcomes. Am J Obstet Gynecol 1999;181:1185–7.
71. Schiff E, Friedman SA, Zolti M, et al. A matched controlled study of Kielland's forceps for transverse arrest of the fetal vertex. J Obstet Gynaecol 2001;21:576–9.
72. Al-Suhel R, Gill S, Robson S, et al. Kielland forceps in the new millennium. Maternal and neonatal outcomes of attempted rotational forceps delivery. Aust N Z J Obstet Gynaecol 2009;49:510–4.
73. Neri A, Kaplan B, Rabinerson D, et al. The management of persistent occipito-posterior position. Clin Exp Obstet Gynecol 1995;22:126–31.
74. Riethmuller D, Ramanah R, Maillet R, et al. Ventouses: description, mecanique, indications et contre-indications. J Gynecol Obstet Biol Reprod 2008;37: S210–21 [in French].

75. Traub AI. A continuing use for Kielland's forceps? Br J Obstet Gynaecol 1984; 91:894–8.

76. Yeomans ER. Operative vaginal delivery. Obstet Gynecol 2010;115:645–53.

77. Schmitz T, Meunier E. Mesures a prendre pendant le travail pour reduire le nombre d'extractions instrumentals. J Gynecol Obstet Biol Reprod 2008;37:S179–87 [in French].

78. Royal Australian and New Zealand College of Obstetricians and Gynaecologists. Guidelines for use of rotational forceps. College Statement No. C-Obs 13. Melbourne (Australia): RANZCOG; 2004. Available at: www.ranzcog.edu.au/publications/statements/C-obs13.pdf. Accessed October 5, 2010.

79. Murphy DJ, Liebling RE, Patel R, et al. Cohort study of operative delivery in the second stage of labour and standard of obstetric care. BJOG 2003;110:610–5.

80. Vacca A. Operative vaginal delivery: clinical appraisal of a new vacuum extraction device. Aust N Z J Obstet Gynaecol 2001;41:156–60.

81. Gopalani S, Bennett K, Critchlow C. Factors predictive of failed operative vaginal delivery. Am J Obstet Gynecol 2004;191:896–902.

82. Al-Kadri H, Sabr Y, Al-Saif S, et al. Failed individual and sequential instrumental vaginal delivery: contributing risk factors and maternal-neonatal complications. Acta Obstet Gynecol Scand 2003;82:642–8.

83. Damron D, Capeless EL. Operative vaginal delivery: a comparison of forceps and vacuum for success rate and risk of rectal sphincter injury. Am J Obstet Gynecol 2004;191:907–10.

84. Whitby EH, Griffiths PD, Rutter S, et al. Frequency and natural history of subdural hemorrhages in babies and relation to obstetric factors. Lancet 2004;363:846–51.

85. Sadan O, Ginath S, Gomel A, et al. What to do after a failed attempt of vacuum delivery? Eur J Obstet Gynecol Reprod Biol 2003;107:151–5.

86. Ezenagu LC, Kakaria R, Bofill JA. Sequential use of instruments at operative vaginal delivery: is it safe? Am J Obstet Gynecol 2000;183:515–6.

87. Bailey PE. The disappearing art of instrumental delivery: time to reverse the trend. Int J Gynaecol Obstet 2005;91:89–96.

88. Hillier CE, Johanson RB. Worldwide survey of assisted vaginal delivery. Int J Gynaecol Obstet 1994;47:109–14.

89. Althabe F, Belizan JM, Villar J, et al. Mandatory second opinion to reduce rates of unnecessary caesarean sections in Latin America: a cluster randomised controlled trial. Lancet 2004;363:1934–40.

90. Signorello LB, Harlow BL, Chekos AK, et al. Postpartum sexual functioning and its relationship to perineal trauma: a retrospective cohort study of primiparous women. Am J Obstet Gynecol 2001;184:881–8.

91. Pirttiniemi P, Gron M, Alvesalo L, et al. Relationship of difficult forceps delivery to dental arches and occlusion. Pediatr Dent 1994;16:289–93.

92. Gillean JR, Coonrod DV, Russ R, et al. Big infants in the neonatal intensive care unit. Am J Obstet Gynecol 2005;192:1948–55.

93. Johnson JH, Figueroa R, Garry D, et al. Immediate maternal and neonatal effects of forceps and vacuum-assisted deliveries. Obstet Gynecol 2004;103: 513–8.

94. Lucas RM, McMichael AJ. Association or causation: evaluating links between "environment and disease". Bull World Health Organ 2005;83:792–5.

95. Carmona F, Martinez-Roman S, Manau D, et al. Immediate maternal and neonatal effects of low-forceps delivery according to the new criteria of the American College of Obstetricians and Gynecologists compared with

spontaneous vaginal delivery in term pregnancies. Am J Obstet Gynecol 1995; 173:55–9.

96. Nichols CM, Pendlebury LC. Chart documentation of informed consent for operative vaginal delivery: is it adequate? South Med J 2006;99:1337–9.

97. Yancey MK, Herpolsheimer A, Jordan GD, et al. Maternal and neonatal effects of outlet forceps delivery compared with spontaneous vaginal delivery in term pregnancies. Obstet Gynecol 1991;78:646–50.

98. Operative vaginal delivery. Consent Advice 11. RCOG; 2010. Available at: http://www.rcog.org.uk/operative-vaginal-delivery-consent-advice-11. Accesssed October 5, 2010.

99. An assisted birth (operative vaginal delivery): information for you. Published. RCOG; 2007. Avilable at: http://www.rcog.org.uk/files/rcog-corp/uploaded-files/PIAssistedBirth2007.pdf. Acccessed October 5, 2010.

100. Murphy DJ, Pope C, Frost J, et al. Women's views on the impact of operative delivery in the second stage of labour: qualitative interview study. BMJ 2003; 327:1132.

101. Menage J. Post-traumatic stress disorder after childbirth: the phenomenon of traumatic birth. CMAJ 1997;156:831–5.

102. Fisher J, Astbury J, Smith A. Adverse psychological impact of operative obstetric interventions: a prospective longitudinal study. Aust N Z J Psychiatry 1997;31:728–38.

103. Creedy DK, Shochnet IM, Horsfall J. Childbirth and the development of acute trauma symptoms: incidence and contributing factors. Birth 2000;27:104–11.

104. Jolly J, Walker J, Bhabra K. Subsequent obstetric performance related to primary mode of delivery. Br J Obstet Gynaecol 1999;106:227–32.

105. Bahl B, Strachan B, Murphy DJ. Outcome of subsequent pregnancy three years after previous operative delivery in the second stage of labour: cohort study. BMJ 2004;328(7435):311.

106. Zupan J. Perinatal mortality in developing countries. N Engl J Med 2005;352: 2047–8.

107. Cook RJ, Dickens BM, Syed S. Obstetric fistula: the challenge to human rights. Int J Gynaecol Obstet 2004;87:72–7.

Antenatal Exposure to Magnesium Sulfate and Neuroprotection in Preterm Infants

Maged M. Costantine, MD*, Nathan Drever, MD

KEYWORDS

- Pregnancy • Magnesium sulfate • Cerebral palsy
- Neuroprotection

INTRODUCTION: PREVALENCE AND BURDEN OF CEREBRAL PALSY

Cerebral palsy (CP) is the most common cause of motor disability in childhood. CP is a complex disease characterized by aberrant control of movement or posture that is nonprogressive and permanent, appearing early in life and not the result of recognized progressive disease.[1] The prevalence of CP is estimated to be 3.6 per 1000, or about 1 in 276 children.[2] These numbers have been stable, despite the advances in neonatal and perinatal care that have resulted in improved survival of extremely premature infants and secondary increase in the morbidities and neurosensory disabilities associated with extreme prematurity (such as blindness, deafness, developmental delay, CP, and others).[3,4] Although preterm birth is a major risk for CP, nearly half of CP cases occur in term infants, with an incidence of 1 in 1500 at term versus 4% to 8% among those born with very low birth weight.[5]

Both economically and emotionally, the burden of CP is enormous. The Centers of Disease Control and Prevention estimates the lifetime costs, including direct medical (physician visits, hospital stays, medication, assistive devices, long-term care), direct nonmedical (home and automobile modifications, special education), and indirect (productivity loses), for all people born with CP in 2000 to be $11.5 billion. The estimated lifetime cost of CP is $1 million per case (2003 US dollars).[6] There have been recent improvements in surgical care and rehabilitation that can improve quality of life and functional outcomes in patients with CP; however, there has been limited

Conflict of interest: The authors have nothing to disclose.
Division of Maternal Fetal Medicine, Department of Obstetrics and Gynecology, The University of Texas Medical Branch, 301 University Boulevard, Galveston, TX 77555-0587, USA
* Corresponding author.
E-mail address: mmcostan@utmb.edu

progress in understanding the causes of CP and in developing primary prevention strategies.

The focus of this article is to review the current understanding of CP, with emphasis placed on the role of antenatal exposure to magnesium sulfate ($MgSO_4$) as a neuroprotectant in the setting of anticipated premature birth.

ETIOLOGY OF CEREBRAL PALSY

In the 1860s, British surgeon William Little stated that all cases of CP were caused by intrapartum events.[7] It is now believed that CP is the result of neuronal injury or insult to the developing brain secondary to inflammatory, hypoxic, excitatory, or oxidative injury; and that the timing of that insult is in the prenatal or perinatal period in about 70% of the cases in infants born preterm and 85% in those born at term, with only 10% to 28% cases of CP being due to birth asphyxia.[1,8,9] Preterm delivery, low birth weight, infection/inflammation, multiple gestation, thrombophilias, obstetric hemorrhage, and preeclampsia have all been associated with CP, and are reviewed elsewhere.[4] This section focuses specifically on the association of preterm delivery and low birth weight with CP.

Preterm delivery and very low birth weight (VLBW), defined as less than 1500 g, poses the highest risk for CP.[3,10] It is estimated that the risk of developing CP is 60 times higher for neonates born at less than 28 weeks compared with those born at term.[3] The most significant morbidities in VLBW infants are associated with white matter injury (WMI), intraventricular hemorrhage (IVH), periventricular leukomalacia (PVL), and intraparenchymal echodensities.[11,12] These conditions are directly linked to the degree of brain immaturity and are inversely associated with the gestational age at birth. In addition, research focusing on the pathology of brain damage as it is related to the timing and stage of brain development may be useful in providing clinical insight into possible antenatal factors that are present at the time of injury. Hagberg and colleagues[1] published findings from a Swedish population-based CP report that included their findings from neuroimaging in 90% of children diagnosed with CP. Their results indicate that cerebral malformations originate early in fetal life no later than 20 to 24 weeks' gestation, periventricular atrophy occurs between 24 and 34 weeks' gestation, and cortical/subcortical atrophy occurs after 34 weeks.[1] Although these results do not enhance the clinical diagnosis of CP, it is possible that silent early third-trimester PVL lesions and late third-trimester cortical lesions may play a major role in CP, a role that could not be otherwise explained by hypoxic events at the time of delivery.[1]

PATHOGENESIS OF NEURONAL INJURY AND POTENTIAL THERAPEUTIC EFFECTS OF MAGNESIUM SULFATE

Because of the many possible causes of CP, animal models are difficult to develop. However, several inflammatory, hypoxic-ischemic (HI), and excitatory animal models have been used to generate insight into the pathogenesis of CP as well as the potential neuroprotectant role of magnesium sulfate ($MgSO_4$). $MgSO_4$ has been proposed to act as a neuroprotectant through one or many of the following mechanisms:

1. Hemodynamic stability. Although the data are not consistent, $MgSO_4$ has been shown to have beneficial hemodynamic effects by stabilizing the blood pressure, reducing the constriction in the cerebral arteries, and restoring cerebral perfusion in the preterm neonate.[13–15]

2. Prevention of excitatory injury and neuronal stabilization. In the acute phase after an HI injury, oxygen is depleted and the fetus switches to anaerobic metabolism, causing an inability to maintain cellular functions, rapid depletion of adenosine triphosphate (ATP), and accumulation of lactic acid.[16] This process results in intracellular accumulation of sodium, calcium, chloride, and water (cytotoxic edema) caused by a disruption in transcellular ion pumping. Excitatory neurotransmitters, such as glutamate, are then released from axon terminals as a function of membrane depolarization, causing an increase of calcium and sodium into post-synaptic neurons.[17,18] $MgSO_4$ has been shown to block this postsynaptic influx of Na^+ current in rat hippocampal neurons,[19] and to act as membrane stabilizer to prevent the persistent membrane depolarization resulting from failure of the Na^+-K^+ ATP-dependent pump.[15] In addition, $MgSO_4$ in lamb fetuses caused restoration of the blood-brain barrier permeability after an HI injury.[20] Moreover, glutamate causes an influx of calcium to the intracellular milieu by activating the N-methyl-D-aspartate (NMDA) receptors, and Mg^{2+} is known to noncompetitively bind and inhibit this influx.[17,18] A protective role of $MgSO_4$ against excitatory damage has been demonstrated in murine HI models.[21,22]

3. Antioxidant properties. The counterregulatory measure of calcium efflux through plasma membrane is inhibited by energy depletion. Calcium is also released from the mitochondria and endoplasmic reticulum. Increased intracellular calcium inhibits the activation of lipases, proteases, endonucleases, and phospholipases, leading to neuronal cell injury and irreversible brain damage.[17,18] Membrane phospholipid turnover is increased, producing an increase in free fatty acids in the cytoplasm, which then undergo peroxidation by oxygen free radicals within the mitochondria.[17,18] The two main contributors of oxygen free radical formation are xanthine, a byproduct of ATP metabolism, and prostaglandin, a by-product of free fatty acid metabolism. In addition, the intracellular accumulation of calcium induces the production of nitric oxide (NO), a free radical with cytotoxic effects.[17,18] The combination of superoxide and NO produces peroxynitrate, which activates lipid peroxidation. NO also enhances glutamate release.[23] Under normal conditions, antioxidants (superoxide dismutase, catalase, endoperoxidase) and scavengers (cholesterol, α-tocopherol, ascorbic acid, glutathione) protect against the generation of free radicals. However, after an HI injury the balance tips in favor of oxidative injury as there is increased generation of free radicals, which overcome the protective effects of antioxidants and scavengers. Free oxygen radicals attack the cellular membrane causing fragmentation and cell death.[18,23] In a rat model of HI injury, $MgSO_4$ reduced the brain damage in 7-day-old pups as compared with controls.[24,25]

4. Anti-inflammatory properties. The expression of inflammatory mediators, specifically interleukin-1β and tumor necrosis factor α, are increased within 1 to 4 hours after HI injury. These cytokines may contribute to the cytotoxicity of HI injury by increasing the expression of inducible NO synthase, cyclooxygenase, and release of free radicals, as well as the production of excitatory amino acids from glial cells.[26,27] $MgSO_4$ has been shown to decrease these proinflammatory cytokines.[28] Recently, Burd and colleagues[29] showed a direct role of $MgSO_4$ in preventing neuronal injury in a murine model of inflammation-induced preterm delivery.

In summary, the progression of cellular injury and death in HI injury is a product of energy failure, acidosis, glutamate release, intracellular accumulation of calcium, lipid peroxidation, oxidative and inflammatory injury, as well as direct neuronal injury. $MgSO_4$ has been shown to restore perfusion and to protect against excitatory, oxidative, and inflammatory insults, as well as to have direct neuroprotectant properties. However, despite these studies, the exact mechanism of how MgSO$_4$ protects against CP is not yet clear.

HUMAN OBSERVATIONAL STUDIES

A link between MgSO$_4$ and a reduction in the risk of CP was first suggested in 1995 by Nelson and Grether[30] in a case-control analysis from the California Cerebral Palsy project. In that study, infants born weighing less than 1500 g who survived until the age of 3 years with CP were less likely to have been exposed in utero to MgSO$_4$ than those without CP (odds ratio [OR] 0.14, 95% confidence interval [CI] 0.05–0.51).[30] Subsequent to this publication there have been numerous observational studies evaluating the association of MgSO$_4$ and cerebral palsy or other neurologic outcomes, with conflicting results.[30–40] These studies were limited by their design (most were case-control or retrospective cohort), small sample size, and many confounding factors such as maternal obstetric complications and the fact that MgSO$_4$ was not used primarily for neuroprotective purposes. Most of these studies are summarized in **Table 1**.

RANDOMIZED CONTROLLED TRIALS

Five prospective randomized controlled trials (RCTs) have examined and reported the long-term neurologic outcomes of infants exposed antenatally to MgSO$_4$.[41–46] MgSO$_4$ was used for fetal neuroprotection in 3 trials (Beneficial Effects of Antenatal Magnesium Sulfate [BEAM],[45] the Australasian Collaborative Trial of Magnesium Sulfate [ACTOMgSO$_4$],[42] and PREMAG[44,46]), and in the neuroprotection arm of the Magnesium and Neurological Endpoints Trial (MagNET) study.[41] MgSO$_4$ was used for prevention of eclampsia in the Magnesium Sulfate for the Prevention of Eclampsia (Magpie) trial[43] and for tocolysis in MagNET.[41] These studies differed in many aspects including patients' characteristics, magnesium protocol, and others. The studies' details (including MgSO$_4$ regimen), their primary and secondary outcomes, and their long-term infant follow-up are summarized in **Tables 2–4**. Although none of these trials demonstrated significant improvements in their primary outcome, most found significant benefit in some of their prespecified secondary outcomes.

The Magnesium and Neurological Endpoints Trial (MagNET)

MagNET[41] consisted of two tandem trials in which MgSO$_4$ was given for either neuroprotection or tocolysis based on the maternal cervical dilatation status at entry into the study. Patients between 24 and 33 weeks' gestation, with cervical dilatation less than 4 cm, were randomized in the treatment or tocolysis arm to either MgSO$_4$ (n = 46 women, 55 babies) or other tocolytic (nonblinded; n = 46 women, 51 babies). Those women with cervical dilatation greater than 4 cm were not deemed candidates for tocolysis and were enrolled in the preventive or neuroprotectant arm to either 4 g MgSO$_4$ bolus (n = 29 women, 30 babies) or placebo (n = 28 women, 29 babies). The primary outcome was a composite of "adverse pediatric health outcomes" and included neonatal or infant mortality, PVL, IVH, or CP. In the tocolysis arm, there was no difference in the rate of adverse events, 29% (16/55) in neonates exposed to MgSO$_4$ versus 18% (9/51) in those exposed to placebo; $P = .18$. In the preventive neuroprotection arm, 37% (11/30) of the newborns whose mother had received MgSO$_4$ experienced an adverse event as compared with 21% (6/29) of those who had received placebo ($P = .25$). When these two arms were combined, 32% (27/85) of infants whose mother received MgSO$_4$ experienced adverse events compared with 19% (15/80) of those

Table 1
Summary of observational studies

Study	Inclusion		Effects of Antenatal Exposure to Magnesium Sulfate
Nelson and Grether,[30] 1995	Singleton, Bwt <1500 g, survived until 3 y	Reduction in CP at 3 y	For CP: OR 0.14, 95% CI 0.05–0.51
Hauth et al,[31] 1995	Bwt 500–1000 g	Reduction of CP at 1 y	For CP: OR 0.35, 95% CI 0.16–0.99
Schendel et al,[32] 1996	Bwt <1500 g	Reduction of CP at 3–5 y	For CP: OR 0.11, 95% CI 0.02–0.81
		No effect on infant mortality	(Lost significance after controlling for confounding variables)
Finesmith et al,[33] 1997	Bwt <1750 g	Less likely to develop PVL	OR 0.196, 95% CI 0.039–0.988
Canterino et al,[34] 1999	Bwt 500–1750 g	No effect on PVL or IVH	OR 1.01, 95% CI 1.7–1.44
O'Shea et al,[35] 1998	Bwt 500–1500 g	No effect on CP	OR 0.7, 95% CI 0.4–1.3
Paneth et al,[36] 1997	Bwt <2000 g	No benefit on CP (2 y)	OR 1, 95% CI 0.53–1.88
		No association with intraventricular hemorrhage or parenchymal brain lesions	
Leviton et al,[37] 1997	Bwt 500–1500 g	No effect on WMI	OR 1, 95% CI 0.7–1.5
		No effect on IVH	OR 1, 95% CI 0.7–1.3
		No effect on ventriculomegaly	OR 1.1, 95% CI 0.7–1.7
Boyle et al,[38] 2000	Singleton, Bwt <1750 g	No association with CP	OR 0.9, 95% CI 0.3–2.6
Grether et al,[39] 2000	GA <33 wk, Bwt <1999 g	No benefit on CP	OR 0.84, 95% CI 0.56–1.26
Wiswell et al,[40]	GA <33 wk	Intracranial hemorrhage, large cystic periventricular leukomalacia (>5 mm) and long-term neurodevelopmental outcome	No-MgSO4 group increased risk of grade III–IV IVH, cystic PVL: OR 4.1, 95% CI 2.0–8.5 No-MgSO4 group increased risk of adverse neurodevelopmental outcomes, OR 4.0, 95% CI 1.6–9.7

Abbreviations: Bwt, birth weight; CI, confidence interval; CP, cerebral palsy; GA, gestational age; OR, odds ratio; PVL, periventricular leukomalacia; IVH, intraventricular hemorrhage; OR, odds ratio; WMI, white matter injury.

Table 2
Characteristics of randomized controlled trials

Study	Inclusion	Exclusion	Magnesium Sulfate Regimen	Patient Characteristics	Follow-up (months)
BEAM, Rouse/MFMU 1997–2004 USA	24–31 wk Singleton or twins High risk for spontaneous delivery (PPROM, PTL (4–8 cm), or indicated)	Delivery anticipated <2 h Dilatation >8 cm PROM <22 wk Major fetal anomalies IUFD HTN/Preeclampsia MgSO$_4$ C/I or received it in prior 12 h	6 g bolus over 20–30 min then 2 g/h for 12 h	2241 women 2444 fetuses 9% twins 87% PPROM 10% PTL	24
ACTOMgSO$_4$, Crowther 1996–2000 Australia/New Zealand	<30 wk Singleton or higher order pregnancy Delivery expected in 24 h	Second stage of labor Received MgSO$_4$ this pregnancy MgSO$_4$ C/I	4 g bolus over 20 min then 1 g/h until birth or up to 24 h, whichever was first	1062 women 1255 fetuses alive 1061 survivors at 2 y 17% multiple 63% PTL 15% preeclampsia 9% PPROM	24
PREMAG, Marret 1997–2003 France	<33 wk Singleton, twin, or triplet Delivery expected in 24 h	Severe congenital or chromosomal abnormalities Indication for emergency CD Pregnancy-associated vascular disease CCB, digitalins, or indocin in prior 24 h Betamimetics, aminoglycosides, or steroids in prior 1 h MgSO$_4$ C/I	4 g bolus over 30 min	564 women 688 fetuses 22% multiple 85% PTL 61% PPROM	24

| Magpie, 1998–2001 International | Undelivered Singleton or higher order pregnancy Preeclampsia Clinical uncertainty whether MgSO$_4$ would be beneficial | Hypersensitivity to magnesium Hepatic coma Myasthenia gravis | IV: 4 g bolus over 10–15 min then 1 g/h for 24 h. IM: 4 g IV bolus with 10 g IM, followed by 5 g every 4 h for 24 h | 1544 women <37 wk 1593 fetuses 2%–3% multiple[a] | 18 |
| MagNET, Mittendorf 1995–1997 USA | 24–33 wk Singleton or twins PTL | NRFHT Clinical evidence of infection or preeclampsia (did not exclude congenital anomalies) | Preventive arm if cervix >4 cm; 4 g bolus only Tocolytic arm if cervix ≤4 cm; 4 g bolus then 2–3 g/h vs other tocolytic | Preventive arm: 57 women 3.5% twins 59 fetuses 100% PTL Tocolytic arm: 92 women 15% twins 106 fetuses 100% PTL | 18 |

Abbreviations: CCB, calcium channel blockers; CD, cesarean delivery; CI, contraindication; HTN, hypertension; IUFD, intrauterine fetal demise; IM, intramuscular; IV, intravenous; NRFHT, nonreassuring fetal heart tracing; (P)PROM, (preterm) premature rupture of membrane; PTL, preterm labor.

[a] Estimate—uncertain from published data.

From Costantine MM, Weiner SJ, Eunice Kennedy Shriver NICHD Maternal-Fetal Medicine Units Network. Effects of antenatal exposure to magnesium sulfate on neuroprotection and mortality in preterm infants. Obstet Gynecol 2009;114:356; with permission.

Table 3
Definitions of primary and secondary neonatal outcomes of individual trials and infant follow-up

	Primary and Secondary Neonatal Outcome	Definitions of Selected Outcomes	Miscellaneous, Infant Follow-up
BEAM	*Primary*: combined outcome of stillbirth or infant death by 1 y old or moderate or severe CP at 2 y *Secondary*: neonatal complications, mild, moderate, and severe CP, stillbirth and infant death, Bayley Scales of Infant Development—II	CP: presence of at least 2 out of the following 3 criteria: minimum 30% delay in gross motor developmental milestones; abnormalities in muscle tone, movement, or deep tendon reflexes; or persistence of primitive, or absence of protective reflexes	Primary outcome reported for 95.6% of fetuses
ACTOMgSO₄	*Primary*: total pediatric mortality, CP, and a combined outcome of death or CP at 2 y *Secondary*: IVH (grade III or IV), cystic PVL, neurosensory disability	CP: tone abnormalities and loss of motor function	Developmental pediatrician and psychologist Outcomes available for 99% of fetuses 1047/1061 survivors at 2 y
PREMAG	*Primary*: fetal or neonatal mortality before hospital discharge, severe WMI, combined outcome of death or severe WMI *Secondary*: severe or moderate WMI, nonparenchymal hemorrhage, periventricular cavitary lesions and their extensions, neonatal complications, motor and cognitive development at 2 y	Severe WMI: cystic PVL, periventricular parenchymal hemorrhage, or large single unilateral porencephalic cyst (caused by ischemic–hemorrhagic infarction)	Developmental questionnaire and pediatric examination or phone call
Magpie	*Primary*: combined outcome of death or neurosensory disability (blind, deaf, severe CP, or developmental quotient <−2 standard deviations) at 18 mo *Secondary*: death, neurosensory disability, delayed speech, other disability	Severe CP: not walking or unlikely to walk unaided at 24 mo	Not all surviving children followed up (outcomes of 73% of a group of predetermined centers)
MagNET	*Primary*: composite of "adverse pediatric health outcomes" (neonatal IVH, PVL, CP, or death) by 18 mo old	—	No criteria for CP diagnosis In tocolytic arm, crossover allowed

Abbreviations: CP, cerebral palsy; IVH, intraventricular hemorrhage; PVL, periventricular leukomalacia; WMI, white matter injury.
Modified from Costantine MM, Weiner SJ, Eunice Kennedy Shriver NICHD Maternal-Fetal Medicine Units Network. Effects of antenatal exposure to magnesium sulfate on neuroprotection and mortality in preterm infants. Obstet Gynecol 2009;114:358; with permission.

whose mother received placebo (OR 2.0, 95% CI 0.99–4.1; P = .07). Despite being statistically not significant, these findings led to premature termination of the study because of safety concerns of increased pediatric mortality and adverse outcomes.[41]

The Australasian Collaborative Trial of Magnesium Sulfate (ACTOMgSO₄)

Patients at less than 30 weeks' gestation with expected (indicated or spontaneous) delivery in less than 24 hours were included. This study excluded patients if they were in the second stage of labor, previously received $MgSO_4$ in the current pregnancy, or had other contraindications. A total of 1062 women were randomized to $MgSO_4$ (4 g loading infusion over 20 minutes, followed by a maintenance infusion of 1 g/h for 24 hours or until birth, whichever was first; n = 535 women) or equal infusion volume of normal saline as placebo (n = 527 women). The primary outcomes of the study were total pediatric mortality, CP, and a combined outcome of death or CP at 2 years of corrected age. The criteria for CP included abnormalities of tone and loss of motor function, and the investigators reported that its diagnosis was reflective of "usual clinical practice." "Substantial gross motor dysfunction," one of the secondary outcomes, was defined as "inability to walk independently" at 2 years, which corresponds to a Gross Motor Function Classification System (GMFCS) score of at least 2 out of 5 using the Palisano criteria.[47] This criterion is consistent with what other studies used to diagnose moderate to severe CP (see later discussion). There was no difference in the composite neonatal outcome of death or CP (19.8% vs 24.0%, relative risk [RR] 0.83, 95% CI 0.66–1.03; P = .09), or CP (6.8% vs 8.2%, RR 0.83, 95% CI 0.54–1.27; P = .38), or total pediatric mortality (13.8% vs 17.1%, RR 0.83, 95% CI 0.64–1.09; P = .19) in those exposed to $MgSO_4$ or placebo, respectively. However, the secondary outcomes of substantial gross motor dysfunction (3.4% vs 6.6%, RR 0.51, 95% CI 0.29–0.91; P = 0 .02) and the combined outcome of death or substantial gross motor dysfunction (17.0% vs 22.7%, RR 0.75, 95% CI 0.59–0.96; P = .02) were decreased in infants exposed in utero to $MgSO_4$ or placebo, respectively.[42]

The Magnesium Sulfate for the Prevention of Eclampsia (Magpie) Trial

The Magpie[43] study was an international study evaluating the benefit of $MgSO_4$ in preventing eclampsia. It also had a planned follow-up of longer than 18 months to assess the long-term effect of in utero exposure to $MgSO_4$. The primary outcome was a combined outcome of death or neurosensory disability at 18 months of corrected age. There were no differences in the primary outcome (15.0% vs 14.1%, RR 1.06, 95% CI 0.90–1.25), neurosensory disability (1.3% vs 1.9%, RR 0.72, 95% CI 0.40–1.29), or death (13.8% vs 12.5%, RR 1.11, 95% CI 0.93–1.32) among those exposed to $MgSO_4$ or placebo, respectively.[43]

PREMAG

Women with singleton or multiple gestations at less than 33 weeks' gestation with anticipated delivery in 24 hours were included. Those with need for emergency delivery, had pregnancy-associated vascular disease, received calcium channel blockers or indocin in the prior 24 hours, or had various maternal/fetal complications such as preeclampsia or intrauterine growth restriction, were excluded. Women were randomized to intravenous $MgSO_4$ 4 g infusion bolus or saline as placebo. The primary outcomes were severe WMI, infant death before hospital discharge, or their combined outcome.[44] A 2-year follow-up of these infants was done to evaluate the long-term morbidities and mortality, including CP, motor and cognitive retardation, pediatric mortality, and combined outcomes.[46] The study was terminated before achieving its

Table 4
Magnesium sulfate regimen variations between individual trials

Study	Magnesium Regimen	Actual Amount Received (in the Magnesium Group)
BEAM	6 g bolus over 20–30 min then 2 g/h maintenance Maintenance stopped if delivery had not occurred in 12 h and was no longer considered imminent Infusion resumed when delivery was deemed imminent again; if ≥6 h from last infusion, another loading dose given	996/1096 (90.9%) received magnesium for ≥3 h 82/1096 (7.5%) received magnesium <3 h 18/1096 (1.6%) did not receive magnesium 27 (2.5%) received magnesium for other indications magnesium dose median (IQR): 31.5 (29.0–44.6) g
ACTOMgSO$_4$	4 g bolus over 20 min then 1 g/h maintenance until birth or up to 24 h, whichever was first Treatment was not repeated	13/535 (2.4%) did not receive magnesium 38/535 (7.1%) received partial loading dose only 33/535 (6.2%) received full loading dose only 381/535 (71.2%) received full loading + partial maintenance 70/535 (13.1%) received full loading + full maintenance dose 4 (0.7%) received magnesium for clinical reasons after enrollment magnesium dose, median (IQR): 6.5 (4.5–14) g
PREMAG	4 g bolus over 30 min	20/286 (7.0%) did not receive magnesium 7/286 (2.4%) received partial dose only 259/286 (90.6%) received full dose None received magnesium for other indications
Magpie	IV: 4 g bolus over 1–15 min then 1 g/h for 24 h IM: 4 g IV bolus combined with 10 g IM, given as 5 g into each buttock, followed by 5 g every 4 h for 24 h	4% did not receive magnesium Magnesium dose, median (IQR): 18 (9–29) g[a] Time to delivery, median (IQR): 12 (4–46) h[a]
MagNET	Preventive arm: 4 g bolus Tocolytic arm: 4 g bolus then 2–3 g/h	Did not report

[a] Estimate—uncertain from published data.

From Costantine MM, Weiner SJ, Eunice Kennedy Shriver NICHD Maternal-Fetal Medicine Units Network. Effects of antenatal exposure to magnesium sulfate on neuroprotection and mortality in preterm infants. Obstet Gynecol 2009;114:359; with permission.

sample size because of poor recruitment. There were no differences in the primary outcomes: total mortality (9.4% vs 10.4%; OR 0.79, 95% CI 0.44–1.44), severe WMI (10.0% vs 11.7%; OR 0.78, 95% CI 0.47–1.31), and their combined outcome (16.5% vs 17.9%; OR 0.86, 95% CI 0.55–1.34) between those exposed to MgSO$_4$

or placebo, respectively. At the 2-year follow-up of 606 infants, perinatal mortality (9.7% vs 11.3%, RR 0.74, 95% CI 0.42–1.32; P = .47), CP (7.0% vs 10.2%, OR 0.63, 95% CI 0.35–1.15; P = .13), and death or CP (16.1% vs 20.2%, RR 0.65, 95% CI 0.42–1.03; P = .07) were similar between those exposed to $MgSO_4$ or placebo, respectively. However, death or gross motor dysfunction (25.6% vs 30.8%, OR 0.62, 95% CI 0.41–0.93; P = .02) and death or motor/cognitive delay (34.9% vs 40.5%, OR 0.68, 95% CI 0.47–0.99; P = .05) were reduced in the group exposed to $MgSO_4$.[44,46]

The Beneficial Effects of Antenatal Magnesium Sulfate (BEAM) Trial

The Eunice Kennedy Shriver National Institute of Child Health and Human Development Maternal-Fetal Medicine Units (MFMU) Network conducted this study at 20 centers in the United States from 1997 to 2004. The study randomized women at imminent risk of delivery between 24 and 31 weeks' gestation to either $MgSO_4$ (6 g bolus of $MgSO_4$ followed by a continuous infusion of 2 g/h for 12 hours) or placebo.[45] The study allowed retreatment if the patient did not deliver after 12 hours. A total of 2241 women were randomized, and their neonates were followed up and assessed at 2 years of age. CP was determined by a certified pediatrician or pediatric neurologist using prespecified criteria of gross motor delay and tone, movement, and reflex abnormalities, and its severity was assessed using GMFCS criteria with the diagnosis of moderate to severe CP defined by a GMFCS score of 2 or more.[47] The primary outcome was a composite of moderate or severe CP or death. There was no difference in the primary outcome between those exposed to $MgSO_4$ versus placebo (11.3% vs 11.7%, RR 0.97, 95% CI 0.77–1.23). There was also no difference in the risk of perinatal mortality (9.5% vs 8.5%, RR 1.12, 95% CI 0.85–1.47). However, moderate or severe CP was significantly less likely to occur among children exposed to $MgSO_4$ compared with placebo (1.9% vs 3.5%, RR 0.55, 95% CI 0.32–0.95; P = .03) as well as overall cerebral palsy (4.2% vs 7.3%, P = .004).[45]

META-ANALYSES

After the publication of the BEAM trial, several systematic reviews and meta-analyses were published.[48–51] These reviews showed similarly that magnesium reduced the rate of CP by approximately 30% (RR 0.68; 95% CI 0.54–0.87) and moderate to severe CP (by ≈40%–45%) without increasing the rate of death in 6145 infants (RR 1.04, 95% CI 0.92–1.17).[48] Moderate or severe CP in the BEAM study was defined as "inability to walk independently at age 2 years," which corresponded to what other studies reported as substantial gross motor dysfunction. Both correspond at 2 years of age to a severity level of 2 or greater on the GMFCS, developed by Palisano and colleagues.[47]

When all studies were pooled according to the gestational age at randomization of less than 30 (3107 fetuses/infants) and less than 32 to 34 weeks' (n = 5235 fetuses/infants) gestation, $MgSO_4$ did not reduce the risk of the composite outcome of CP or death. However, the benefit of $MgSO_4$ was seen in reducing CP as well as moderate to severe CP without increasing the risk of death.[48,50,51] In infants exposed to $MgSO_4$ in utero before 32 to 34 weeks' gestation and who survive until age 18 to 24 months, the number needed to treat (NNT) to prevent one case of CP is 56 (95% CI 34–164); similarly, in those exposed prior to 30 weeks' gestation the NNT to prevent one case of CP is 46 (95% CI 26–187).[50]

Studies designed for neuroprotection were MagNET preventive arm, ACTOMgSO4, PREMAG, and BEAM. Their gestational age upper limits for inclusion were 34, 30, 33, and 32 weeks, respectively. The majority of patients in these studies were admitted or enrolled with a diagnosis of preterm labor or preterm premature rupture of membranes (PPROM). When these studies were pooled together (n = 4446 fetuses/infants), ante-natal exposure to $MgSO_4$ was associated with a reduction in the combined outcome of death or CP (RR 0.85, 95% CI 0.74–0.98) as well as that of death or moderate to severe CP.[48,51] In addition, antenatal exposure to $MgSO_4$ was found to decrease the risk of CP (RR = 0.71, 95% CI 0.55–0.91) and moderate to severe CP (RR 0.60, 95% CI 0.43–0.84) without increasing the risk of perinatal or infant death (RR 0.95, 95% CI 0.80–1.13) or any other maternal or pediatric adverse events. In this subgroup the NNT to prevent one case of CP, in infants exposed to $MgSO_4$ in utero and who survive until age 18 to 24 months, is 52 (95% CI 30–184).[50]

LIMITATION OF THE STUDIES AND META-ANALYSES

The studies and meta-analyses previously described led the American Congress of Obstetricians and Gynecologists and the Society for Maternal-Fetal Medicine to publish a committee opinion stating:

> ...none of the individual studies found a benefit with regard to their primary outcome. However, the available evidence suggests that magnesium sulfate given before anticipated early preterm birth reduces the risk of cerebral palsy in surviving infants. Physicians electing to use magnesium sulfate for fetal neuropro-tection should develop specific guidelines regarding inclusion criteria, treatment regimens, concurrent tocolytics, and monitoring in accordance with one of the larger trials.[52]

This statement was necessary, as there remain many questions that need to be answered because the available data lack consensus support in the obstetric community:

1. Although the meta-analyses reported no statistical heterogeneity between the studies, they suffered from clinical heterogeneity in patient selection and character-istics (see **Table 2**). All patients in the Magpie trial[43] were enrolled with a diagnosis of preeclampsia. However, in the other trials preterm labor (PTL) and PPROM were the main indications for admission/delivery: 87% of patients in the BEAM[45] trial had PPROM, and 63% of those in ACTOMgSO4[42] had PTL. In the PREMAG[44,46] trial the majority of the patients had either PTL or PPROM. All patients of the MagNET trial[41] were enrolled in PTL. Different maternal diseases and intrauterine environments leading to preterm delivery (eg, premature rupture of the membranes and intra-uterine infection/inflammation) have been shown to modify the risk of CP. It is plau-sible that the impact of $MgSO_4$ neuroprotection may be different according to the indication for preterm birth. Nevertheless, the studies that were dominated by patients with PPROM and by PTL demonstrated similar findings in this regard. In addition, because only Magpie[43] specifically provides outcomes up to 37 weeks' gestational age, and none of the other 4 trials randomized anyone beyond 34 weeks, it is inappropriate to include these studies in any analysis beyond the upper end of their gestational age limit for randomization. Therefore, the benefit of using $MgSO_4$ beyond 32 to 34 weeks for fetal neuroprotection is unproven.
2. The magnesium regimen used and the actual dosage received varied between different studies and between patients within individual studies (see **Table 4**). Moreover, although most of the studies included women with anticipated delivery within 24 hours, not all patients delivered within that time frame, which raises the issue of the timing of $MgSO_4$ infusion for fetal neuroprotection. Thus, the

appropriate dosage and therapeutic window for neuroprotection is not known. The MFMU Network trial also analyzed the relation of $MgSO_4$ dose received to the studied outcomes. The OR for fetal or infant death in the highest $MgSO_4$ total dose quartile (dose range, 44–201 g) and the highest quartile of cord blood magnesium at birth, relative to the lowest quartiles, were 1.01 (95% CI 0.48–2.10) and 0.82 (95% CI 0.36–1.84), respectively. This result refutes the suggestion of a "toxic" dose or fetal concentration of $MgSO_4$.[53]

3. The use of a composite outcome of death or CP (or gross motor dysfunction) in these studies is expected for both logistic reasons (power/sample size and feasibility issues) and the fact that these are competing outcomes: if the infant dies, he or she cannot be evaluated for diagnosis of CP. The results from all the RCTs were negative for the primary outcome. Only the meta-analysis of neuroprotective trials demonstrates a reduction in the composite outcome with $MgSO_4$. This finding has reignited the debate on the appropriate use of meta-analytical studies of well-designed and powered individual RCTs.[54]

4. Other questions that are not answered in these studies involve the concomitant use of tocolytics with $MgSO_4$ given in the setting of neuroprotection. Of note, the BEAM trial included patients who were not candidates for tocolysis (PPROM, advanced cervical dilatation, or indicated deliveries). Therefore, the findings of the trials should not be extrapolated to $MgSO_4$ use as a tocolytic. The combination of both may have serious adverse effects.

SUMMARY

$MgSO_4$ has been used extensively either as a tocolytic or for eclampsia prevention and treatment. Based on the available data from meta-analyses, 46 to 56 (95% confidence limits range from 26 to 187) would need to be exposed to $MgSO_4$ in utero before 30 or 32 weeks of gestation, respectively, to prevent one case of CP.[50] Cerebral palsy is permanent, can result in severe sequelae for the infant, and can significantly affect the family and society as a whole. The NNT to prevent one case of CP appears justifiable and comparable (or better) with those for eclampsia prevention. Given the relative safety of $MgSO_4$ for the mother, the lack of evident risk regarding infant mortality, and the familiarity of most obstetricians with its use, $MgSO_4$ should be considered for use as a neuroprotectant in the setting of anticipated preterm birth, after discussing the risks and benefits with the patient and obtaining her approval. Significant questions remain unanswered, in particular the ideal candidate and the dosage/timing of $MgSO_4$. Until then, it is preferable to follow a specific protocol that should be decided upon at the institution level.[54,55]

REFERENCES

1. Hagberg B, Hagberg G, Beckung E, et al. Changing panorama of cerebral palsy in Sweden. VIII. Prevalence and origin in the birth year period 1991–94. Acta Paediatr 2001;90:271–7.
2. Yeargin-Allsopp M, Van Naarden Braun K, Doernberg NS, et al. Prevalence of cerebral palsy in 8-year-old children in three areas of the United States in 2002: a multisite collaboration. Pediatrics 2008;121:547–54.
3. Jacobsson B, Hagberg G, Hagberg B, et al. Cerebral palsy in preterm infants: a population-based case-control study of antenatal and intrapartal risk factors. Acta Paediatr 2002;91:946–51.

4. Clark SM, Ghulmiyyah LM, Hankins GD. Antenatal antecedents and the impact of obstetric care in the etiology of cerebral palsy. Clin Obstet Gynecol 2008;51: 775–86.

5. Nelson KB, Grether JK. Causes of cerebral palsy. Curr Opin Pediatr 1999;11: 487–91.

6. Honeycutt A, Dunlap L, Chen H, et al. Economic costs associated with mental retardation, cerebral palsy, hearing loss, and vision impairment—United States 2003. MMWR Morb Mortal Wkly Rep 2004;53:57–9.

7. Hankins GD, Speer M. Defining the pathogenesis and pathophysiology of neonatal encephalopathy and cerebral palsy. Obstet Gynecol 2003;102:628–36.

8. Keogh JM, Badawi N. The origins of cerebral palsy. Curr Opin Neurol 2006;19: 129–34.

9. Stanley F, Blair E, Alberman E. Cerebral palsies: epidemiology and causal pathways. London: MacKeith Press; 2000. p. 22–39.

10. Murphy DJ, Sellers S, MacKenzie IZ, et al. A case-control study of antenatal and intrapartum risk factors for cerebral palsy in very preterm singleton babies. Lancet 1995;346:1449–54.

11. Kent A, Lomas F, Hurrion, et al. Antenatal steroids may reduce adverse neurologic outcome following chorioamnionitis: neurodevelopmental outcome and chorioamnionitis in premature infants. J Paediatr Child Health 2005;41:186–90.

12. Ribiani E, Rosati A, Romanelli M, et al. Perinatal infections and cerebral palsy. Minerva Ginecol 2007;59:151–7.

13. de Hann HH, Gunn AJ, Williams CE, et al. Magnesium sulfate therapy during asphyxia in near-term fetal lambs does not compromise the fetus but does not reduce cerebral injury. Am J Obstet Gynecol 1997;176:18–27.

14. MacDonald RL, Curry DJ, Aihara Y, et al. Magnesium and experimental vasospasm. J Neurosurg 2004;100:106–10.

15. Schiff SJ, Somjen GG. Hyperexcitability following moderate hypoxia in hippocampal tissue slices. Brain Res 1985;337:337–40.

16. Wyatt JS, Edwards AD, Azzopardi D, et al. Magnetic resonance and near infrared spectroscopy for investigation of perinatal hypoxic-ischaemic brain injury. Arch Dis Child 1989;64:953–63.

17. Volpe JJ. Perinatal brain injury: from pathogenesis to neuroprotection. Ment Retard Dev Disabil Res Rev 2001;7:56–64.

18. Grow J, Barks JD. Pathogenesis of hypoxic-ischemic cerebral injury in the term infant: current concepts. Clin Perinatol 2002;29:585–602.

19. Sang N, Meng Z. Blockade by magnesium of sodium currents in acutely isolated hippocampal CA1 neurons of rat. Brain Res 2002;952:218–21.

20. Goñi-de-Cerio F, Alvarez A, Alvarez FJ, et al. $MgSO_4$ treatment preserves the ischemia-induced reduction in S-100 protein without modification of the expression of endothelial tight junction molecules. Histol Histopathol 2009;24: 1129–38.

21. McDonald JW, Silverstein FS, Johnston MV. Magnesium reduces N-methyl-D-aspartate (NMDA)-mediated brain injury in perinatal rats. Neurosci Lett 1990; 109:234–8.

22. Marret S, Gressens P, Gadisseux JF, et al. Prevention by magnesium of excitotoxic neuronal death in the developing brain: an animal model for clinical intervention studies. Dev Med Child Neurol 1995;37:473–84.

23. Palmer C. Hypoxic-ischemic encephalopathy. Therapeutic approaches against microvascular injury, and role of neutrophils, PAF, and free radicals. Clin Perinatol 1995;22:481–517.

24. Thordstein M, Bågenholm R, Thiringer K, et al. Scavengers of free oxygen radicals in combination with magnesium ameliorate perinatal hypoxic-ischemic brain damage in the rat. Pediatr Res 1993;34:23–6.

25. Spandou E, Soubasi V, Papoutsopoulou S, et al. Neuroprotective effect of long-term $MgSO_4$ administration after cerebral hypoxia-ischemia in newborn rats is related to the severity of brain damage. Reprod Sci 2007;14:667–77.

26. Hagan P, Barks JD, Yabut M, et al. Adenovirus-mediated over-expression of interleukin-1 receptor antagonist reduces susceptibility to excitotoxic brain injury in perinatal rats. Neuroscience 1996;75:1033–45c.

27. Yamasaki Y, Shozurhara H, Onodera H, et al. Blocking of interleukin-1 activity is a beneficial approach to ischemia brain edema formation. Acta Neurochir Suppl 1994;60:300–2.

28. Shogi T, Miyamoto A, Ishiguro S, et al. Enhanced release of IL-1beta and TNF-alpha following endotoxin challenge from rat alveolar macrophages cultured in low-Mg(2+) medium. Magnes Res 2003;16:111–9.

29. Burd I, Breen K, Friedman A, et al. Magnesium sulfate reduces inflammation-associated brain injury in fetal mice. Am J Obstet Gynecol 2010;202:292. e1–9.

30. Nelson KB, Grether JK. Can magnesium sulfate reduce the risk of cerebral palsy in very low birth weight infants? Pediatrics 1995;95:263–9.

31. Hauth JC, Goldenberg RL, Nelson KG, et al. Reduction of cerebral palsy with maternal $MgSO_4$ treatment in newborns weighing 500–1000 g. Am J Obstet Gynecol 1995;172:419.

32. Schendel DE, Berg CJ, Yeargin-Allsopp M, et al. Prenatal magnesium sulfate exposure and the risk of CP or mental retardation among very-low-birth-weight children aged 3 to 5 years. JAMA 1996;276:1805–10.

33. Finesmith RB, Roche K, Yellin PB, et al. Effect of magnesium sulfate on the development of cystic periventricular leukomalacia in preterm infants. Am J Perinatol 1997;14:303–7.

34. Canterino JC, Verma UL, Visintainer PF, et al. Maternal magnesium sulfate and the development of neonatal periventricular leukomalacia and intraventricular hemorrhage. Obstet Gynecol 1999;93:396–402.

35. O'Shea TM, Klinepeter KI, Dillard RG. Prenatal events and the risk of cerebral palsy in very low birth weight infants. Am J Epidemiol 1998;147:362–9.

36. Paneth N, Jetton J, Pinto-Martin J, et al. The Neonatal Brain Hemorrhage Study Analysis Group. Magnesium sulfate in labor and risk of neonatal brain lesions and cerebral palsy in low birth weight infants. Pediatrics 1997;99:E1.

37. Leviton A, Paneth N, Susser M, et al. Maternal receipt of magnesium sulfate does not seem to reduce the risk of neonatal white matter damage. Pediatrics 1997; 99:E2.

38. Boyle CA, Yeargin-Allsopp MM, Schendel DE, et al. Tocolytic magnesium sulfate exposure and risk of cerebral palsy among children with birth weights less than 1,750 grams. Am J Epidemiol 2000;152:120–4.

39. Grether JK, Hoogstrate J, Walsh-Greene E, et al. Magnesium sulfate for tocolysis and risk of spastic cerebral palsy in premature children born to women without preeclampsia. Am J Obstet Gynecol 2000;183:717–25.

40. Wiswell TE, Graziani LJ, Caddell JL, et al. Maternally administered magnesium sulfate protects against early brain injury and long term adverse neurodevelopmental outcomes in premature infants: a prospective study. Pediatr Res 1996;39:253A.

41. Mittendorf R, Dambrosia J, Pryde PG, et al. Association between the use of antenatal magnesium sulfate in preterm labor and adverse health outcomes in infants. Am J Obstet Gynecol 2002;186:1111–8.

42. Crowther CA, Hiller JE, Doyle LW, et al. Australasian Collaborative Trial of Magnesium Sulphate (ACTOMgSO$_4$) Collaborative Group. Effect of magnesium sulfate given for neuroprotection before preterm birth: a randomized controlled trial. JAMA 2003;290:2669–76.

43. Magpie Trial Follow-Up Study Collaborative Group. The Magpie Trial: a randomised trial comparing magnesium sulphate with placebo for pre-eclampsia. Outcome for children at 18 months. BJOG 2007;114:289–99.

44. Marret S, Marpeau L, Zupan-Simunek V, et al, PREMAG Trial Group. Magnesium sulphate given before very-preterm birth to protect infant brain: the randomised controlled PREMAG trial. BJOG 2007;114:310–8.

45. Rouse DJ, Hirtz DG, Thom E, et al, Eunice Kennedy Shriver NICHD Maternal-Fetal Medicine Units Network. A randomized trial of magnesium sulfate for the prevention of cerebral palsy. N Engl J Med 2008;359:895–905.

46. Marret S, Marpeau L, Follet-Bouhamed C, et al, PREMAG Trial Group. Effect of magnesium sulphate on mortality and neurologic morbidity of the very-preterm newborn with two-year neurologic outcome: results of the prospective PREMAG trial. Gynecol Obstet Fertil 2008;36:278–88 [in French].

47. Palisano R, Rosenbaum P, Walter S, et al. Development and reliability of a system to classify gross motor function in children with cerebral palsy. Dev Med Child Neurol 1997;39:214–23.

48. Doyle LW, Crowther CA, Middleton P, et al. Magnesium sulphate for women at risk of preterm birth for neuroprotection of the fetus. Cochrane Database Syst Rev 2009;1:CD004661.

49. Doyle LW, Crowther CA, Middleton P, et al. Antenatal magnesium sulfate and neurologic outcome in preterm infants: a systematic review. Obstet Gynecol 2009;113:1327–33.

50. Costantine MM, Weiner SJ, Eunice Kennedy Shriver NICHD Maternal-Fetal Medicine Units Network. Effects of antenatal exposure to magnesium sulfate on neuroprotection and mortality in preterm infants. Obstet Gynecol 2009;114:354–64.

51. Conde-Agudelo A, Romero R. Antenatal magnesium sulfate for the prevention of cerebral palsy in preterm infants less than 34 weeks' gestation: a systematic review and metaanalysis. Am J Obstet Gynecol 2009;200:595–609.

52. American College of Obstetricians and Gynecologists. Magnesium sulfate before anticipated preterm birth for neuroprotection. Committee Opinion No. 455. Obstet Gynecol 2010;115:669–71.

53. Rouse DJ, Hirtz DG, Thom EA. Magnesium sulfate for the prevention of cerebral palsy. Reply to Mittendorf R, Pryde P. N Engl J Med 2009;360:190.

54. Cahill AG, Caughey AB. Magnesium for neuroprophylaxis: fact or fiction? Am J Obstet Gynecol 2009;200:590–4.

55. Scott J. Magnesium sulfate for neuroprotection. What do we do now? Obstet Gynecol 2009;114:500–1.

Clinical Management of the Short Cervix

Julio Mateus, MD

KEYWORDS

- Short cervix • Progesterone • Cervical cerclage
- Cervical length

Preterm birth (PTB), defined as a birth before 37 weeks of gestation or 259 days from the first day of the last normal menstrual period or 245 days after conception,[1] is responsible of major perinatal and infant morbidity and mortality.[2–4] PTB contributes to approximately one-third of the infant deaths in the United States.[2] More than one-half of all infant deaths in this country in 2005 occurred in infants born at less than 32 weeks of gestation.[3] Mortality and morbidities are inversely proportional to the gestational age at delivery. Morbidities associated with prematurity include respiratory distress syndrome, bronchopulmonary dysplasia, necrotizing enterocolitis, intraventricular hemorrhage, retinopathy, and sepsis. Compared with children born at term, infants born preterm have higher rates of major complications at 5 years of age including cerebral palsy, learning disabilities, sensory deficits, and other serious neurologic disabilities.[4] The most recent preliminary data from the National Center for Health Statistics in the United States showed that the rate of PTB declined 0.3% from 12.7% of all births in 2007 to 12.3% of all births in 2008.[5] The downturn in preterm births in 2007 to 2008 was mostly in pregnancies at late preterm gestational ages or 34 to 36 weeks (down from 9.0% to 8.8%), whereas the percentage of infants delivered at very low birth weight (VLBW; <1500 g) who are at the highest risk of early death or disability declined very slightly, from 1.48% to 1.46%. Although the decline is promising and could be the result of new preventive actions and changes in medical practice, efforts should continue to focus on the prevention of the extreme premature birth associated with significant immediate and long-term consequences. Recent studies on predictive factors suggest that cervical length (CL) measured by transvaginal ultrasonography (TVU) is among the best predictors of preterm birth, particularly in the high-risk population. Thus, ultrasonography of the cervix is gaining more acceptance among obstetricians. Based on its high accuracy to predict PTB, recent clinical trials assessed the efficacy of clinical interventions such as progesterone and cervical cerclage in the prevention of PTB. This article summarizes the most relevant data on the clinical strategies for pregnant women diagnosed with shortening cervix in the mid-trimester. The

There is no any conflict of interest.

Division of Maternal Fetal Medicine, Department of Obstetrics and Gynecology, The University of Texas Medical Branch at Galveston, 301 University Boulevard, Galveston, TX 77555, USA

E-mail address: jfmateus@utmb.edu

Obstet Gynecol Clin N Am 38 (2011) 367–385

doi:10.1016/j.ogc.2011.02.020

0889-8545/11/$ – see front matter © 2011 Elsevier Inc. All rights reserved.

obgyn.theclinics.com

study is focused on the effects of progesterone and cervical cerclage in the reduction of PTB and perinatal morbidity and mortality in 3 subgroups: (1) low-risk, defined as nulliparous and women with no history of PTB, (2) women with prior PTB, and (3) twin gestation. Other interventions proposed for the management of women with a short cervix, such as indomethacin and vaginal pessary, are also discussed.

TRANSVAGINAL ULTRASOUND EXAMINATION OF THE CERVIX

Digital cervical examination has been the most traditional method to assess early cervical changes that precede PTB. However, this method is a poor predictor of preterm delivery, because is not reliable, is subjective, and has greater than 50% inter-observer variability.[6] Manual cervical examination is also nonspecific, as 15% to 16% of primiparous women and 17% to 35% of multiparous women who are delivered at term have had a cervical dilation between 1 and 2 cm in the late second trimester.[7] In the last 3 decades, measurement of CL using TVU has become an accurate screening tool for preterm delivery. The superiority of this method over the traditional manual cervical examination has been consistently demonstrated.[8,9] Compared with manual cervical examination, measurement of CL on TVU between 14 and 30 weeks of gestation is a better predictor of preterm delivery at less than 35 weeks of gestation in a high-risk population such as women with a history of preterm delivery, mullerian anomaly, 2 or more voluntary terminations, diethylstilbestrol (DES) exposure, history of cone biopsy, and Ehler-Danlos syndrome.[9] The predictive values are particularly high when the CL is measured between 14 and 22 weeks of gestation. The high accuracy of TVU CL is attributed to the ability to measure the total cervical length including the internal os, where early changes are highly predictive of PTB, and the low interobserver and intraobsever variability with adherence to proper technique, both estimated at less than 10%.[9]

The technique to assess the CL by ultrasonography has been well described.[10] Measurements are performed using a transvaginal probe after the patient has emptied her bladder. The CL is measured from the internal os to the external os along the endocervical canal. At least 3 measurements are obtained and the shortest best measurement is recorded in millimeters. It is recommended to apply fundal pressure for 15 seconds to observe any changes in the CL or funneling. The length of the closed cervix or functional cervix is the most useful measurement to predict PTB.[10] When the internal os is opened, the funnel length is measured from the upper portion of the cervix to the internal os. The total cervical length is equivalent to the sum of the functional cervix and the funnel length, and the percent funneling is defined as funnel length divided by total cervical length.[9] If funneling is present, the shape of the funneling needs to be recorded from the normal T shape, to Y, then V, and finally U,[11] as funneling is a continuous process that seems to be associated with the risk of PTB.[9] In a high-risk population study, minimal funneling defined as less than 25% at 14 to 22 weeks of gestation was not associated with PTB, whereas moderate (25%–50%) and severe (more than 50%) funneling were associated with a risk greater than 50% for PTB.[9] A recent secondary analysis of a randomized trial of cerclage showed that compared with a V-shaped funnel, a U-shaped funnel was more associated with PTB at less than 24, 28, 35, and 37 weeks of gestation.[12] The earlier in gestation the cervical shortening is detected, the higher the risk of PTB.[13,14] Furthermore, the risk of PTB at a gestational age of less than 35 weeks decreases by approximately 6% for each additional millimeter of CL and by approximately 5% for each additional week of pregnancy at which the CL is measured.[14] The best cervical parameter found in most studies to have the best predictive accuracy has been a CL less than 25 mm. Besides the CL cutoff, other factors such as the study population, the gestational age at screening, the prevalence of preterm birth, and single versus serial screening influence the sensitivity and specificity of this test.

PREDICTION OF SPONTANEOUS PTB IN LOW-RISK WOMEN WITH A SHORT CERVIX ON TVU IN THE SECOND TRIMESTER

In asymptomatic pregnant women without any recognizable risk factor for PTB, CL is a continuous variable with a mean of 35 to 40 mm from 14 to 30 weeks. For this range of gestational age, the CL lower 10th percentile is 25 mm, whereas the upper 10th percentile or 90th percentile is 50 mm.[13,15] A progressive shortening of the cervix is noted after 30 weeks of gestation in this population even in women destined to deliver at term.[16] Using a different CL cutoff from 15 mm to 34 mm, several studies have reported that the shorter the cervix, the higher the risk of PTB.[13,15,17] However, the positive predictive values (PPVs) reported in these studies are low, 44% being the highest.[17] In a well-designed large study in low-risk women, the PPV for preterm delivery before 35 weeks was only 18%, which means that 82% of women diagnosed with shortening cervix in fact delivered by 35 weeks.[13] Based on these data, CL should not be used a screening predictor of PTB in low-risk women.

CLINICAL MANAGEMENT OF LOW-RISK WOMEN WITH A SHORT CERVIX

Clinical management of cervical shortening in asymptomatic low-risk women is under much investigation. Progesterone used in different compounds and routes of delivery is one of the most studied agents in recent years for the prevention of PTB. Progesterone's biologic effects on the cervix, myometrium, and chorioamniotic membranes can have potential beneficial effects in women with a short cervix. The actions of progesterone on the pregnant myometrium include relaxation of myometrial smooth muscle, blocking of oxytocin action, and inhibition of gap junctions formation.[18,19] In sheep and other mammals, a decrease in plasma progesterone and an increase in circulating estrogen precede the onset of labor.[20] In humans, there is not such large alteration in the ratio of plasma estrogen to progesterone before the onset of labor. However, there is evidence that local changes in the progesterone level or the ratio of progesterone to estrogen in the placenta, decidua, or fetal membranes may be important in the initiation of labor.[21] Recent data suggest that 17α-hydroxyprogesterone (17-P) may prevent PTB by inhibiting inflammatory cytokines in the cervix.[22] Conversely, administration of progesterone antagonists in women at term results in an increased rate of spontaneous labor.[23] It is noteworthy that epidemiologic and animal studies have found no significant relationship between clinically administered progestational drugs and congenital malformations.[24]

Only one clinical trial has investigated the effect of progesterone in the reduction of PTB in women with a short cervix on ultrasonography in the mid-trimester.[25] Of these, only one study analyzed a separate subgroup of women considered to be at low risk for PTB, nulliparous women, and women with no history of PTB.[25] A secondary analysis was intended for women without history of PTB and a short cervix (CL ≤25 mm) enrolled in a clinical trial of progesterone for prevention of PTB in a high-risk population.[26] However, there were only 9 patients (1.3%) who met these criteria out of 609 women enrolled in the original trial. Instead, this group of investigators conducted a secondary analysis of women with history of PTB and a short cervix enrolled in the clinical trial.[27] In this secondary analysis, the rate of spontaneous PTB ≤32 weeks was significantly lower in women with a CL ≤28 mm in the mid-trimester who received 90 mg of vaginal progesterone gel daily compared with those assigned to placebo (0% vs 29.6; $P = 0.01$).[27] In the largest existent randomized clinical trial, 250 women with singleton or twin pregnancies who had a CL 15 mm or less on TVU at 20 to 25 weeks of gestation were randomized to receive either 200 mg of micronized progesterone or identical-appearing capsules of placebo vaginally each night from day 24 to 33 completed weeks.[25] Spontaneous delivery at less than 34 weeks was less frequent in the progesterone group than in the placebo group (19.2% vs 34.4%; relative risk [RR], 056; 95% confidence interval [CI], 0.36–0.86). There were no significant differences in the rate of perinatal mortality or morbidity between the two groups. In women without a history of PTB, there was a significant reduction of spontaneous delivery before 34 weeks in the progesterone group compared with the placebo group (20% vs 31.2%). However, it was not possible to discern whether the reduction was in singleton or twin gestations, or in both.[25] At present there are two ongoing clinical trials investigating the role of progesterone in the reduction of PTB in women with a short cervix. One of these, conducted by Spong and colleagues, assesses the effect of 17-P in nulliparous women with a short cervix (**Table 1**). This trial is of paramount importance, as it will determine the role of 17-P in the reduction of PTB in this subgroup of low-risk women.

Cervical cerclage is the other intervention that has been extensively studied in women with a risk of PTB. It has been proposed that once the cervix is short, reinforce-ment the cervix and keeping at least the bottom half of the endocervical canal closed with a stitch (cerclage) can be beneficial. Thus, among women with a high risk of PTB, those with a short cervix may have the best benefit from cervical cerclage. Five clinical trials investigated the efficacy of cervical cerclage in preventing PTB in asymptomatic pregnant women with a short cervix on TVU in the second trimester.[28–32] A meta-analysis of the first 4 trials using patient-individual data was recently reported.[33] The screening population, gestational age at screening, CL cutoff, type of cerclage, type of suture, and primary outcome, among other factors, vary considerably between these trials (**Table 2**). The meta-analysis of Berghella and colleagues[33] is the only study that investigated the efficacy of cervical cerclage in low-risk women with a short cervix. In this study, cervical cerclage did not reduce the rate of PTB before 35 weeks in women with a short cervix in the mid-trimester and without history of prior PTB, and no other risks for PTB (RR 0.84, 95% CI 0.80–1.17 and RR 0.76, 95% CI 0.53–1.15, respectively). In addition, this intervention did not decrease the rate of perinatal mortality in either subgroup (RR 0.94, 95% CI 0.46–1.90 and RR 1.18, 95% CI 0.48–2.88). Thus, the evidence regarding the efficacy of cervical cerclage is limited, but suggests that cerclage is not efficacious in preventing PTB and improving perinatal outcomes in this low-risk population. Until more data are available, the use of cervical cerclage in nulliparous women and in multiparous women with no history of PTB or any other risks factors for preterm delivery should be discouraged.

Management of low-risk women with a short cervix is still uncertain. Data reported in the trial of Fonseca and colleagues[25] support the use of vaginal progesterone in singleton gestations with a short cervix, but the study population was a mix of nulliparous and multiparous women with and without risk factors for PTB, and twin gestations. Although after controlling for these factors the protective effect of vaginal progesterone persisted, the potential benefit of this treatment in low-risk women remains unclear. Data in agreement are scarce regarding the effects of cervical cerclage in low-risk women with a short cervix, but it is suggested that it does not prevent preterm birth and does not improve perinatal outcomes.[33] Therefore, progesterone supplementation, but no cerclage, may be considered for such women with a short cervix. These pregnancies certainly benefit from antenatal steroids[34] once the limit of viability is reached (**Fig. 1**).[34]

Table 1
Ongoing clinical trials investigating the effect of progesterone in pregnant women with a short cervix

Registry	Title	Principal Investigator	Inclusion Criteria	Primary Outcome	Progesterone Compound
NCT00615550	PREGNANT Short Cervix Trial	George W. Creasy, Roberto Romero, Sonia Hassan	Singleton gestation with CL 10–20 mm on TVU at $19^{0/7}$–$23^{6/7}$ wk	Spontaneous PTB at less than $32^{6/7}$ wk	8% vaginal gel, 1.125 g
NCT00439374	RCT of Progesterone to Prevent Preterm Birth in Nulliparous Women with a Short Cervix	Catherine Y. Spong	Nulliparous with singleton gestation and CL <30 mm on TVU at $16^{0/7}$–$22^{6/7}$ wk	Spontaneous PTB at less than $37^{0/7}$ wk	17α-Hydroxyprogesterone caproate

Abbreviations: CL, cervical length; PTB, preterm birth; RCT, randomized controlled trial; TVU, transvaginal ultrasonography.

Table 2
Descriptive characteristics of trials that compare cerclage with no cerclage in women with a short cervix

Study	Randomized Sample Size	Population	GA at Screening (wk)	CL Cutoff (mm)	Funneling (%)	Cerclage Type	Cerclage Suture	Primary Outcome
Rust et al[28]	113	All singleton and multiple gestations	16–24	<25	≥25	McDonald	Permanent monofilament	PTB <34 wk
Althuisius et al[29]	35	All singleton with prior PTB, risk factors of PTB, and suspected cervical incompetence	14–27	<25	NR	McDonald	Braided polyester thread	PTB <34 wk
To et al[30]	243	All singleton	22–24	≤15	NR	Shirodkar	Mersilene tape	PTB <33[6/7] wk
Berghella et al[31]	61	Singleton with risk factors of PTB and twins	14–25	<25	>25	McDonald	Braided tape	PTB <35 wk
Owen et al[32]	302	Singleton with prior PTB	16–23	<25	NR	McDonald	NR	PTB <35 wk

Abbreviations: GA, gestational age; NR, not reported.

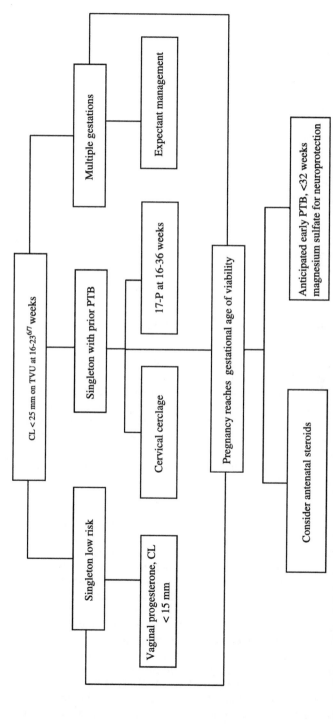

Fig. 1. Evidence-based clinical management of women with a short cervix on ultrasound in the second trimester.

PREDICTION OF SPONTANEOUS PTB IN SINGLETON PREGNANCIES WITH PRIOR PTB AND A SHORT CERVIX

Contrary to the low predictive accuracy of CL TVU screening in low-risk women, CL is a good predictor of PTB in women at high risk, such as those who have history of PTB. In a well-designed blinded multicenter observational study of women with prior PTB at less than 32 weeks, serial measurements of CL by TVU had a good prediction of PTB before 35 weeks of gestation. With this method and using a CL cutoff of 25 mm, the sensitivity, specificity, and PPV of an abnormal test were 69%, 80%, and 55%, respectively.[35] The accuracy of TVU depends also on the gestational age. Thus, in women with clinical risk factors for PTB, the PPV for PTB of a CL less than 25 mm at 14 to 18 weeks is 70%, whereas it drops to 40% when the abnormal test is found between 18 and 20 weeks.[9] Of importance, high-risk women with a normal CL between 18 and 22 weeks have only a 4% risk of delivering preterm, which represents an 80% reduction in risk. Furthermore, PTB in high-risk women with a short cervix is preceded by preterm premature rupture of membranes (preterm PROM) instead of preterm labor in approximately 50% of the cases.[9,36] Although TVU of the cervix since 14 to 16 weeks of gestation in women with a prior PTB could be a good strategy that allows to detect early cervical changes that can predict PTB with high accuracy, there are no randomized trials that evaluate the effectiveness of TVU CL for preventing PTB in asymptomatic women. Serial measurements of the cervix every 2 weeks if the length remains normal and every week if shortening is noted (<30 mm) from 14 to 24 weeks are advocated by some experts.[37]

CLINICAL MANAGEMENT OF SHORT CERVIX IN SINGLETON PREGNANCIES WITH PRIOR PRETERM BIRTH

Previous randomized studies have demonstrated that progestational agents may prevent PTB in high risk women, particularly in those with a prior spontaneous PTB.[38,39] In a randomized placebo-controlled trial, 142 women at high risk of PTB, 90% of whom had a previous spontaneous PTB, were randomly assigned to receive vaginal progesterone or placebo.[38] This study showed a significant reduction of PTB before 34 weeks in women allocated to progesterone treatment compared with those receiving placebo (2.7% vs 18.6%).[38] The National Institute of Child Health and Human Development (NICHD) Maternal-Fetal Medicine Units Networks conducted a randomized controlled trial that evaluated the ability of 17-P to decrease recurrent preterm delivery in women with history of spontaneous PTB. In this study, 17-P was administered since the second trimester (16–20 weeks) before signs or symptoms of preterm labor, and continued until delivery or 36 weeks of gestation.[39] This trial demonstrated a significant reduction in the preterm birth rate at less than 37 weeks from 55% to 36% in women who were assigned randomly to receive 17-P.[39] In addition, infants of women treated with 17-P had significantly lower rates of necrotizing enterocolitis, intraventricular hemorrhage, and need for supplemental oxygen. Based on this trial, the use of progesterone for patients with previous preterm delivery is advocated by the American Congress of Obstetricians and Gynecologists.[40] The use of progesterone for the prevention of spontaneous PTB has also been tested in women with a short cervix.[25,27] As mentioned earlier, the population enrolled in these studies is heterogenous. In the recent study conducted by Fonseca and colleagues,[25] 38 of 250 women (15.2%) who had a CL of 15 mm or less also had a history of PTB. Analysis of this subgroup showed that vaginal progesterone supplementation did not reduce the rate of spontaneous delivery at less than 34 weeks of gestation. The small number of women with prior

PTB in the other study does not allow one to discern the role of progesterone in women with a short cervix and history of PTB.[27] Recently, Berghella and colleagues[41] performed a secondary analysis of the Eunice Kennedy Shriver NICHD-sponsored randomized trial to estimate the effect of 17-P for the prevention of PTB in women with a prior spontaneous PTB, and a short cervix, with and without ultrasound-indicated cerclage. This study showed that 17-P in women with a CL less than 25 mm at 16 to 22$^{6/7}$ weeks who did not undergo cervical cerclage reduced the rate of spontaneous PTB at less than 24 weeks (odds ratio [OR] 0.08, 95% CI 0.01–0.60) and perinatal death (OR 0.14, 95% CI 0.03–0.61). Of importance, birth at less than 24 weeks and perinatal mortality were significantly less frequent in women with a CL at 15 to 24 mm assigned to no cerclage who received 17-P than in those who did not (OR 0.11, 95% CI 0.15–0.88 and OR 0.18, 95% CI 0.05–0.81). These differences were abolished with a CL less than 15 mm. Therefore it seems that 17-P may be beneficial for women with a lesser degree of cervical shortening, as shown in this study. However, the effect of 17-P in women with a short cervix is still uncertain, and further investigation is needed.

The role of cervical cerclage in the prevention of spontaneous PTB in women with prior PTB and a short cervix has been specifically studied in one individual trial and one meta-analysis using individual data (**Table 3**).[33,35] Another individual trial that studied women with risk of PTB, including women with a prior PTB, showed beneficial effects of cervical cerclage.[29] In this study, 35 high-risk women with cervical incompetence defined as history of preterm delivery less than 34 weeks, previous preterm PROM less than 32 weeks, history of cold knife conization, diethylstilbestrol exposure, and uterine anomaly who had a CL on TVU less than 25 mm before 27 weeks of gestation were randomized to either cervical cerclage with bed rest or bed rest alone.[29] Spontaneous preterm delivery less than 34 weeks was significantly lower in the cerclage and bed-rest group than in the bed-rest group (0% vs 43.7%). In addition, there was a significant reduction in perinatal morbidity in women treated with cervical cerclage and bed rest than in those managed with only bed rest (5.2% vs 50.0%).[29] These findings agree with the findings of a recent meta-analysis of randomized trials.[33] In this study, women with a prior spontaneous PTB and a short cervix who underwent cervical cerclage had a significantly lower rate of spontaneous PTB before 35 and 37 weeks of gestation. The number needed to treat with cervical cerclage to prevent one PTB less than 35 weeks was approximately 8. Conversely, this meta-analysis showed no significant reduction of the perinatal mortality in these high-risk women treated with cerclage. The most powered data, however, are provided by the most recent randomized trial conducted in 15 United States centers.[39] Three hundred and two women with a prior spontaneous delivery at 17 to 33$^{6/7}$ weeks and a CL less than 25 mm on TVU at 16 to 22$^{6/7}$ weeks were randomized to cerclage or no cerclage. Although there was no significant difference in the rate of PTB at less than 35 weeks between the cerclage and no-cerclage groups, spontaneous PTB less than 24 weeks and perinatal mortality was significantly less frequent in the cerclage group than in the no-cerclage group. Significant interaction was noted between cerclage and CL. Birth less than 35 weeks was significantly lower in women with a CL less than 15 mm who had cerclage compared than in those who did not (OR 0.23, 95% CI 0.08–0.66).

Existing data support the placement of cervical cerclage in women with prior PTB who have cervical shortening on TVU in current pregnancy. The protective effects of progesterone for these high-risk women are still unknown; however, vaginal progesterone may prevent PTB, particularly at CL less than 15 mm.[25] A recent small randomized trial compared the two strategies.[42] In this study, 70 singleton pregnancies with

Table 3
Effects of cervical cerclage in the prevention of PTB and perinatal mortality in singleton gestations with a short cervix and prior PTB

Study	Inclusion Criteria	CL Cutoff	Outcome	Cerclage (%)	No Cerclage (%)	Statistical Test Results
Berghella et al[33]	Prior PTB <37 wk Prior delivery at 16–23 wk	<25 mm (3 studies) ≤15 mm (1 study)	PTB <35 wk	23.4	38.6	RR, 0.61; 95% CI, 0.40–0.92
			Perinatal death	8.4	13.8	RR, 0.62; 95% CI 0.29–1.30
			PTB <35 weeks	22.1	39.2	RR, 0.57; 95% CI 0.33–0.99
			Perinatal death	5.9	9.8	RR, 0.62; 95% CI, 0.19–2.06
Owen et al[35]	At least one prior PTB at 17–33[6/7] wk	<25 mm <15 mm <25 mm	PTB <35 wk PTB <35 wk Perinatal mortality	32 NR 8.8	42 NR 16	OR, 0.67; 95% CI, 0.42–1.07 OR, 0.23; 95% CI, 0.08–0.66 P = .46

Abbreviations: CI, confidence interval; OR, odds ratio; RR, relative risk.

a CL on TVU of less than 25 mm were randomly assigned to cervical cerclage or weekly injections with 17-P. Spontaneous PTB less than 35 weeks did not differ significantly between women on 17-P and those with cerclage (43.2% vs 38.1%). Analysis of women with a prior history of PTB did not show a significant difference on the rate of spontaneous PTB between the two groups. Conversely, women with a CL 15 mm or less who received cerclage had a significantly lower rate of spontaneous PTB less than 35 weeks than women treated with 17-P (RR 0.48, 95% CI 0.24–0.97). It is noteworthy that this study did not enroll the planned sample size, as it was thought impractical and unethical to withhold 17-P from women with a prior spontaneous PTB. Another important issue to elucidate is whether the use of progesterone and cerclage together has additive benefits in women with a short cervix and prior PTB. In a recent secondary analysis of the Owen's multicenter trial, Berghella and colleagues[41] reported that administration of 17-P to women with a CL of less than 25 mm and prior spontaneous PTB had no additional effect in the group that received cervical cerclage. This study, however, was underpowered, as the calculated sample size was based on the planned primary outcome for the original study.

The clinical management of singleton gestations in women with a short cervix and prior PTB is dictated by several factors. The number of women with a prior PTB undergoing TVU screening of the cervix seems to be low, as many of them opt for history-indicated cerclage, particularly when previous spontaneous delivery has occurred in the second trimester. In the United States, 17-P should be offered to singleton gestations with at least one prior spontaneous PTB,[40] whereas CL on TVU is not a routine practice based on that history. The only scenario in which the cervix should be assessed on ultrasonography is when women with a prior second trimester delivery due to spontaneous preterm labor or preterm PROM decline history-indicated cerclage. The cervix is then serially measured on TVU at 16 to 23$^{6/7}$ weeks. The frequency of testing depends on the CL. If this remains normal (>30 mm) TVU is performed every 2 weeks, but if cervical shortening starts the frequency is reduced to every week. The CL cutoff at which ultrasound-indicated cerclage should be placed is still debatable. The most recent data indicate that cerclage is more beneficial at the greater degrees of cervical shortening (<15 mm).[32] Many of us would agree that continuing to measure the cervix once shortening is noted can result in pregnancy loss or cervical dilation, and bulging membranes that would make impossible or extremely risky cerclage placement. Thus, cerclage can be both safe and beneficial once the CL is less than 25 mm. Based on the data provided in the randomized trial of Fonseca and colleagues,[25] women should be counseled on vaginal progesterone in special circumstances, such as when cerclage is declined or the procedure is technically impossible to perform. The use of progesterone and cerclage together is understudied and therefore not recommended, unless the patient is already receiving 17-P because of her history of prior PTB (see **Fig. 1**). It is also not recommended to use different progesterone compounds together. Other factors should be taken into consideration in the clinical management of these patients, such as the presence of other risk factors including smoking, history of cervical conization, mullerian anomalies, and the presence of cervicovaginal infection. The efficacy of cerclage and progesterone in women with these and other risk factors has not been studied in powered trials. Factors still unknown at present include the optimal dose and the best route of administration of progesterone supplementation, the best strategy for screening the cervix on ultrasonography, and the optimal follow-up of pregnancies after cerclage is placed.

PREDICTION OF SPONTANEOUS PTB IN TWIN GESTATIONS IN WOMEN WITH A SHORT CERVIX

Twin gestations are at elevated risk of spontaneous PTB. In the United States, the rates of PTB less than 37 and less than 32 weeks for twin gestations are estimated at 60.4% and 12.1%, respectively.[43] Individual studies[44–46] and more recently a meta-analysis[47] have assessed the accuracy of TVU in the second trimester to predict PTB in twin gestations. Goldenberg and colleagues[44] estimated the sensitivity, specificity, PPV, and negative predictive value (NPV) of PTB less than 35 weeks in twin gestations with a CL less than 25 mm at 22 to 24 weeks of gestation in 30%, 88%, 55%, and 74%, respectively. In another study,[45] only 4% of pregnancies with a TVU CL greater than 35 mm delivered before 35 weeks of gestation. Others have reported a PPV of 100% for PTB less than 28 weeks in twin gestations with a CL less than 20 mm in the mid-trimester.[46] A recent meta-analysis of 16 studies found that TVU in the second trimester is a good predictor of PTB in asymptomatic twin gestations.[47] A CL less than 20 mm at 20 to 24 weeks was the most accurate parameter to predict preterm delivery at less than 32 and 34 weeks of gestation. The respective pooled sensitivities, specificities, and positive and negative likelihood ratios were 39% and 29%, 96% and 97%, 10.1 and 9.0, and 0.64 and 0.74. A CL less than 25 mm at 20 to 24 weeks of gestation had a pooled positive likelihood ratio of 9.6 to predict PTB at less than 28 weeks of gestation.[47] In contrast to a previous individual study,[45] this meta-analysis demonstrated that TVU CL has a low NPV.[47] Nevertheless, second-trimester TVU is a good predictor of PTB in twin gestation. The applicability of the test is, however, questionable, as the implementation of available clinical interventions has not been shown to prevent PTB in twin gestations.

CLINICAL MANAGEMENT OF TWIN GESTATIONS IN WOMEN WITH A SHORT CERVIX

Previous studies on medical therapies for the prevention of PTB in twin gestations have shown disappointing results. The use of progesterone for this purpose has been examined in two recent randomized controlled trials in Europe and the United States (**Table 4**).[48,49] A randomized, multicenter double-blind placebo-controlled trial in the United Kingdom[48] compared the efficacy of progesterone in the prevention of spontaneous PTB and the improvement in perinatal outcomes. Five hundred women were randomly assigned to either vaginal progesterone gel 90 mg or to placebo gel from 24 to 34 weeks. The study found that spontaneous preterm delivery less than 34 weeks or intrauterine death did not differ significantly between the progesterone and the placebo groups (see **Table 4**): 24.7% and 19.4%; OR 1.36, 95% CI 0.89–2.09. The investigators also performed a meta-analysis of the published and unpublished data with the aim of determining the efficacy of progesterone in the prevention of PTB. The results were similar to the individual trial, as progesterone did not reduce spontaneous PTB before 34 weeks of gestation (OR 1.16, 95% CI 0.89–1.51). A recent randomized, double-blind placebo-controlled trial in 14 United States centers was performed to assess the efficacy of 17-P in the reduction of PTB in twin gestations.[49] Six hundred and sixty-one women with twin gestations were allocated randomly to weekly intramuscular (IM) injections of 17-P 250 mg or its equivalent placebo from 16 to 20 weeks to 35 weeks. In agreement with the United Kingdom trial,[48] this study showed that 17-P did not prevent PTB or fetal death before 35 weeks of gestation (see **Table 4**). In addition, there were no differences in the rate of adverse fetal or neonatal events between the 17-P and the placebo groups. Findings of the United States trial in twins were similar to those reported in triplets by the same group of investigators (see **Table 4**).[50] One hundred and thirty-four triplet gestations

Table 4
Effect of progesterone in the prevention of PTB in multiple gestations: data from randomized trials

Study	Population	Primary Outcome	Progesterone Preparation	Progesterone (%)	Placebo (%)	Reported Statistical Results
Norman et al[48]	Twins	PTB or fetal death <34 wk	Vaginal progesterone 90 mg	61/247 (24.7)	48/247 (19.4)	OR, 1.36; 95% CI 0.89–2.09
Rouse et al[49]	Twins	PTB or fetal death <35 wk	17-P 250 mg IM	135/325 (41.5)	123/330 (37.3)	RR, 1.1; 95% CI 0.9–1.3
Caritis et al[50]	Triples	PTB of fetal death <35 wk	17-P 250 mg IM	59/71 (83.1)	53/63 (84.1)	RR, 1.0; 95% CI 0.9–1.1

Abbreviations: IM, intramuscular; 17-P, 17α-hydroxyprogesterone.

were randomly assigned to either 17-P or placebo. The primary outcome, which was the composite of spontaneous preterm delivery less than 35 weeks or fetal loss, did not vary significantly between the 17-P and the placebo groups (83% vs 84%; RR 1.0, 95% CI 0.9–1.0).[50]

There are no clinical trials that assess the efficacy of progesterone in the prevention of PTB specifically in twin gestations in women with a short cervix. A small subgroup of the population were twins in the trial of Fonseca and colleagues,[25] 24 (9.6%) sets of twins out of 250 randomized women. The investigators reported that the use of vaginal progesterone in this subgroup reduced, but not significantly, the rate of preterm delivery before 34 weeks of gestation. These findings do not agree with the results reported in the other large multicenter trials.[48,49] One plausible explanation of this is that the efficacy of progesterone depends on the dose and route of delivery, and varies between singleton and twin gestation. As mentioned earlier, the trial of Fonseca and colleagues used 200 mg micronized progesterone vaginally,[25] whereas the other two trials chose 90 mg of progesterone gel vaginally[48] and 250 mg 17-P IM,[49] respectively. The absorption and bioavailability of the different preparations may explain the variation of results between these trials.

Data are limited on the efficacy of cervical cerclage in the prevention of preterm delivery in twin gestations. However, there is evidence indicating that cervical cerclage can cause detrimental effects in twin pregnancies. In a small randomized trial, 50 twin gestations that occurred after induction of ovulation were randomly assigned to elective cervical cerclage or no cerclage.[51] There were no differences in the incidence of preterm delivery (45.4% vs 47.8%) and in the neonatal death rate (18.2% vs 15.2%) between the cerclage and no-cerclage groups.[51] These women were not randomized based on cervical shortening on TVU. An observational study assessed the efficacy of cervical cerclage to prolong gestation in twins with shortened cervix.[52] This study enrolled 128 twin gestations and cervical cerclage was offered to women with a CL of 25 mm or less on TVU. Neither the incidence of PTB less than 34 weeks of gestation nor the rate of selected perinatal outcomes varied between 21 women who underwent cerclage compared with 12 women who did not.[52] The recent meta-analysis of Berghella and colleagues[33] showed that cervical cerclage in twins (n = 49) was associated with a significantly higher incidence of preterm birth less than 35 weeks (RR 2.15, 95% CI 1.15–4.01) and showed a trend toward increasing perinatal mortality (RR 2.66, 95% CI 0.83–8.54).

The clinical management of twins in women with a short cervix is a major dilemma. Although TVU is one of the best risk-assessment methods for prediction of preterm delivery in twin gestations, its use may not be justified as there are no efficacious clinical interventions that can prevent PTB. Vaginal progesterone at the dose used by Fonseca and colleagues[25] in their recent trial may play a role in the prevention of PTB in twin gestations in women with a short cervix, but the sample size in this trial was very small. There are several ongoing trials assessing the efficacy of progesterone supplementation at different doses and delivery routes in multiple gestations. The results of these studies will contribute information in the future. On the other hand, cervical cerclage seems to be associated with increased morbidity in twins.[33] A randomized trial is urged to clarify the effects of cerclage for women with a short cervix carrying twins, but at present cervical cerclage is discouraged for these pregnancies. Based on existing evidence, expectant management becomes the best clinical approach for women with twin gestations even though cervical shortening is noted on TVU. These pregnancies benefit from antenatal steroids after the gestational age of viability is reached[40] and from magnesium sulfate for neuroprotection if early PTB is anticipated.[53]

INDOMETHACIN FOR THE PREVENTION OF SPONTANEOUS PTB IN ASYMPTOMATIC WOMEN WITH A SHORT CERVIX

There are some studies showing an association between uterine contractions and short cervix in asymptomatic women.[54,55] Indomethacin is a nonselective, nonsteroid anti-inflammatory agent that inhibits the transformation of arachidonic acid into prostaglandins. These hormone-like substances are implicated in uterine contractility during labor, but more importantly in the induction of cervical ripening. Indomethacin may play a role in the prevention of PTB in women with a short cervix. A recent meta-analysis of 4 randomized trials showed that indomethacin therapy for asymptomatic women with a short CL less than 25 mm on TVU between 14 and 27 weeks of gestation did not prevent PTB before 35 weeks.[56] However, it reduced the incidence of PTB less than 24 weeks from 7.5% in women without therapy to 1.0% in women receiving indomethacin (RR 0.14, 95% CI 0.02–0.92). Indomethacin also decreased the rate of preterm PROM (10% with therapy vs 38% without it). In this study, indomethacin did not have any impact on the perinatal death rate. An important point is that women with cervical cerclage were excluded from this study. A more recent retrospective cohort study assessed the effects of indomethacin administered around the time of cerclage placement due to a short cervix on TVU.[57] This study showed no difference in the incidence of PTB less than 35 weeks between women treated with and without indomethacin (39% vs 34%).[57]

The use of indomethacin in pregnancy has been associated with potential adverse effects in the fetus. In a recent Cochrane systematic review of randomized trials,[58] there was only one case of antenatal closure of ductus arteriosus in 403 women who received short-course tocolysis (up to 48 hours) with cyclooxygenase inhibitors, mainly indomethacin. This study, however, did not have enough power to assess maternal and fetal adverse effects associated with indomethacin therapy. Another systematic review and meta-analysis[59] reported no cases of intraventricular hemorrhage, bronchopulmonary dysplasia, patent ductus arteriosus, necrotizing enterocolitis, and perinatal mortality in 1621 fetuses exposed to indomethacin. Asymptomatic women with a short cervix in the second trimester may benefit from a short course (48 hours) of indomethacin. However, this intervention needs to be assessed in a randomized trial.

VAGINAL PESSARY IN ASYMPTOMATIC WOMEN WITH A SHORT CERVIX

Pessaries have been used to treat cervical insufficiency for more than 50 years. However, their use has been less frequent, probably due to the popularity of cervical cerclage. Because it is noninvasive, a pessary carries much lower risks than cervical cerclage.[60,61] The efficacy of vaginal pessary in the prevention of spontaneous PTB has been recently addressed. In a cohort study, 32 women carrying singleton and multiple gestations with a short cervix (≤25 mm) on TVU before 30 weeks of gestation were treated with a vaginal pessary.[61] Analysis was limited to 29 women in whom delivery was not medically indicated. The mean interval between pessary and delivery was 10.4 (range 2–19) weeks and the mean gestational age at delivery was 34 (range 22–42) weeks. There are currently two ongoing clinical trials in Europe assessing the efficacy of vaginal pessary in the prevention of PTB in singleton pregnancies in women with a short cervix. Their information will be very valuable.

In summary, CL on TVU is a useful screening tool, but only in specific pregnant populations. TVU CL should not be measured in singleton low-risk pregnancies and multiple gestations. Women with a prior early spontaneous preterm delivery who have not undergone history-indicated cerclage may be the only candidates for this screening test. If the decision is made to perform it, the gestational age range for testing should be 14 to 16 weeks to $23^{6/7}$ weeks. The frequency of TVU is dictated mainly by the measurement of CL. If the length of the cervix remains normal ($\geq$30 mm), ultrasonography can be repeated every 2 weeks, otherwise it should be performed weekly. Singleton women with a prior PTB benefit from cervical cerclage when cervical shortening is detected, a CL of 15 mm or less being that at which cerclage seems to be more beneficial. As most women with singleton pregnancies and prior spontaneous PTB are receiving 17-P in the United States, this therapy should continue regardless of the evidence of cervical shortening later in pregnancy. Progesterone supplementation may be beneficial in the specific subgroup of singleton gestations in women with a short cervix; however, its efficacy as well as the dose and route of administration remain to be elucidated. Based on available evidence, progesterone and cervical cerclage are not recommended in twin gestations. Ongoing clinical trials will probably provide some of the answers to help fill the current gaps in the clinical management of women at different risk levels with a short CL on TVU during the mid-trimester.

REFERENCES

1. International statistical classification of diseases and related health problems. 10th revision. Geneva (Switzerland): World Health Organization; 2007.
2. Callaghan WD, MacDorman MF, Rasmussen SA, et al. The contribution of preterm birth to infant mortality rates in the United States. Pediatrics 2006;118: 1566–73.
3. Matthews TJ, MacDorman MF. Infant mortality statistics from the 2005 period linked birth/infant death data set. Natl Vital Stat Rep 2008;57(2):1–32.
4. Larroque B, Ancel PY, Marret S, et al. Neurodevelopmental disabilities and special care of 5-year-old children born before 33 weeks of gestation (the EIPAGE study): a longitudinal cohort study. Lancet 2008;371(9615):813–20.
5. Hamilton BE, Martin JA, Ventura SJ, et al. Births: preliminary data for 2008. Natl Vital Stat Rep 2010;58(6):1–5.
6. Phelps JY, Higby K, Smityth H, et al. Accuracy and intraobserver variability of simulated cervical dilatation measurements. Am J Obstet Gynecol 1995;173: 942–5.
7. Michaels WH, Montgomery C, Karo J, et al. Ultrasound differentiation of the competent and incompetent cervix: prevention of preterm delivery. Am J Obstet Gynecol 1986;154:537–46.
8. Sonek JD, Iams JD, Blumenfeld M. Measurement of cervical length in pregnancy: comparison between vaginal ultrasonography and digital examination. Obstet Gynecol 1990;76:172–5.
9. Berghella V, Tolosa JE, Kuhlman K, et al. Cervical ultrasonography compared to manual examination as a predictor of preterm delivery. Am J Obstet Gynecol 1997;177:723–30.
10. Berghella V, Bega G, Tolosa JE, et al. Ultrasound assessment of the cervix. Clin Obstet Gynecol 2003;46(4):947–62.
11. Zilianti M, Azuaga A, Calderon F, et al. Transperineal sonography in the second trimester to term pregnancy and early labor. J Ultrasound Med 1991;10:481–5.
12. Mancuso MS, Szychowski JM, Owen J, et al. Cervical funneling: effect on gestational length and ultrasound-indicated cerclage in high-risk women. Am J Obstet Gynecol 2010;203:259, e1–5.

13. Iams JD, Goldenberg RL, Meis PJ, et al. The length of the cervix and the risk of spontaneous premature delivery. N Engl J Med 1996;334:567–72.
14. Berghella V, Roman A, Daskalakis C, et al. Gestational age at cervical length measurement and incidence of preterm birth. Obstet Gynecol 2007;110: 311–7.
15. Andersen HF, Nugent CE, Wanty CD, et al. Prediction risk for preterm delivery by ultrasonographic measurement of cervical length. Am J Obstet Gynecol 1990; 163:859–67.
16. Andersen HF. Transvaginal and transabdominal ultrasonography of the uterine cervix during pregnancy. J Clin Ultrasound 1991;19:77–81.
17. Hibbard JU, Tart M, Moawad AT. Cervical length at 18-22 weeks' gestation and risk of preterm delivery. Obstet Gynecol 2000;96:972–8.
18. Siiteri PK, Serón-Ferré M. Some new thoughts on the feto-placental unit and parturition in primates. In: Novy MJ, Resko JA, editors. Fetal endocrinology. New York: Academic Press; 1981. p. 1–34.
19. Garfield RE, Kannan MS, Daniel EE. Gap junction formation in myometrium: control by estrogens, progesterone, and prostaglandins. Am J Physiol 1980; 238:C81–9.
20. Challis JRG. Sharp increases in free circulating oestrogens immediately before parturition in sheep. Nature 1971;229:208.
21. Mitchell B, Cruickshank B, McLean D, et al. Local modulation of progesterone production in human fetal membranes. J Clin Endocrinol Metab 1982;55: 1237–9.
22. Facchineti F, Dante G, Venturini P, et al. 17alpha-hydroxy-progesterone effects on cervical proinflammatory agents in women at risk for preterm delivery. Am J Perinatol 2008;25:503–6.
23. Frydman R, LeLaider C, Baton-Saint-Mleux C, et al. Labor induction in women at term with mifepristone (RU 486): a double-blind, randomized, placebo-controlled study. Obstet Gynecol 1992;80:972–5.
24. Brent RL. Nongenital malformations following exposure to progestational drugs: the last chapter of an erroneous allegation. Birth Defects Res A Clin Mol Teratol 2005;73:906–18.
25. Fonseca EB, Celik E, Parra M, et al. Progesterone and the risk of preterm birth among women a short cervix. N Engl J Med 2007;357:462–9.
26. O'Brien JM, Adair CD, Lewis DF, et al. Progesterone vaginal for the reduction of recurrent preterm birth: primary results from a randomized, double-blinded, placebo-controlled trial. Ultrasound Obstet Gynecol 2007;30:687–97.
27. DeFranco EA, O'Brien JM, Adair CD, et al. Vaginal progesterone is associated with a decrease in risk for early preterm birth and improved neonatal outcome in women with a short cervix: a secondary analysis from a randomized, double-bind, placebo-controlled trial. Ultrasound Obstet Gynecol 2007;30: 697–705.
28. Rust OA, Atlas RO, Reed J, et al. Revision the short cervix detected by transvaginal ultrasound in the second trimester: why cerclage therapy may not help. Am J Obstet Gynecol 2001;185:1098–105.
29. Althuisius SM, Dekker GA, Hummel P, et al. Final results of the cervical incompetence prevention randomized cerclage trial (CIPRACT): therapeutic cerclage with bed rest versus bed rest alone. Am J Obstet Gynecol 2001;185:1106–12.
30. To MS, Alfirevic Z, Heath VC, et al. Cervical cerclage for prevention of preterm delivery in women with a short cervix: randomized controlled trial. Lancet 2004; 363:1849–53.

31. Berghella V, Odibo AO, Tolosa JE. Cerclage for prevention of preterm birth in women with a short cervix found on transvaginal ultrasound examination: a randomized trial. Am J Obstet Gynecol 2004;191:1311–7.
32. Owen J, Hankins G, Iams JD, et al. Multicenter randomized trial of cerclage for preterm birth prevention in high-risk women with shortened midtrimester cervical length. Am J Obstet Gynecol 2009;201:375, e1–8.
33. Berghella V, Odibo AO, To MS, et al. Cerclage for short cervix on ultrasonography. Meta- analysis of trials using individual patient-level data. Obstet Gynecol 2005; 106:181–9.
34. Crowley P. Prophylactic corticosteroids for preterm birth. Cochrane Database Syst Rev 2000;(2).
35. Owen J, Yost N, Berghella V, et al. Mid-trimester sonography in women at high risk for spontaneous preterm birth. JAMA 2001;286(11):1340–8.
36. Odibo AO, Berghella V, Reddy U, et al. Does transvaginal ultrasound of the cervix predict preterm premature rupture of membranes in a high-risk population? Ultrasound Obstet Gynecol 2001;18:223–7.
37. Grimes-Dennis J, Berghella V. Cervical length and prediction of preterm delivery. Curr Opin Obstet Gynecol 2007;19:191–5.
38. Da Fonseca EB, Bittar RE, Carvalho MH, et al. Prophylactic administration of progesterone by vaginal suppository to reduce the incidence of spontaneous preterm birth in women at increased risk: a randomized placebo-controlled double-blind study. Am J Obstet Gynecol 2003;188:419–24.
39. Meiss PJ, Klebanoff M, Thom E, et al. Prevention of recurrent preterm delivery by 17 alpha-hydroxyprogesterone caproate. N Engl J Med 2003;348:2379–85.
40. American Congress of Obstetricians and Gynecologists. ACOG committee opinion: use of progesterone to reduce preterm birth. Obstet Gynecol 2003;102:1115–6.
41. Berghella V, Figueroa D, Szychowski JM, et al. 17-alpha hydroxyprogesterone caproate for the prevention of preterm birth in women with prior preterm birth and a short cervical length. Am J Obstet Gynecol 2010;202:351.e1–6.
42. Keeler SM, Kiefer D, Rochon M, et al. A randomized trial of cerclage vs 17 α-hydroxyprogesterone caproate for treatment of short cervix. J Perinat Med 2009;37:473–9.
43. Martin JA, Hamilton BE, Sutton PD, et al. Births: final data for 2006. Natl Vital Stat Rep 2009;57:1–102.
44. Goldenberg RL, Iams J, Miodovnik M, et al. The preterm prediction study: risk factors in twin gestation. Am J Obstet Gynecol 1996;175:1047–53.
45. Yang JH, Kuhlman K, Daly S, et al. Prediction of preterm birth by second trimester cervical sonography in twin pregnancies. Ultrasound Obstet Gynecol 2000;15:288–91.
46. Skentou C, Souka A, To MS, et al. Prediction of preterm delivery in twins by cervical assessment at 23 weeks. Ultrasound Obstet Gynecol 2001;17:7–10.
47. Conde-Agudelo A, Romero R, Hassan S, et al. Transvaginal sonographic cervical length for the prediction of spontaneous preterm birth in twin pregnancies: a systematic review and metaanalysis. Am J Obstet Gynecol 2010;203:128, e1–128.
48. Norman JE, Mackenzi F, Owen P, et al. Progesterone for the prevention of preterm birth in twin pregnancy (STOPPIT): a randomized, double-blind, placebo-controlled study and meta-analysis. Lancet 2009;373:2034–40.
49. Rouse D, Caritis SN, Peaceman AM, et al. A trial of 17 alpha-hydroxyprogesterone caproate to prevent prematurity in twins. N Engl J Med 2007;357:454–61.

50. Caritis SN, Rouse FJ, Peaceman AM, et al. Prevention of preterm birth in triplets using 17 alpha-hydroxyprogesterone caproate. Obstet Gynecol 2009;113: 285–92.

51. Dor J, Shalev J, Mashiach S, et al. Elective cervical suture of twin pregnancies diagnosed ultrasonically in the first trimester following induced ovulation. Gynecol Obstet Invest 1982;13:55–60.

52. Newman RB, Krombach RS, Myers MC, et al. Effect of cerclage on obstetrical outcome in twin gestations with a shortened cervical length. Am J Obstet Gynecol 2002;186:634–40.

53. American Congress of Obstetricians and Gynecologists. ACOG committee opinion: magnesium sulfate before anticipated preterm birth for neuroprotection. Obstet Gynecol 2010;115:669–71.

54. Berghella V, Iams JD, Newman RB, et al. Frequency of uterine contractions in asymptomatic pregnant women with and without a short cervix on transvaginal ultrasound scan. Am J Obstet Gynecol 2004;191:1253–6.

55. Lewis D, Pelham JJ, Done E, et al. Uterine contractions in asymptomatic women with a short cervix on ultrasound. J Matern Fetal Neonatal Med 2005;18:325–8.

56. Berghella V, Rust OA, Althuisius SM. Short cervix on ultrasound: Does indomethacin prevent preterm birth? Am J Obstet Gynecol 2006;195:809–13.

57. Visintine J, Airoldi J, Berghella V. Indomethacin administration at the time of ultrasound-indicated cerclage; is there any association with a reduction in spontaneous preterm birth? Am J Obstet Gynecol 2008;198:643, e1–3.

58. King J, Flenady V, Cole S, et al. Cyclo-oxygenase (COX) inhibitors for treating preterm labour. Cochrane Database Syst Rev 2005;(3).

59. Loe SM, Sanchez-Ramos L, Kaunitz A. Assessing the neonatal safety of indomethacin tocolysis: a systematic review with metaanalysis. Obstet Gynecol 2005;106: 173–9.

60. Dharan VB, Ludmir J. Alternative treatment for a short cervix: the cervical pessary. Semin Perinatol 2009;33:338–42.

61. Acharya G, Eschler B, Grønberg M. Noninvasive cerclage for the management of cervical incompetence: a prospective study. Arch Gynecol Obstet 2006;273: 283–7.

Management of Oligohydramnios in Pregnancy

Mary B. Munn, MD

KEYWORDS

- Oligohydramnios • Ultrasound • Amniotic fluid volume
- Amniotic fluid index • Deepest vertical pocket

Amniotic fluid plays an important role in fetal health and development, and is far from the "stagnant pool" it was once thought to be. Amniotic fluid physiology is a highly dynamic process. Studies looking at the amount of turnover when proteins were injected into amniotic fluid indicate that a significant amount of fluid enters and leaves the amniotic cavity.[1] Amniotic fluid allows for proper growth and development of the fetal lung and musculoskeletal system, has bacteriostatic and anti-inflammatory properties, and aids in thermoregulation, to name but a few of the important functions. Abnormal amounts of amniotic fluid in either direction are associated with potential problems with pregnancy. Oligohydramnios is most often thought to be associated with a variety of fetal abnormalities and ruptured membranes, and may reflect uteroplacental insufficiency and hypoxemia. However, the diagnosis and management of oligohydramnios remains somewhat enigmatic for many reasons, including the inherent difficulties in accurately assessing the amount of amniotic fluid noninvasively, a standardized definition of oligohydramnios, and convincing data that all cases of oligohydramnios require intervention to reduce adverse perinatal outcomes. Although many disorders associated with oligohydramnios will prompt logical and beneficial interventions (eg, termination for renal agenesis, antibiotics for preterm premature rupture of membranes [PPROM], shunt procedures for lower urinary tract obstruction), often this finding is isolated and idiopathic. At present, controversy exists regarding the best way to manage oligohydramnios, especially when it is the only finding at or near term in an otherwise normal pregnancy, to ensure fetal well-being without incurring maternal morbidities.

AMNIOTIC FLUID PRODUCTION AND DYNAMICS

During the first trimester, the amniotic fluid is isotonic with the maternal plasma.[2] This fluid more than likely arises as a transudate from fetal skin or from maternal plasma

---

The author has nothing to disclose.

Division of Maternal Fetal Medicine, University of Texas Medical Branch, 301 University Boulevard Route 0587, Galveston, TX 77555, USA

E-mail address: mbmunn@utmb.edu

across the decidua and/or placental surface.[3] As the gestation advances, the amniotic fluid becomes more hypotonic than the maternal plasma. Despite large fluid shifts, the amniotic fluid volume remains relatively stable.[4] In the second half of pregnancy, the amniotic fluid is derived from two major sources: fetal urine and fetal lung liquid. The amount of human fetal urine produced has been estimated from ultrasound assessment of the fetal bladder and, although these results have varied, is thought to be 250 to 300 mL/d per kilogram of the fetus.[5–7] Pulmonary fluid contributes approximately 60 to 100 mL/d per kilogram of the fetus near term.[8] Fetal swallowing accounts for the most of the removal of amniotic fluid throughout gestation, and has been estimated to be approximately 210 to 760 mL/d at term.[9] The amount of fluid swallowed by the fetus does not equal the sum of what is produced by the fetal lung and kidneys. Other routes thought to play a role are the transmembranous and intramembranous pathways. The transmembranous pathway, where amniotic fluid moves from the fetal membranes into the maternal circulation, contributes very little to amniotic fluid homeostasis.[10] However, the intramembranous pathway may transfer up to 500 mL/d and accounts for the difference seen between the amount of fluid produced and swallowed. This pathway allows direct absorption of amniotic fluid water and solutes directly into the fetal vasculature via microvessels on the fetal surface of the placenta. The particular mechanism of intramembranous flow has not been fully elucidated. An osmotic gradient between the hypotonic amniotic fluid and isotonic fetal plasma does favor this flow.[11] Esophageal ligation studies in sheep demonstrate this process. The amniotic fluid volume returns to normal despite the inability of the fetus to swallow. The exact mechanism of water absorption is the subject of investigation. The role of vascular endothelial growth factor (VEGF) and hormonal regulation through Prolactin have been suggested as mechanisms for controlling the permeability of the membranes. Water channel proteins known as aquaporins may also play a role in this process.[12]

DEFINITION OF OLIGOHYDRAMNIOS

Oligohydramnios is thought to complicate 0.5% to 5.5% of all pregnancies, depending on the definition that is used and the population under study.[13] It is usually thought to be a result of decreased production of fluid from urinary tract or other fetal abnormalities, or uteroplacental insufficiency. PPROM, maternal hydration status, maternal medications, and even altitude may cause a decreased amount of amniotic fluid. Various methods have been employed to assess the amount of fluid present. In the assessment of amniotic fluid volumes, the dye-dilution test is considered the gold standard.[14] However, as this requires amniocentesis with its inherent complications, it is not often used clinically to determine the amniotic fluid volume. Fetal magnetic resonance imaging (MRI) has been used to assess the amniotic fluid volume, largest pocket, and the amniotic fluid index (AFI). Zaretsky and colleagues[15] compared the actual amniotic fluid volume with the largest vertical pocket, the AFI derived from ultrasound, and the amniotic fluid volume determined from MRI measurements. None of the techniques were sensitive for detecting oligohydramnios. Three-dimensional ultrasound techniques have also been used to determine fluid volumes.[16,17] None of these techniques have proven to be superior to the current modality used to assess amniotic fluid, 2-dimensional ultrasonography. However, assessing the amniotic fluid with ultrasonography has proven difficult for many reasons. The ability to evaluate a 3-dimensional entity in 2 dimensions limits the accuracy. Also, confusion exists as to what constitutes a normal amount of amniotic fluid and which technique is the most accurate for measuring the amount of fluid present. Several different techniques have been described to quantify the amount of fluid by ultrasound. These methods include the single deepest vertical pocket (SDVP), the 2-diameter pocket, and the AFI.[18–20] In addition, a variety of cutoff threshold points for low amniotic fluid have also been proposed, but there seems to be no consensus on the definition of oligohydramnios.

Controversy exists over whether the currently accepted normal ranges for AFI throughout gestation are even accurate and reproducible.[21,22] When the AFI and SDVP were compared with dye-dilution techniques, neither technique appeared to be superior to the other for detecting abnormal amniotic fluid volumes, and both were very poor predictors of abnormal amniotic fluid volumes.[23] Color Doppler has been investigated as a tool to aid in the diagnosis of oligohydramnios. When color Doppler was used to exclude areas containing umbilical cord, the diagnosis of oligohydramnios increased.[24,25] However, when the actual amniotic fluid volume was calculated using dye-dilution techniques, the addition of color Doppler did not enhance the diagnosis of true oligohydramnios, and actually labeled 21% of patients as having low fluid when the amniotic of amniotic fluid was normal.[26] Therefore it appears that the current modalities for diagnosing oligohydramnios are somewhat imprecise.

ASSOCIATION OF OLIGOHYDRAMNIOS WITH ADVERSE OUTCOMES

Oligohydramnios traditionally has been associated with adverse perinatal outcomes. Studies published in the early 1980s found an association between low amniotic fluid and fetal growth restriction. Hypoxemia was thought to decrease renal blood flow, which reduced urine output and the amniotic fluid volume[27] A relationship was also found between low fluid and fetal compromise as a component of the biophysical profile.[18] Reports associating oligohydramnios and adverse outcomes began to appear throughout the literature.[28–31] A meta-analysis of 18 studies describing more than 10,000 patients reported an increased incidence of cesarean section for "fetal distress" and low Apgar scores at 5 minutes in the oligohydramnios group.[32] This study, as well as many of the others relating oligohydramnios with poor outcomes, are limited by their retrospective nature, as well as lack of stratification for maternal or fetal conditions. It may be that the adverse outcomes are related to conditions that affect the pregnancy and not necessarily to the low fluid itself. However, even in high-risk pregnancies, some studies suggest that the amniotic fluid volume is not a good predictor of adverse outcome. Magann and colleagues[33] looked at high-risk patients with an AFI of 5 cm or less and compared this group to high-risk women whose AFI was greater than 5 cm; they saw no difference in adverse outcomes. A similar conclusion was drawn by Ott,[34] who also found that the AFI was a weak predictor of perinatal outcomes in high-risk patients.

ISOLATED IDIOPATHIC OLIGOHYDRAMNIOS

Even less clear is the association of isolated idiopathic oligohydramnios with perinatal outcomes. In a recent study, Schwartz and colleagues[35] surveyed members of the Society of Maternal Fetal Medicine about practice patterns and opinions regarding isolated oligohydramnios. Although 92% of respondents thought that isolated oligohydramnios was a strong enough risk factor to warrant delivery before 39 weeks, only 33% believed that delivery would decrease adverse outcomes. The confusion is understandable given the conflicting data. Morris and colleagues[36] reported an observational study of women of 40 weeks' gestation or greater who had an AFI measured, and reported that an AFI less than 5 cm was associated with adverse outcomes. Zhang and colleagues,[37] however, found no evidence of adverse outcomes in patients with isolated oligohydramnios when compared with patients with a normal AFI. Even if a low AFI is associated with adverse outcomes, given the low sensitivity for detecting poor outcomes, there appears to be limitations on using it as a screening test.[35,36] There has been one prospective randomized trial that has looked at addressing the issue of idiopathic oligohydramnios. Ek and colleagues[38] randomized 54 patients who were found to have an amniotic fluid index less than 5.0 cm to labor induction versus expectant management. These investigators found no difference in umbilical artery pH, Apgar scores, or neonatal intensive care unit between the two groups. However, caution must be exercised in interpreting these findings, as this study was limited by its small numbers.

INTERVENTION FOR OLIGOHYDRAMNIOS

Therapeutic options for oligohydramnios depend largely on the etiology of the low fluid volume. There are some fetal abnormalities causing oligohydramnios that may be amenable to therapy for the prevention the sequelae of significant oligohydramnios (pulmonary hypoplasia, limb contractures). This mode of treatment includes procedures such as shunting for a bladder outlet obstruction. There are others that will not be amenable (aneuploidy, renal agenesis), and pregnancy termination in these cases may be a reasonable option. For oligohydramnios related to PPROM, delivery or expectant management with steroids and/or antibiotics may be the safest option for the fetus depending on the gestational age. Very early PPROM (<22 weeks) presents a significant dilemma. Given the poor prognosis in very early PPROM, termination may be reasonable. A variety of interventions have been attempted to improve outcomes. Attempts to seal the fetal membranes using platelets, cryoprecipitate, fibrin, or gelatin sponge[39–42] have been reported, with some success. However, these studies are limited by small numbers and no comparison group. Amnioinfusion in cases of oligohydramnios from PPROM has also been investigated. Although studies are limited by the small number of patients, there may be some benefit. Recent data suggest that this therapy may decrease the number of neonates with pulmonary hypoplasia[43] and improve perinatal outcome.[44–46] Further studies are needed before this treatment should be adopted for routine practice.

The amniotic fluid volume appears to be influenced by maternal hydration status. Goodlin and colleagues[47] found an increase in the AFI of women who had plasma volume expansion. This finding was also reported by Sherer and colleagues[48] in a case report in 1990, who found an increase in the AFI after rehydrating a severely dehydrated patient. Kilpatrick and Safford[49] found that oral hydration could increase the AFI in patients with oligohydramnios. The success of hydration on raising the AFI may depend on the type of fluid that is used, as Doi and colleagues[50] found that only hypotonic and not isotonic fluids improved the AFI. Flack and colleagues[51] suggested that the mechanism for increasing the amniotic fluid may lie with improved uteroplacental function. These investigators found improved AFI and improved uterine Doppler studies in patients undergoing hydration. However, this may not be applicable to low-risk patients at term. Yan-Rosenberg and colleagues[52] did not find a difference between the patients with oligohydramnios who received intravenous fluids and those who received placebo. It was concluded that the changes seen in AFI may be a result of normal diurnal variation, change in fetal position, or even inaccuracies in the AFI measurement.

Other less studied therapies to improve amniotic fluid have included administration of the arginine vasopressin-selective agonist 1-deamnio-[8-D-arginine]vasopressin (DDAVP). Studies by Ross and colleagues[53,54] showed an increase in amniotic fluid when DDAVP was given to sheep and human subjects. However, the long-term maternal and fetal consequences have yet to be determined, and this therapy remains under investigation.

AMNIOTIC FLUID VOLUME VERSUS SINGLE DEEPEST VERTICAL POCKET

Given the uncertainty of the significance of isolated oligohydramnios, it is difficult to judge the superiority of one technique over the other when measuring the amniotic fluid with ultrasonography. If the goal is to determine which comes closer to reflecting the true volume of fluid, then each should be compared with a technique that directly measures the fluid by dye-dilution techniques or direct measurement. Unfortunately, most of the data indicate that both are poor predictors of oligohydramnios.[23,55,56] Because it appears that neither method measures the actual amniotic fluid volume very well, the next question then becomes: which is the most reliable for predicting adverse outcomes and improving neonatal outcomes? Various nonrandomized studies have reached differing conclusions. Myles and Santolaya-Forgas[57] found that AFI performed slightly better in predicting the adverse outcomes of meconium, cesarean section for fetal distress, and admission to the neonatal intensive care unit. Youssef and colleagues[58] also found the AFI to be a better predictor of adverse outcome when compared with the deepest pocket measurement. By contrast, others have found the SDVP to be a better prediction of complications. Fischer and colleagues[59] found the largest vertical pocket to have a better correlation with the abnormal outcomes of operative delivery for fetal distress, low Apgar scores, low umbilical artery pH, admission to the neonatal intensive care unit, and birth weight less than 10th percentile. Most of the studies comparing AFI with SDVP have found neither to be superior and both to be of limited value for predicting adverse outcomes.[38,60,61] Recently, randomized controlled trials have been performed comparing AFI with the SDVP and evaluating the outcomes.[62–65] A meta-analysis of these studies concluded that the SDVP was the method of choice for evaluating the amniotic fluid volume. There was no difference in the outcomes measured (admission to neonatal intensive care unit, acidosis, meconium, low Apgar scores). When AFI was used, this resulted in more labor inductions and more cesarean sections for fetal distress.[66]

SUMMARY

Oligohydramnios remains somewhat enigmatic. Our understanding of what controls the amount of amniotic fluid, as well as our ability to precisely measure it, are limited. The significance of oligohydramnios is unclear in high-risk and especially low-risk populations, and may lead to interventions that increase morbidity and mortality, especially in the mother. Although therapies exist to treat oligohydramnios, many remain experimental and investigational. In the case of idiopathic oligohydramnios, they may not even be necessary. Given the various ways to measure amniotic fluid, measuring the SDVP rather than the AFI should be the method of choice for determining oligohydramnios. The SDVP performs no worse than the AFI regarding outcome, but does result in less iatrogenic prematurity as well as fewer inductions, which certainly increase the incidence of cesarean section. What is sorely needed is a prospective randomized trial of idiopathic oligohydramnios at or near term with patients randomized to delivery or expectant management. The outcomes assessed should be the most important outcomes, such as stillbirth and acidosis. The number of patients needed to complete a study of this magnitude would require a multicenter collaboration, as more than 20,000 patients would probably be needed. Given that this is a clinical conundrum faced by obstetricians on almost a daily basis, it is a worthwhile area of investigation.

REFERENCES

1. Gitlin D, Kumate J, Morales C, et al. The turnover of amniotic fluid protein in the human conceptus. Am J Obstet Gynecol 1972;113:632–45.
2. Campbell J, Wathen N, Macintosh M, et al. Biochemical composition of amniotic fluid and extraembryonic coelomic fluid in the first trimester of pregnancy. Br J Obstet Gynaecol 1992;99:563–5.
3. Anderson DF, Faber JJ, Parks CM. Extraplacental transfer of water in the sheep. J Physiol 1988;406:75–84.
4. Underwood MA, Gilbert WM, Sherman MP. Amniotic fluid: not just fetal urine anymore. J Perinatol 2005;25(5):341–8.
5. Rabinowitz R, Peters MT, Vyas S, et al. Measurement of fetal urine production in normal pregnancy by real-time ultrasonography. Am J Obstet Gynecol 1989; 161(5):1264–6.
6. Wladimiroff JW, Campbell S. Fetal urine-production rates in normal and complicated pregnancy. Lancet 1974;1(7849):151–4.
7. Hedriana HL, Moore TR. Accuracy limits of ultrasonographic estimation of human fetal urinary flow rate. Am J Obstet Gynecol 1994;171(4):989–92.
8. Brace RA, Wlodek ME, Cock ML, et al. Swallowing of lung liquid and amniotic fluid by the ovine fetus under normoxic and hypoxic conditions. Am J Obstet Gynecol 1994;171(3):764–70.
9. Pritchard JA. Fetal swallowing and amniotic fluid volume. Obstet Gynecol 1966; 28(5):606–10.
10. Sherer DM. A review of amniotic fluid dynamics and the enigma of isolated oligohydramnios. Am J Perinatol 2002;19(5):253–66.
11. Gilbert WM, Brace RA. The missing link in amniotic fluid volume regulation: intramembranous absorption. Obstet Gynecol 1989;74(5):748–54.
12. Liu H, Zheng Z, Wintour EM. Aquaporins and fetal fluid balance. Placenta 2008; 29(10):840–7.
13. Peipert JF, Donnenfeld AE. Oligohydramnios: a review. Obstet Gynecol Surv 1991;46(6):325–39.
14. Magann EF, Bass JD, Chauhan SP, et al. Amniotic fluid volume in normal singleton pregnancies. Obstet Gynecol 1997;90:524–8.
15. Zaretsky MV, McIntire DD, Reichel TF, et al. Correlation of measured amniotic fluid volume to sonographic and magnetic resonance predictions. Am J Obstet Gynecol 2004;191(6):2148–53.
16. Gadelha PS, Da Costa AG, Filho FM, et al. Amniotic fluid volumetry by three-dimensional ultrasonography during the first trimester of pregnancy. Ultrasound Med Biol 2006;32(8):1135–9.
17. Mann SE, Grover J, Ross MG. Novel technique for assessing amniotic fluid volume: use of a three-dimensional bladder scanner. J Matern Fetal Med 2000; 9(5):308–10.
18. Manning FA, Platt LD, Sipos L. Antepartum fetal evaluation: development of a fetal biophysical profile. Am J Obstet Gynecol 1980;136(6):789–95.
19. Magann EF, Isler CM, Chauhan SP, et al. Amniotic fluid volume estimation and the biophysical profile: a confusion of criteria. Obstet Gynecol 2000;96(4):640–2.
20. Phelan JP, Ahn MO, Smith CV, et al. Amniotic fluid index measurements during pregnancy. J Reprod Med 1987;32(8):601–4.

21. Chauhan SP, Magann EF, Morrison JC. Invalid equation to describe the amniotic fluid index in normal pregnancy [letter]. Am J Obstet Gynecol 1994;170(4): 1209–10.
22. Nwosu EC, Welch CR, Manasse PR, et al. Longitudinal assessment of amniotic fluid index. Br J Obstet Gynaecol 1993;100(9):816–9.
23. Magann EF, Chauhan SP, Barrilleaux PS, et al. Amniotic fluid index and single deepest pocket: weak indicators of abnormal amniotic volumes. Obstet Gynecol 2000;96(5 Pt 1):737–40.
24. Bianco A, Rosen T, Kuczynski E, et al. Measurement of the amniotic fluid index with and without color Doppler. J Perinat Med 1999;27(4):245–9.
25. Zlatnik MG, Olson G, Bukowski R, et al. Amniotic fluid index measured with the aid of color flow Doppler. J Matern Fetal Med 2003;13:242–5.
26. Magann EF, Chauhan SP, Barrilleaux PS, et al. Ultrasound estimate of amniotic fluid volume; color Doppler overdiagnosis of oligohydramnios. Obstet Gynecol 2001;98(1):71–4.
27. Manning FA, Hill LM, Platt LD. Qualitative amniotic fluid volume determination by ultrasound: antepartum detection of intrauterine growth retardation. Am J Obstet Gynecol 1981;139(3):254–8.
28. Chamberlain PF, Manning FA, Morrison I, et al. Ultrasound evaluation of amniotic fluid volume. I. The relationship of marginal and decreased amniotic fluid volumes to perinatal outcome. Am J Obstet Gynecol 1984;150(3):245–9.
29. Rutherford SE, Phelan JP, Smith CV, et al. The four-quadrant assessment of amniotic fluid volume: an adjunct to antepartum fetal heart rate testing. Obstet Gynecol 1987;70(3 pt 1):353–6.
30. Chauhan SP, Washburne JF, Magann EF, et al. A randomized study to assess the efficacy of the amniotic fluid index as a fetal admission test. Obstet Gynecol 1995;86(1):9–13.
31. Casey BM, McIntire DD, Bloom SL, et al. Pregnancy outcomes after antepartum diagnosis at or beyond 34 weeks gestation. Am J Obstet Gynecol 2000;182(2): 909–12.
32. Chauhan SP, Sanderson M, Hendrix NW, et al. Perinatal outcomes and amniotic fluid index in the antepartum and intrapartum periods: a meta-analysis. Am J Obstet Gynecol 1999;181(6):1473–8.
33. Magann EF, Kinsella MJ, Chauhan SP, et al. Does an amniotic fluid volume index of <5 cm necessitate delivery in high-risk pregnancies? A case-control study. Am J Obstet Gynecol 1999;180(6 Pt 1):1354–9.
34. Ott WJ. Reevaluation of the relationship between amniotic fluid volume and perinatal outcome. Am J Obstet Gynecol 2005;192(6):1803–9.
35. Schwartz N, Sweeting R, Young BK. Practice patterns in the management of isolated oligohydramnios: a survey of perinatologists. J Matern Fetal Med 2009; 22(4):357–61.
36. Morris JM, Thompson K, Smithey J, et al. The usefulness of ultrasound assessment of amniotic fluid in predicting adverse outcome in prolonged pregnancy: a prospective blinded observational study. Br J Obstet Gynaecol 2003;110(11): 989–94.
37. Zhang J, Troendle J, Meikle S, et al. Isolated oligohydramnios is not associated with adverse perinatal outcomes. Br J Obstet Gynaecol 2004;111(3): 220–5.
38. Ek S, Andersson A, Johansson A, et al. Oligohydramnios in uncomplicated pregnancies beyond 40 completed weeks. A prospective, randomized, pilot study on maternal and neonatal outcomes. Fetal Diagn Ther 2005;20(3):182–5.

39. Uchide K, Terada S, Hamasaki H, et al. Intracervical fibrin instillation as an adjuvant to treatment for second trimester rupture of membranes. Arch Gynecol Obstet 1994;255(2):95–8.

40. Reddy UM, Shah SS, Nemiroff RL, et al. In vitro sealing of punctured fetal membranes: potential treatment for midtrimester premature rupture of membranes. Am J Obstet Gynecol 2001;185(5):1090–3.

41. Quintero RA, Morales WJ, Allen M, et al. Treatment of iatrogenic previable premature rupture of membranes with intra-amniotic injection of platelets and cryoprecipitate (amniopatch): preliminary experience. Am J Obstet Gynecol 1999;181(3):744–9.

42. Sciscione AC, Manley JS, Pollock M, et al. Intracervical fibrin sealants: a potential treatment for early preterm premature rupture of the membranes. Am J Obstet Gynecol 2001;184(3):368–73.

43. Locatelli A, Vergani P, Di Pirro G, et al. Role of amnioinfusion in the management of premature rupture of the membranes <26 weeks gestation. Am J Obstet Gynecol 2000;183(4):878–82.

44. Ogunyemi D, Thompson W. A case controlled study of serial transabdominal amnioinfusions in the management of second trimester oligohydramnios due to premature rupture of membranes. Eur J Obstet Gynecol Reprod Biol 2002;102(2):167–72.

45. Tranquilli AL, Giannubilo SR, Bezzeccheri V, et al. Transabdominal amnioinfusion in preterm premature rupture of membranes: a randomized controlled trial. Br J Obstet Gynaecol 2005;112(6):759–63.

46. Singla A, Yadav P, Vaid NB, et al. Transabdominal amnioinfusion in preterm premature rupture of membranes. Int J Gynaecol Obstet 2010;108(3):199–202.

47. Goodlin R, Anderson J, Gallagher T. Relationship between amniotic fluid volume and maternal plasma expansion. Am J Obstet Gynecol 1983;146:505–10.

48. Sherer DM, Cullen JB, Thompson HO, et al. Transient oligohydramnios in a severely hypovolemic gravid woman at 35 weeks' gestation with fluid reaccumulating after intravenous hydration. Am J Obstet Gynecol 1990;162(3):770–1.

49. Kilpatrick SJ, Safford KL. Maternal hydration increases amniotic fluid index in women with normal amniotic fluid. Obstet Gynecol 1993;81(1):49–52.

50. Doi S, Osada H, Seki K, et al. Effect of maternal hydration on oligohydramnios: a comparison of three volume expansion methods. Obstet Gynecol 1998;92:525–9.

51. Flack NJ, Sepulveda W, Bower S, et al. Acute maternal hydration in third-trimester oligohydramnios: effects on amniotic fluid volume, uteroplacental perfusion, and fetal blood flow and urine output. Am J Obstet Gynecol 1995;173(4):1186–91.

52. Yan-Rosenberg L, Burt B, Bombard AT, et al. A randomized clinical trial comparing the effect of maternal intravenous hydration and placebo on the amniotic fluid index in oligohydramnios. J Matern Fetal Med 2007;20(10):715–8.

53. Ross MG, Nijland MJ, Kullama LK. 1-Deamnio-[8-D-arginine] vasopressin-induced maternal plasma hypoosmolality increases ovine amniotic fluid volume. Am J Obstet Gynecol 1996;174(5):1118–25.

54. Ross MG, Cedars L, Nijland MJ, et al. Treatment of oligohydramnios with maternal 1-deamnio-[8-D-arginine] vasopressin-induced plasma hypoosmolality. Am J Obstet Gynecol 1996;174(5):1608–13.

55. Dildy GA III, Lira N, Moise KJ, et al. Amniotic fluid volume assessment: comparison of ultrasonographic estimates versus direct measurements with a dye-dilution technique in human pregnancy. Am J Obstet Gynecol 1992;167(4 Pt 1):986–94.

56. Sepulveda W, Flack NJ, Fisk NM. Direct volume measurement at midtrimester amnioinfusion in relation to ultrasonographic indexes of amniotic fluid volume. Am J Obstet Gynecol 1994;170:1160–3.

57. Myles TD, Santolaya-Forgas J. Normal ultrasonic evaluation of amniotic fluid volume in low risk patients at term. J Reprod Med 2002;47(8):621–4.

58. Youssef AA, Abdulla SA, Sayed EH, et al. Superiority of amniotic fluid index over amniotic fluid pocket measurement for predicting bad fetal outcome. South Med J 1993;86(4):426–9.

59. Fischer RL, McDonnell M, Bianculli KW, et al. Amniotic fluid volume estimation in post dates pregnancy: a comparison of techniques. Obstet Gynecol 1993; 81(5 Pt 1):698–704.

60. Magann EF, Chauhan SP, Martin JN. Is the amniotic fluid volume predictive of fetal acidosis at delivery? Aust N Z J Obstet Gynaecol 2003;43(2):129–33.

61. Verrotti C, Bedocchi L, Piantelli G. Amniotic fluid index versus largest vertical pocket in the prediction of perinatal outcome in post-term pregnancies. Acta Biomed 2004;75(Suppl 1):67–70.

62. Alfirevic Z, Luckas M, Walkinshaw SA, et al. A randomised comparison between amniotic fluid index and maximum pool depth in the monitoring of post-term pregnancy. Br J Obstet Gynaecol 1997;104(2):207–11.

63. Chauhan SP, Doherty DD, Magann EF, et al. Amniotic fluid index vs single deepest pocket technique during modified biophysical profile: a randomized clinical trial. Am J Obstet Gynecol 2004;191(2):661–7.

64. Magann EF, Doherty DA, Field K, et al. Biophysical profile with amniotic fluid volume assessments. Obstet Gynecol 2004;104(1):5–10.

65. Moses J, Doherty DA, Magann EF, et al. A randomized clinical trial of the intrapartum assessment of amniotic fluid volume: amniotic fluid index versus the single deepest pocket technique. Am J Obstet Gynecol 2004;190(6):1564–9.

66. Nabhan AF, Abdelmoula YA. Amniotic fluid index versus single deepest vertical pocket: a meta-analysis of randomized controlled trials. Int J Gynaecol Obstet 2009;104(3):184–8.

Optimization of Gestational Weight Gain in the Obese Gravida: A Review

Gayle Olson, MD[a],*, Sean C. Blackwell, MD[b]

KEYWORDS

• Pregnancy • Gestational weight gain • Lifestyle modification

"The diet should be abundant and nourishing . . .a diet poor in carbohydrates and fluids exerts a marked influence upon the weight of the child without otherwise affecting it."[1]

Improving pregnancy outcome via gestational weight gain has been a focal point of many areas in obstetrics including prenatal care, research, and child health and development.

In the past century, recommendations for weight gain during pregnancy have changed from 15 to 20 pounds in general to specific ranges tailored for prepregnancy body mass index (BMI). The Centers for Disease Control and Prevention (CDC) uses overweight and obese as terms for weights that are greater than what is generally considered healthy for a given height. The body mass index (BMI), determined by dividing the weight by height (kg/m^2), is used as a descriptor of weight and is viewed as one of the most practical, noninvasive indicators of the amount of body fat.[2]

The most recent guidelines for gestational weight gain (GWG), as suggested by the Institute of Medicine (IOM), benefit from new knowledge related to the contributions of maternal weight to birth outcome as well as consistent weight classification schemes between agencies.[3]

Maternal weight, depicted both as BMI and GWG, has been positively associated with increased infant,[4] child,[5,6] and adolescent[7] BMI. This was most recently studied

Disclosure: The author has nothing to disclose.
[a] Division of Maternal Fetal Medicine, Department of Obstetrics and Gynecology, The University of Texas Medical Branch, 301 University Boulevard, Galveston, TX 77555-0587, USA
[b] Department of Obstetrics, Gynecology and Reproductive Sciences, University of Texas Health Science Center at Houston, 6431 Fannin, Suite 3.283, Houston, TX 77030, USA
* Corresponding author.
E-mail address: golson@utmb.edu

Obstet Gynecol Clin N Am 38 (2011) 397–407
doi:10.1016/j.ogc.2011.03.003
0889-8545/11/$ – see front matter. Published by Elsevier Inc.

by Ludwig and Currie,[4] who used birth certificate data linking 513,501 mothers with their 1,164,750 offspring. They were able to demonstrate that infants whose mothers gained 20 to 22 kg and more than 24 kg were 103 g and 149 g heavier respectively when compared with infants whose mothers maintained gestational weight gain at 8 to 10 kg. In a retrospective cohort study of more than 8400 children born in the 1990s, Whitaker[8] reported that children who were born to obese mothers (based on BMI in the first trimester) had double the rate of obesity at age 2. In women with BMI of 30 or higher, the prevalence of childhood obesity (BMI >95th percentile) at ages 2, 3, and 4 years was 15.1%, 20.6%, and 24.1%, respectively. Oken and colleagues[5] analyzed data from Project Viva. This prospective study of 1000 predominantly non–low-income pregnant women and their children in Massachusetts revealed the rate of excessive GWG to be 51%. When adjusted for key covariates and compared with inadequate GWG, excessive gain was associated with odds ratios of 4.35 (1.69, 11.24) for obesity at 3 years of age (BMI >95th percentile vs <50th percentile). In addition, the investigators found higher BMI z-score, sum of triceps and subscapular skinfold thicknesses, and systolic blood pressure for each 5-kg increment in total GWG. In a later study including nearly 12,000 participants in the Growing Up Today Study, Oken and colleagues[7] found a strong, nearly linear association between total GWG and obesity (BMI >95th vs <85th percentile) at the age group of 9 to 14 years after adjusting for maternal BMI and other covariates. Overall, each 5-lb increment in GWG was associated with an odds ratio of 1.09 (95% confidence interval [CI]: 1.06–1.13) for obesity.

Cardiovascular parameters in childhood and adulthood may also be influenced by maternal BMI and GWG. A recent study was designed to examine the association of adherence to the updated GWG recommendations by the IOM and offspring outcome to include BMI, fat mass, waist circumference, blood pressure, lipids, and other cardiovascular risk factors.[9] Using a prospective population-based parent-child cohort, these investigators confirmed that offspring of mothers with high prepregnancy weight or excess GWG before 14 weeks, had greater BMI, waist circumference, fat mass, leptin, and systolic blood pressure.[9] These findings begin to provide supportive evidence for the role of fetal developmental programming in obesity, and metabolic and cardiovascular disease.[3] Studies focusing on determinants of GWG related to fetal programming, role of DNA sequence variation, and epigenetics may yet shed light on the modulation of weight gain during pregnancy and its effects on child and adult obesity, but are beyond the scope of this review. The remainder of this article will focus on the updated IOM GWG recommendations and measures directed at maintaining those guidelines and improving pregnancy outcome.

COMPLICATIONS OF OBESITY

The epidemic increase in obesity is obvious from the CDC's Behavioral Risk Factor Surveillance System.[2] In 1990, few areas in the United States had a prevalence of obesity greater than 25%. This dramatically contrasts with the data from 2007, at which time 30 states had a prevalence of obesity of 25% or higher.[2] In general, overweight and obesity result from an energy imbalance, taking in more energy than one expends. Behavior and environment are major modifiable factors in this imbalance. Behavior and environment have been identified by the Surgeon General as areas with the greatest promise in prevention and treatment and, therefore, areas for research. During pregnancy, excessive GWG is an example of such an energy imbalance, and as such is modifiable and a target for research influencing pregnancy outcomes. Excessive gestational weight gain contributes to rising obesity, with implications for the overall health care burden.

Increased morbidity for both the mother and infant are potentially related to excessive GWG. Gravidas with excessive GWG more often demonstrate gestational diabetes, preeclampsia, cesarean section, postpartum wound infection, and postpartum weight retention. The infant may have alterations in birth weight as well as increased risks for childhood obesity.[3] Obesity, independent of GWG, is also associated with increased adverse pregnancy outcomes including miscarriage,[10] fetal congenital anomaly,[11] thromboembolism,[12,13] gestational diabetes,[14] preeclampsia,[15] dysfunctional labor,[16] postpartum hemorrhage,[14] wound infections,[14] stillbirth,[17] induced labor,[18] caesarean section,[19] anesthetic complications,[20,21] and neonatal death.[17,22–24] Obese women may be less likely to initiate and maintain breastfeeding.[25] Finally, evidence suggests that obesity may increase the risk for maternal death.[26]

GESTATIONAL WEIGHT GAIN

The 1990 IOM recommendations for weight gain during pregnancy were based on prepregnancy BMI and the mean weight gain for women delivering full-term infants weighing between 3 and 4 kg.[27] The 4 prepregnancy BMI categories used in the 1990 recommendations were selected from the 1959 Metropolitan Life Insurance Company's ideal weight-for-height standards. The updated recommendations of 2009 have adopted the World Health Organization (WHO) BMI categories. In addition, WHO further stratifies obesity into 3 classes: BMI 30.0 to 34.9 (Class I); BMI 35.0 to 39.9 (Class II); and BMI 40 and over (Class III or morbid obesity). This stratification recognizes the continuous relationship between BMI and morbidity and mortality.[28]

Table 1 is a synopsis of the current IOM recommendations.[3] The calculations for GWG also assumed there would be a 1.1- to 4.4-lb weight gain in the first trimester.[3]

Table 1
Synopsis of GWG recommendations

Prepregnancy BMI		Total GWG, lb		2nd and 3rd Trimester Mean (Range) Gain (lb)/wk	
Weight	kg/m²	Singleton	Twin	Singleton	Twin
Under	<18.5	28–40		1 (1–1.3)	
Normal	18.5–24.9	25–35	37–54	1 (0.8–1)	
Over	25.0–29.9	15–25	31–50	0.6 (0.5–0.7)	
Obese	>30.0	11–20	25–42	0.5 (0.4–0.6)	
Category I	30.0–34.9				
Category II	35.0–39.9				
Category III	≥40				
Short stature					
Adolescent					
Ethnicity					

Abbreviations: BMI, body mass index; GWG, gestational weight gain.
Data from Rasmussen KM, Yaktine AL, editors. Weight gain during pregnancy: reexamining the guidelines. Institute of Medicine (US) and National Research Council (US) Committee to Reexamine IOM Pregnancy Weight Guidelines. Washington, DC: National Academies Press; 2009.

The IOM had previously recommended (1990) that women of short stature (<157cm) should maintain their GWG at the lower end of their prepregnancy BMI range.[27] The updated guidelines have maintained this recommendation. Similarly, the 1990 strategy was maintained for adolescents who were felt to be adequately categorized using cutoffs for adults. There was insufficient evidence to stratify recommendations further on the basis of ethnicity.[27] Assumptions for twin gestations, listed in **Table 1**, were based on cumulative weight gain among women who delivered between 37 and 42 weeks with twins weighing greater than or equal to 2500 g on average.[3]

Historically, adherence to any of the IOM guidelines has been difficult. Chu and colleagues,[29] in a population-based study assessing gestational weight gain for 52,988 women, demonstrated that the 1990 IOM guidelines were difficult to achieve. Approximately 40% of the normal-weight women and 60% of the overweight women gained more weight during pregnancy than recommended. Obese women gained less weight as a group compared with the normal and overweight groups, but approximately 25% still exceeded IOM recommendations.[29] These investigators also noted that GWG was increased for women younger than 19 years, women who were white, and women with more than 12 years of education. Importantly, the finding that there is a correlation between excessive GWG and weight retention postpartum, as well as increased BMI in later life, established a link between GWG and later obesity.[29] Similarly, Nohr and colleagues,[30] in an examination of 60,892 pregnancies from the Danish National Birth Cohort, found that more than half of the subjects in the overweight/obese categories (BMI $\geq$25 kg/m^2) gained more than 10 kg (22 lbs). An important finding was that 54% of overweight and 66% of obese women with gestational weight gain less than 10 kg were more than 2 kg below their prepregnancy weight at 6 months after delivery. GWG was such an important determinant of long-term obesity that approximately 25% of overweight and 30% of obese women with GWG less than 10 kg actually moved down a BMI category at 6 moths postpartum. By contrast, with a gestational weight gain of 16 to 19 kg, 12% and 14% of overweight and obese women respectively, moved up a BMI category.

Poor eating habits have been attributed to obesity. Surveys show that adults eat at restaurants on average 7.5 $\pm$ 8.5 times per month.[31] After controlling for age and gender, the frequency of consuming restaurant food was positively associated with body fat. Likewise, a survey conducted among participants in the Pound of Prevention study showed that 21% of adults reported eating fast food more than 3 times a week.[32] The frequency of fast food consumption was associated with higher total energy and fat intake, and greater body weight. Such eating habits increase the risk of obesity and thereby also increase the risk of developing diabetes. It is imperative that women who are pregnant gain knowledge about the nutritional requirements during pregnancy.

NUTRITION DURING PREGNANCY

Pregnant women should eat a variety of foods to meet the increased nutritional requirements during pregnancy, which increase approximately 300 to 400 kcal in the second and third trimester, respectively. Most pregnant women will need a diet containing 2200 to 2900 kcal per day preferably individualized for maternal age, trimester and activity.[33] Considering the increased requirements of pregnancy and individual needs, a breakdown of nutrients for a meal plan is considered as follows: $\leq$40% carbohydrate, $\pm$30% fat, $\pm$30% protein.

In addition to the increased caloric requirement during pregnancy, the dietary allowances for most nutrients increase.[34] For example, requirements for folic acid, vitamin D, and iron double, whereas the amounts of the following additional macronutrients and micronutrients increase more than 20% over nonpregnant requirements: protein, calcium, phosphorus, thiamin, zinc, and pyridoxine.[34]

Additional dietary supplements for women who are obese (BMI $\geq$30 kg/m^2) may need to be considered also. Women with this BMI range have been shown to have an increased risk for neural tube defects compared with women with a normal weight (odds ratio 1.7, 95% CI 1.34–2.15).[11] These findings would suggest additional folic acid supplement would be beneficial for women in this weight category.

Meal plans created during pregnancy not only must account for the increased macronutrient and micronutrient requirements but also need to be tailored to the cultural factors influencing the patient. For example, Gutierrez[35] demonstrated that cultural foods contributed significantly to the energy and nutrient intake of the pregnant Mexican American adolescent. In addition to traditional dietary staples, the participants added even more corn tortillas, beans, and rice to their diets during pregnancy and on average consumed approximately 300 calories more during the third trimester compared with second-trimester dietary intake (2390 vs 2619 kcal). Gutierrez[35] concluded that acculturation affects nutritional knowledge, attitudes about weight gain during pregnancy, and the psychosocial and educational levels of pregnant Mexican American adolescents during pregnancy. Successful diet counseling, also addressed in studies by Kittler and Sucher, emphasizes the need for culturally sensitive communication strategies to identify food adaptations for each client.[36]

OPTIMIZING GESTATIONAL WEIGHT GAIN AND REDUCING OBESITY

The Surgeon General has targeted behavioral modification as one of the most promising areas for prevention and treatment of obesity. In studies performed in nonpregnant adults, lifestyle interventions were the most cost-effective means of treatment of obesity and obesity-related disorders. Education alone was not successful as an intervention for weight loss.[37] Powell and colleagues[37] summarized the evidence relating to the effects of lifestyle modification, pharmacotherapy, and surgery on sustained weight loss in adults. They identified 9 lifestyle modification trials that consistently produced an approximately 7-lb sustainable weight loss for 2 years. What was remarkable was the impact of even modest levels of weight reduction on clinical outcome. For example, even a weight loss of 5.9 lb (2.7 kg) in obese, glucose-intolerant individuals was associated with a 58% reduction in diabetes when compared with controls. Frequency of interventions also affects weight loss. Weekly visits were associated with the greatest weight reduction. As the frequency of visits decreased, the weight loss similarly decreased. However, even monthly or bimonthly contacts following a more intensive phase of treatment appeared sufficient to maintain 60% to 80% of the weight loss achieved in the intensive phase.[37,38] Interestingly, 20% to 65% of the participants in the studies reviewed by Powell and colleagues sought additional diets after their study participation was concluded, suggesting continued motivation to maintain lifestyle interventions for weight control.[37,39]

LIFESTYLE INTERVENTION DURING PREGNANCY

Lifestyle modification and education trials have been conducted during pregnancy with the aim of affecting gestational weight gain and pregnancy outcome. Pregnancy may be the perfect time to introduce lifestyle modification strategies.

Teachable moments occur during significant life transitions that motivate people to adopt risk-reducing health behaviors. The characteristics of teachable moments have best been described as follows: personal risk and the potential for adverse outcome are perceived as increased, a strong emotional response occurs, and the environment promotes redefining self-concepts and social roles. Pregnancy provides a time frame that incorporates all these domains, thus making pregnancy an excellent "teachable moment" and a time to influence women when they are redefining themselves.[40] Examples of such lifestyle modification trials during pregnancy are limited but the few randomized studies suggest these interventions improve pregnancy outcome. Although there are a plethora of observational studies that evaluate prognostic factors for excessive weight gain, to date there are only 4 randomized clinical trials designed to affect GWG and reduce excessive GWG (in nondiabetic women) (see **Table 2**).

Asbee and colleagues[41] randomized 100 pregnant women to routine prenatal care or an intervention consisting of one session with a dietician to receive standardized counseling on nutrition, exercise, and IOM recommendations. Thereafter, the study participants received additional counseling only if their GWG fell outside the IOM guidelines. The study group gained less weight than the control group (28.7 $\pm$ 12.5 lb vs 35.6 $\pm$ 15.5 lb; $P = .01$) and had fewer cesarean sections (14.0% vs 27.9%; $P = .09$). In addition, nulliparous participants gained significantly more weight than did parous participants (36.5 $\pm$ 14.5 lb vs 27.7 $\pm$ 12.7 lb; $P<.01$).[41] Dodd and colleagues[42] conducted a systematic review of randomized controlled trials of overweight or obese pregnant women receiving lifestyle interventions with the intent of improving pregnancy outcomes and showed improvements in overall GWG and

Table 2
Randomized trials of gestational weight gain

Author (Year)	Study Site (n)	Intervention	Results
Polley et al,[52] 2002	Pittsburgh, PA (59 control, 61 intervention)	Stepped-care behavioral intervention with advice on appropriate GWG, exercise, and healthful eating	Reduction in excessive GWG, only among the normal-weight, and not the overweight, women
Wolff et al,[53] 2008	Copenhagen, Denmark (27 control, 23 intervention)	Restriction of GWG to 6–7 kg with 10 1-h dietary consultations; obese women only	Decrease in GWG, decrease in serum insulin, and leptin concentrations at 27 wk gestation, and decrease in serum insulin and fasting blood glucose concentrations at 36 wk gestation
Asbee et al,[41] 2009	Charlotte, NC (43 control, 57 intervention)	Organized, consistent program of intensive dietary and lifestyle counseling	Decrease in GWG
Thornton et al,[54] 2009	New York City, NY area (133 control, 124 intervention)	Prescription for a balanced nutritional regimen with recording of all foods eaten each day; obese women only	Decrease in last weight before delivery and weight at 6 wk postpartum; decrease in gestational HTN

Abbreviations: GWG, gestational weight gain; HTN, hypertension.

decreased rates of excessive GWG, but data were insufficient to show improvements in perinatal or newborn outcomes.

ACTIVITY DURING PREGNANCY

Activity is a key component of a successful lifestyle modification regimen. The American College of Obstetricians and Gynecologists (ACOG) recommends, in the absence of either medical or obstetrical complications, 30 minutes or more of moderate exercise a day on most, if not all, days of the week for pregnant women.[43] This is consistent with recent recommendation from the American College of Sports Medicine and the American Heart Association, which states that all healthy adults aged 18 to 65 years need moderate-intensity aerobic (endurance) physical activity for a minimum of 30 minutes a day on 5 days each week.[44] Studies have shown that the physical activity of most pregnant women does not meet the recommendations from ACOG, and, in fact, demonstrates a low-activity to sedentary lifestyle.[45] In a case-control study of supervised exercise sessions that involved walking or cycling once a week, with unsupervised exercise on the following 6 days in obese women with gestational diabetes, women in the exercise group had significantly less weight gain per week (0.1 ± 0.4 kg vs 0.3 ± 0.4 kg; $P<.05$).[46] Supervised exercise may not always be feasible; however, tools such as pedometers have been shown to be motivators of independent activity.

Pedometers are small meter devices worn either on the wrist or clipped onto the waistband that can measure the number of steps an individual takes per day. Some can even measure distance walked and energy expended over time. The use of pedometers has gained popularity as a tool to measure level of physical activity and to motivate increases in physical activities particularly in obese adults with chronic illnesses.[47,48] An established pedometer-based physical activity guideline indicates that approximately 30 minutes of moderate-intensity physical activity translates into about 3000 to 4000 steps.[49] Categories of physical activity have been defined as sedentary at fewer than 5000 steps, low active at 5000 to 6499 steps, somewhat active at 7500 to 9999 steps, active at 10,000 to 12,499 steps, and highly active at more than12,500 steps per day.[49] In a systematic review of randomized controlled trials, the pedometer users significantly increased their physical activity by more than 2500 steps per day compared with controls.[48] This resulted in a significant decrease in BMI and blood pressure. In pregnancy, pedometers have been used to identify the level of physical activity in pregnant women. In 94 pregnant women, self-reported exercise diaries (minutes of exercise a day) were correlated with pedometer counts (equivalent to 1 mile based on walking measurement) over a 3-day period at 14 weeks and 28 weeks of pregnancy.[45] The mean count was $3.97 +/- 2.4$ and mean minutes of exercise was 10.9 minutes $+/- 16.1$ per day, indicating that many pregnant women have sedentary to low activity during pregnancy. Another study showed that pregnant women were able to use the pedometers without difficulty.[50] These women demonstrated that their levels of activity declined as their pregnancy progressed such that a large proportion of women (73%) were classified as sedentary and low active at 32 weeks of pregnancy compared with 50% at 20 weeks of pregnancy.[50] Finally, in obese low-income women postpartum, pedometers were shown to be an inexpensive motivational tool for weight loss.[51]

SUMMARY

Obesity has risen to epidemic proportions in the United States. GWG during pregnancy contributes to a cycle of obesity for mothers and their offspring. Both obesity and GWG are modifiable through lifestyle interventions and reductions in obesity to positively improve pregnancy outcome. Given the impact of lifestyle modifications for women, their future health, and the health and development of their offspring, the following are recommended during the course of prenatal care:

- Document weight, height, and BMI at the first prenatal visit
- Educate patients about their BMI and set goals for weight gain during the pregnancy
- Provide nutritional counseling tailored for pregnancy, level of BMI, weight gain goals, and ethnic preferences
- Educate and set goals for activity during pregnancy
- Individualize prenatal visits pending adherence to weight gain goals. Discuss weight at each prenatal visit. Increase frequency of visits for women exceeding their goals and repeat nutritional counseling as needed.

Because of the consistent association between GWG and birth weight (along with other maternal and child outcomes such as postpartum weight retention and child obesity),[5] helping women avoid excessive weight gain during pregnancy should be an important objective of prenatal and preconceptional care.

REFERENCES

1. Williams JW. Obstetrics. A text-book for the use of students and practitioners. New York: D. Appleton and Co; 1903.
2. Centers for Disease Control and Prevention. Overweight and obesity. Available at: www.cdc.gov/nccdphp/dnpa/obesity. Accessed February 25, 2011.
3. Rasmussen KM, Yaktine AL, editors. Weight gain during pregnancy: reexamining the guidelines. Institute of Medicine (US) and National Research Council (US) Committee to Reexamine IOM pregnancy weight guidelines. Washington, DC: National Academies Press (US); 2009.
4. Ludwig DS, Currie J. The association between pregnancy weight gain and birthweight: a within-family comparison. Lancet 2010;376(9745):984–90.
5. Oken E, Taveras EM, Kleinman KP, et al. Gestational weight gain and child adiposity at age 3 years. Am J Obstet Gynecol 2007;196:322, e1–8.
6. Wrotniak BH, Shults J, Butts S, et al. Gestational weight gain and risk of overweight in the offspring at age 7y in a multicenter, multiethnic cohort study. Am J Clin Nutr 2008;87:1818–24.
7. Oken E, Rifas-Shima S, Field A, et al. Maternal gestational weight gain and offspring weight in adolescence. Obstet Gynecol 2008;112:999–1006.
8. Whitaker RC. Predicting preschooler obesity at birth: the role of maternal obesity in early pregnancy. Pediatrics 2004;114(1):e29–36.
9. Fraser A, Tilling K, Macdonald-Wallis C, et al. Association of maternal weight gain in pregnancy with offspring obesity and metabolic and vascular traits in childhood. Circulation 2010;121:2557–64.
10. Lashen H, Fear K, Sturdee DW. Obesity is associated with increased risk of first trimester and recurrent miscarriage: matched case-control study. Hum Reprod 2004;19(7):1644–6.
11. Rasmussen SA, Chu SY, Kim SY, et al. Maternal obesity and risk of neural tube defects: a meta-analysis. Am J Obstet Gynecol 2008;198(6):611–9.
12. Jacobsen AF, Skjeldestad FE, Sandset PM. Ante- and postnatal risk factors of venous thrombosis: a hospital-based case control study. J Thromb Haemost 2008;6(6):905–12.

13. Larsen TB, Sorensen HT, Gislum M, et al. Maternal smoking, obesity, and risk of venous thromboembolism during pregnancy and the puerperium: a population-based nested case-control study. Thromb Res 2007;120(4):505–9.

14. Sebire NJ, Jolly M, Harris JP, et al. Maternal obesity and pregnancy outcome: a study of 287,213 pregnancies in London. Int J Obes Relat Metab Disord 2001;25(8):1175–82.

15. O'Brien TE, Ray JG, Chan WS. Maternal body mass index and the risk of preeclampsia: a systematic overview. Epidemiology 2003;14(3):368–74.

16. Nuthalapaty FS, Rouse DJ, Owen J. The association of maternal weight with cesarean risk, labor duration, and cervical dilation rate during labor induction. Obstet Gynecol 2004;103(3):452–6 [erratum appears in Obstet Gynecol 2004;103(5 Pt 1):1019].

17. Kristensen J, Vestergaard M, Wisborg K, et al. Pre-pregnancy weight and the risk of stillbirth and neonatal death. BJOG 2005;112(4):403–8.

18. Usha Kiran TS, Hemmadi S, Bethel J, et al. Outcome of pregnancy in a woman with an increased body mass index. BJOG 2005;112(6):768–72.

19. Chu SY, Kim SY, Schmid CH, et al. Maternal obesity and risk of cesarean delivery: a meta-analysis. Obes Rev 2007;8(5):385–94.

20. Dresner M, Brocklesby J, Bamber J. Audit of the influence of body mass index on the performance of epidural analgesia in labour and the subsequent mode of delivery. BJOG 2006;113(10):1178–81.

21. Saravanakumar K, Rao SG, Cooper GM. The challenges of obesity and obstetric anaesthesia. Curr Opin Obstet Gynecol 2006;18(6):631–5.

22. Cedergren MI. Maternal morbid obesity and the risk of adverse pregnancy outcome. Obstet Gynecol 2004;103(2):219–24.

23. Shah A, Sands J, Kenny L. Maternal obesity and the risk of stillbirth and neonatal death. J Obstet Gynaecol 2006;26(Suppl 1):S19.

24. Weiss JL, Malone FD, Emig D, et al. Obesity, obstetric complication and cesarean delivery rate—a population-based screening study. Am J Obstet Gynecol 2004; 190:1091–7.

25. Amir LH, Donath S. A systematic review of maternal obesity and breastfeeding intention, initiation and duration. BMC Pregnancy Childbirth 2007;7:9.

26. Lewis G, editor. Confidential enquiry into maternal and child health. Saving mothers' lives—reviewing maternal deaths to make motherhood safer 2003–2005. London: CEMACH; 2007.

27. Nutrition during pregnancy. 1. Weight gain. Washington, DC: National Academy Press. Institute of Medicine; 1990. [Ref Type: Report].

28. World Health Organization. Obesity: preventing and managing the global epidemic. Geneva (Switzerland): World Health Organization; 2000.

29. Chu SY, Callaghan WM, Bish CL, et al. Gestational weight gain by body mass index among US women delivering live birth, 2004-2005: fueling future obesity. Am J Obstet Gynecol 2009;200:e1–7.

30. Nohr EA, Bech BH, Vaeth M, et al. Obesity, gestational weight gain and preterm birth: a study within the Danish National Birth Cohort. Paediatr Perinat Epidemiol 2007;21(1):5–14.

31. McCrory MA, Fuss PJ, Hays NP, et al. Overeating in America: association between restaurant food consumption and body fatness in healthy adult men and women ages 19 to 80. Obes Res 1999;7:564–71.

32. French SA, Harnack L, Jeffery RW. Fast food restaurant use among women in the Pound of Prevention study: dietary, behavioral and demographic correlates. Int J Obes Relat Metab Disord 2000;24:1353–9.

33. Kaiser L. Position of the American Dietetic Association: nutrition and life-style for a healthy pregnancy outcome. J Am Diet Assoc 2008;108(3): 553–61.

34. Gabbe SG, Niebyl JR, Simpson JL. In: Obstetrics normal and problem pregnancies. 5th edition. Mosby: Churchill Livingstone/Elsevier; 2007. p. 124.

35. Gutierrez YM. Cultural factors affecting diet and pregnancy outcome of Mexican American adolescents. J Adolesc Health 1999;25(3):227–37.

36. Kittler KG, Sucher KP. Diet counseling in a multicultural society. Diabetes Educ 1990;16:127–31.

37. Powell LH, Calvin JE III, Calvin JE Jr. Effective obesity treatments. Am Psychol 2007;62:234–46.

38. Tuomilehto J, Lindstrom MS, Eriksson JG, et al. Prevention of type 2 diabetes mellitus by changes in lifestyle among subjects with impaired glucose tolerance. N Engl J Med 2001;344:1343–50.

39. Mann T, Tomiyama AJ, Westling E, et al. Medicare's search for effective obesity treatments: diets are not the answer. Am Psychol 2007;62:220–33.

40. Phelan S. Pregnancy: a "teachable moment" for weight control and obesity prevention. Am J Obstet Gynecol 2010;202(2):135, e1–8.

41. Asbee SM, Jenkins TR, Butler JR, et al. Preventing excessive weight gain during pregnancy through dietary and lifestyle counseling. Obstet Gynecol 2009;113: 305–12.

42. Dodd JM, Crowther CA, Robinson JS. Dietary and lifestyle interventions to limit weight gain during pregnancy for obese or overweight women: a systematic review. Acta Obstet Gynecol Scand 2008;87(7):702–6.

43. American College of Obstetricians and Gynecologists. Exercise during pregnancy and the postpartum period. ACOG Committee Opinion No. 267. Obstet Gynecol 2002;99:171–3.

44. Haskell WL, Lee IM, Pate RR, et al. Physical activity and public health: updated recommendation for adults from the American College of Sports Medicine and the American Heart Association. Med Sci Sports Exerc 2007;39(8):1423–34.

45. Lindseth G, Vari P. Measuring physical activity during pregnancy. West J Nurs Res 2005;27(6):722–34.

46. Artal R, Catanzaro R, Gavard J, et al. A lifestyle intervention of weight-gain restriction: diet and exercise in obese women with gestational diabetes mellitus. Appl Physiol Nutr Metab 2007;32:596–601.

47. Decocker KD, De Bourdeaudhuji I, Brown W, et al. Moderators and mediators of pedometer use and step count in the "10,000 Steps Ghent" intervention. Int J Behav Nutr Phys Act 2009;6:1–7.

48. Bravata DM, Smith-Spangler C, Sundaram V, et al. Using pedometers to increase physical activity and improve health. JAMA 2007;298(19):1296–2304.

49. Tudor-Locke C, Hatano Y, Pangrazi RP, et al. Revisiting "how many steps are enough?" Med Sci Sports Exerc 2008;40(7):S537–43.

50. Downs DS, Lemasurier GC, Dinallo JM. Baby steps: pedometer-determined and self-reported leisure-time exercise behaviors of pregnant women. J Phys Act Health 2009;6(1):63–72.

51. Clarke KK, Freeland-Graves J, Klohe-Lehman DM, et al. Promotion of physical activity in low-income mothers using pedometers. J Am Diet Assoc 2007; 107(6):962–7.

52. Polley BA, Wing RR, Sims CJ. Randomized controlled trial to prevent excessive weight gain in pregnant women. Int J Obes Relat Metab Disord 2002;26(11): 1494–502.

53. Wolff S, Legarth J, Vangsgaard K, et al. A randomized trial of the effects of dietary counseling on gestational weight gain and glucose metabolism in obese pregnant women. International Journal of Obesity 2008;32(3):495–501.
54. Thornton YS, Smarkola C, Kopacz SM, et al. Perinatal outcomes in nutritionally monitored obese pregnant women: a randomized clinical trial. J Natl Med Assoc 2009;101(6):569–77.

Index

Note: Page numbers of article titles are in **boldface** type.

Obstet Gynecol Clin N Am 38 (2011) 409–415
doi:10.1016/S0889-8545(11)00059-3
0889-8545/11/$ – see front matter © 2011 Elsevier Inc. All rights reserved.

obgyn.theclinics.com

Moving?

Make sure your subscription moves with you!

To notify us of your new address, find your **Clinics Account Number** (located on your mailing label above your name), and contact customer service at:

Email: journalscustomerservice-usa@elsevier.com

800-654-2452 (subscribers in the U.S. & Canada)
314-447-8871 (subscribers outside of the U.S. & Canada)

Fax number: 314-447-8029

Elsevier Health Sciences Division
Subscription Customer Service
3251 Riverport Lane
Maryland Heights, MO 63043

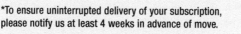

*To ensure uninterrupted delivery of your subscription, please notify us at least 4 weeks in advance of move.

Printed and bound by CPI Group (UK) Ltd, Croydon, CR0 4YY

14/10/2024

01773705-0001